PHARMACY PRACTICE
for technicians

DON A. BALLINGTON, MS
Director, Pharmacy Technician Program
Midlands Technical College
Columbia, South Carolina

D1449819

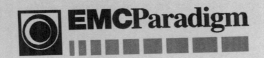
EMCParadigm

Developmental Editors	Sonja M. Brown, Michael Sander
Instructional Designer	Janice C. Johnson
Art Director	Joan D'Onofrio
Cover and Text Designer	Jennifer Wreisner
Copy Editor	Susan T. Gibson
Illustrator	Electronic Illustrators Group
Desktop Production Specialists	Mori Studio
Proofreader	Nancy Sauro
Indexer	Nancy Fulton

Reviewers

The author and publisher wish to thank the following instructors and healthcare professionals for their valuable suggestions during the development of this book: Mary Margaret Laughlin, Pharm.D., Regional Medical Center, Memphis, TN; Mary Ann Jordan, Director, Pharmacy Technician Program, Pima Community College, Tucson, AZ; and Cindy Johnson, Director, Pharmacy Technician Program, Arapahoe Community College, Littleton, CO.

Library of Congress Cataloging-in-Publication Data

Ballington, Don A.
    Pharmacy practice for technicians / Don A. Ballington.
          p.   cm.
    Includes index.
    ISBN 0-7638-0099-6 (text). — ISBN 0-7638-0100-3 (instructor's
guide). — ISBN 0-7638-0098-8 (workbook).
         1. Pharmacy technicians. 2. Medicine—Formulae, receipts,
prescriptions.   I. Title.
         [DNLM: 1. Pharmacy. 2. Pharmacists' Aides. 3. Pharmaceutical
Services—United States.   QV 737B192p 1999]
    RS122.95.B35 1999
    615'.1—dc21
    DNLM/DLC   98-27634
    for Library of Congress   CIP

Text: ISBN 0-7638-0099-6
Instructor's Guide: ISBN 0-7638-0100-3
Workbook: ISBN 0-7638-0098-8

Trademarks

Some of the pharmaceutical product names used in this book have been used for identification purposes only and may be trademarks or registered trademarks of their respective manufacturers.

© 1999 by Paradigm Publishing Inc.
    Published by **EMC**Paradigm
    875 Montreal Way
    St. Paul, MN 55102
    (800) 535-6865
    E-mail: educate@emcp.com
    Web site: www.emcp.com

Printed in the United States of America
10 9 8 7 6 5

contents

CHAPTER 5 — Routes of Drug Administration, 97

CHAPTER 6 — Sources of Information, 111

CHAPTER 7 — Basic Pharmaceutical Measurements and Calculations, 127

CHAPTER 8 — Dispensing, Billing, and Inventory Management, 145

CHAPTER 9 Extemporaneous Compounding, 171

CHAPTER 10 Human Relations and Communications, 187

CHAPTER 11 Hospital and Institutional Pharmacy Practice, 197

CHAPTER 12 Your Future in Pharmacy Practice, 235

preface

The practice of pharmacy is an interesting, challenging, and exciting study of the application of pharmacy knowledge. In this book we hope to guide both students and teachers in an understanding of the pharmacy technician's role working side-by-side with the pharmacist.

Pharmacy Practice introduces you to techniques and procedures necessary to prepare and dispense medications according to physician request. You will become familiar with reading the order/prescription and preparing, packaging, and labeling the medication as well as maintaining the patient profile. Preparing medications involves using sterile and nonsterile techniques to count, measure, and compound drugs for institutional and community practice. Other medication and nonmedication pharmacy-related activities are introduced, including billing and inventory management.

To provide the additional hands-on experience so important to performing the duties of a pharmacy technician, we have included an appendix of laboratory exercises that are coordinated with the appropriate chapters. These exercises allow students to demonstrate their knowledge of preparing and labeling common medications. Two additional appendixes list common categories of drugs, with generic and brand-name examples, and commonly prescribed drugs.

The Pharmacy Technician

1

From its ancient origins in spiritualism and magic, pharmacy has evolved into a scientific pursuit involving not only the compounding and dispensing of medications but also the provision of accurate information and counseling about a wide range of medication-related issues. The contemporary pharmacy technician provides a wide variety of essential services to pharmacy customers and patients, to supervising pharmacists, and to such healthcare professionals as physicians and nurses. In recent years, pharmacy technicians have made tremendous strides toward recognition of their status within the ranks of highly skilled paraprofessionals.

Learning Objectives

- Describe the origins of pharmacy
- Describe three stages of development of the pharmacy profession in the twentieth century
- Enumerate the functions of the pharmacist
- Differentiate among the various subfields within the profession of pharmacy, including pharmaceutics, pharmacognosy, pharmacology, and clinical pharmacy
- Explain the licensing requirements for pharmacists
- Identify the duties and work environments of the pharmacy technician
- Differentiate among the various kinds of pharmacies

TERMS TO KNOW

Apothecary A pharmacist. This term was more commonly used in the past than it is today.

Certified Pharmacy Technician (CPhT) A person who has passed the Pharmacy Technician Certification Examination and who completes the necessary course work for recertification every two years

Clinical pharmacy That part of a pharmacy practice that involves providing information and counseling about medications to patients and to healthcare professionals

Community pharmacy A retail drugstore; the profession of operating or managing a retail drugstore

Compounding The act of preparing a medication to order in a particular dosage form; usually involves combining one or more active ingredients with one or more inert ingredients, or diluents

Druggist A pharmacist

Formulary A list of drugs approved for use by a governmental body or institution

Home health care The provision of health-care services in the home of a patient rather than in an institutional setting

ANCIENT ORIGINS

The word *pharmacy* comes from the ancient Greek word *pharmakon,* meaning "drug." The use of drugs in the healing arts is older than civilization. Modern archaeologists, exploring the five-thousand-year-old remains of the ancient city states of Mesopotamia, have unearthed clay tablets listing hundreds of medicinal preparations from various sources, including plants and minerals. Already, at the dawn of civilization, a traditional pharmacological lore existed, probably reflecting practical experience dating back for centuries or even millennia. The ancient Egyptians compiled lists of drugs, known as **formularies**, **dispensatories**, or **pharmacopeias**, along with directions for creating them from natural sources using such simple equipment as the scale, the sieve, and the mortar and pestle. The peoples of ancient India attributed the miraculous and curative powers of the gods and of their priestly shamans to an intoxicating drug, still unidentified but possibly derived from a mushroom, that they referred to as *soma.* (The word *soma* was picked up by the ancient Greeks and came to mean "body." It is with this meaning that it was later used as a root in such English words as *psychosomatic.*) Predictably, early recipes for drug preparation are freely mixed with incantations, rituals, and imitative magic.

To the ancient Greeks, and particularly to the fathers of medicine, **Hippocrates** and **Galen**, we owe the beginnings of a nonmagical, scientific approach to the arts of healing and to drug use. Hippocrates, who was born on the Greek island of Kos around 430 B.C., established the theory of humors, which was to dominate medicine for almost two thousand years (see Figure 1.1). According to this now long-discredited theory, health involved harmony among four fundamental bodily fluids, known as **humors**. Each humor was associated with particular personality characteristics.

The humors were blood, phlegm, yellow bile, and black bile, and were associated, respectively, with cheerfulness, sluggishness, irritability, and melancholy.

Galen, born around A.D. 129 in Asia Minor, expanded on the theory of humors and produced a systematic classification of drugs for the treatment of pathologies involving want, excess, or corruption of the bodily humors. The greatest of the ancient pharmaceutical texts, however, was *De Materia Medica (On Medical Matters)*, written by **Pedanius Dioscorides** in the first century A.D. Born in what is now Turkey, Dioscorides served in the Roman army during the rule of Nero and traveled widely, gathering knowledge of medicinal herbs and minerals from Persia, Africa, Egypt, Greece, and Rome. His book served as the standard text on drugs, primarily herbal remedies, for fifteen hundred years.

Although drugs from herbal and mineral sources have been used for millennia, *pharmacy* as a distinct professional discipline devoted to creating, storing, dispensing, and providing information about drugs is a relatively young field. Emperor Frederick II of Germany was the first to officially recognize pharmacy as a distinct professional category in 1231. Since that time, the profession of the dispenser of drugs, the **pharmacist**, or, in older terminology, the **apothecary**, **chemist**, or **druggist**, has grown concurrently with that of the modern, scientifically trained physician. Until the nineteenth century, the dispensary that distributed drugs to patients was usually owned by a physician, but gradually it became an independent entity owned and operated by the pharmacist.

THE ROLE OF THE PHARMACIST

Evolution of the Pharmacist's Role in the Twentieth Century

The modern pharmacist has two primary roles. The first of these is to dispense drugs prescribed by physicians and other health practitioners. The second is to provide information to patients, to physicians, and to other healthcare practitioners on the selection, dosages, interactions, and side effects of medications. During the twentieth century, the pharmacy profession evolved through three stages: from the **traditional era**, dominated by the formulation and dispensing of drugs from natural sources; through a **scientific era** in mid-century, dominated by scientific training in the effects of drugs on the body; to a **clinical era** at the end of the century, which combined these traditional roles with a new role as dispenser of drug information.

Prior to the 1940s, the job of the pharmacist/apothecary consisted almost entirely of **pharmaceutics**, the science of preparing and dispensing drugs. Important aspects of the traditional profession included **pharmacognosy**, knowledge of the medicinal functions of natural products of animal, plant, or mineral origin, and **Galenical pharmacy**, knowledge of the techniques for preparing medications from such sources. A nineteenth-century apothecary not only sold drugs but also manufactured them.

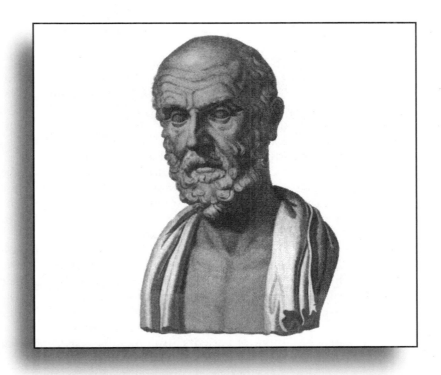

Figure 1.1 To Hippocrates, traditionally viewed as "the father of medicine," the ancients ascribed the creation of approximately 70 works dealing with the identification and treatment of disease. Hippocrates' name is most commonly associated with the Hippocratic Oath, which, among other requirements, pledges physicians "to give no drug . . . for a criminal purpose."

The emergence of the pharmaceutical industry in the twentieth century created a crisis for the profession of the pharmacist. As the manufacturing of drugs moved from the apothecary shop to the labs and factories of the pharmaceutical manufacturers, the pharmacist increasingly became a drugstore operator, a dispenser of drugs who was more a businessperson than a healing arts professional. This situation soon changed, however, as the educational institutions that trained pharmacists turned to scientific studies on drug effects and interactions, researches that were largely funded by pharmaceutical companies. **Pharmacology**, the scientific study of the site and mode of action, the side effects (including the adverse side effects, or **toxicology**), and the metabolism by the body of drugs, became part of the pharmacy curriculum, along with physics, chemistry, and physiology.

By the late 1950s and 1960s, many pharmacists began to feel that their training had shifted too far in the direction of scientific knowledge isolated from actual pharmacy practice. At the same time, many felt that pharmacists were being underutilized. Pharmacists constituted a highly knowledgeable, scientifically trained professional class, with vast pharmacological knowledge, and yet they devoted the bulk of their energies to running businesses rather than interacting with patients and other professionals. Then, in 1973, the American Association of Colleges of Pharmacy established a study commission under **Dr. John S. Millis** to reevaluate the mission of the pharmacy profession. The 1975 **Millis Report**, titled *Pharmacists for the Future,* defined *pharmacy* as a primarily knowledge-based profession and emphasized the role of the pharmacist in sharing knowledge about drug use. This report led to a new emphasis in the profession on what is known as **clinical pharmacy**—the sharing of information about drugs with patients and health practitioners. The modern pharmacist thus carries out the important role of advisor and counselor to physicians and patients, as well as the role of dispenser of drugs.

Functions of the Pharmacist

Today, **compounding**, the mixing of ingredients to create tablets, capsules, ointments, solutions, and the like, is but a small part of the pharmacist's actual practice. The pharmacist who works in a community, or retail, pharmacy (the "drugstore") counsels customers, asking about their medical histories and what other medications they are currently taking, providing information about over-the-counter medications and making recommendations for these, describing possible adverse reactions and drug interactions related to prescriptions, and giving advice about home healthcare supplies and medical equipment. Of course, the pharmacist still compounds and dispenses drugs, and the community pharmacist still commonly functions as a businessperson, hiring and supervising employees, selling merchandise not directly related to health, and otherwise serving as the manager of a retail operation.

The pharmacist who works in a hospital or clinic dispenses medications and advises medical staff on drug selection and effects. Other typical tasks for the hospital pharmacist include preparing sterile solutions, purchasing medical supplies, monitoring drug regimens, and providing prerelease counseling on drugs to patients about to be discharged. The pharmacist who works in home healthcare may prepare medications and **intravenous infusions**, or **IVs**, for home use and may also monitor patients' drug therapies. (For more information on intravenous infusions, see chapters 4, 5, and 6.)

Whether working in community, clinical, long-term care, or home healthcare settings, pharmacists typically keep records of patients' drug therapies, in part to prevent adverse interactions among prescribed medications. Some pharmacists teach and some function as consultants with expertise in particular fields of drug use, such as the diagnostic application of radioactive drugs, intravenous nutrition, or drug therapy for psychiatric, pediatric, or geriatric patients.

Education and Licensing Requirements for Pharmacists

One indication of the professional status of pharmacy is the stringent licensing and educational requirements placed on practitioners. In the United States, all states require pharmacists to be licensed. Obtaining a license involves graduating from an accredited college of pharmacy, passing a state certification examination, and serving an internship under a licensed pharmacist. In addition, in most states, pharmacists must meet continuing education requirements in order to renew their licenses. Most states have reciprocal agreements recognizing licenses granted to pharmacists in other states. Licensing and general professional oversight is carried out by **state pharmacy boards**, self-monitoring professional organizations in each state. Most colleges of pharmacy offer five-year programs, culminating in the **Bachelor of Science (BS) in Pharmacy** degree, and six-year programs, culminating in the **Doctor of Pharmacy (PharmD)** degree. While some colleges of pharmacy admit students with only high school degrees, most require one or two years of prepharmacy education, including chemistry, physics, and biology. The five-year BS program consists of two years of prepharmacy training and three years of pharmacy training. Some colleges require that applicants take the **Pharmacy College Admission Test**, or **PCAT**. Some have master's and PhD programs in pharmacy that prepare pharmacists for specialization and for teaching. In the near future, it is expected that the entry level pharmacy degree will be the PharmD.

THE ROLE OF THE PHARMACY TECHNICIAN

The Technician as Accountable Assistant to the Professional Pharmacist

A **pharmacy technician**, sometimes referred to as a **pharmacy technologist**, **assistant**, **clerk**, or **aide**, is someone who, under the supervision of a licensed pharmacist, assists in a wide variety of skilled activities necessary for the dispensing of drugs and drug information. A central defining feature of the technician's job is **accountability** to the pharmacist for the quality and accuracy of his or her work. While the technician carries out many of the duties carried out by pharmacists, his or her work must always be checked by the pharmacist. As a **paraprofessional**, or skilled assistant to a professional person, the pharmacy technician bears a relationship to the pharmacist similar to that of an X-ray technician to a radiologist or a medical technologist to a pathologist. A pharmacy technician assists the pharmacist with routine technical and nontechnical functions but leaves most judgment calls and decision making to the pharmacist. The technician functions in strict accordance with standard written procedures and guidelines, any deviation from which must be approved by the pharmacist. The pharmacist, in turn, takes final responsibility for the technician's actions.

Work Environments and Conditions

Pharmacy technicians are employed in most of the settings in which pharmacists are, including community pharmacies (drugstores), hospital pharmacies, home healthcare, and long-term care facilities. (For more information on the range of workplaces in pharmacy, see "The Pharmacy Workplace," p. 8.) Pharmacy technicians, like pharmacists, usually work in clean, well-lighted, well-ventilated environments. For the most part, their work requires standing, often for long hours. Because people's health needs know no clock, both pharmacists and pharmacy technicians work days, nights, weekends, and holidays. At any time, 24 hours a day, some number of the estimated 81,000 pharmacy technicians currently employed are on the job.

Characteristics of the Pharmacy Technician

A successful pharmacy technician must possess a wide range of skills, knowledge, and aptitudes. He or she must have a broad knowledge of pharmacy practice and a dedication to providing a critical healthcare service to customers and patients. In addition, the pharmacy technician must have high ethical standards, eagerness to learn, a sense of responsibility toward patients and toward the healthcare professionals with whom he or she interacts, willingness to follow instructions, an eye for detail, manual dexterity, facility in basic mathematics, excellent communication skills, good research skills, and the ability to perform accurately and calmly in hectic or stressful situations.

Training, Certification, Pay, and Job Outlook

At present, no federal requirements and few state requirements exist for the training and licensing of pharmacy technicians, although some states have begun to require registration of pharmacy technicians. In the past, most pharmacy technicians learned their trade on the job, and it is still possible to gain employment as a pharmacy technician with only a high school diploma. However, most pharmacy technicians have Associate degrees or one-year certificates, and roughly a quarter are nationally **Certified Pharmacy Technicians**, or **CPhTs**.

In 1995, several professional organizations, including the American Pharmaceutical Association (APhA), American Society of Health-System Pharmacists (ASHP), Michigan Pharmacists Association, and Illinois Council of Health-System Pharmacists, came together to create the **Pharmacy Technician Certification Board (PTCB)**. This board in turn created the **Pharmacy Technician Certification Examination**, or **PTCE**. It also established guidelines for recertification every two years, which involves ten hours of continuing education each year. Since the creation of the examination, roughly 25,000 people have passed it. Increasingly, hospitals and drugstore chains are requiring technicians to be certified. However, it remains uncertain the extent to which certification will become mandatory across the United States. Most states do not require certification. A few, such as Louisiana, do require certification. Some require taking the PTCE. Some have their own certification examinations. Some require only that pharmacy technicians be registered with the state and undergo supervised on-the-job training.

The job outlook for pharmacy technicians is superb. One school that trains pharmacy technicians estimates that the number of technicians nationwide will grow from about 81,000 in late 1997 to about 109,000 by the year 2005. In 1997, wages for pharmacy technicians ranged from around $11,000 to about $19,000 per year, with hospitals, on the whole, paying higher wages than community pharmacies and higher salaries being paid to certified technicians. Pharmacy technicians can expect to receive additional pay for working off-hours and for overtime. Hospitals and chain store pharmacies tend to have excellent benefits packages, including medical and dental plans, retirement plans, paid sick leave, and tuition reimbursement for those considering pursuing a BS or PharmD degree.

Duties of the Pharmacy Technician

Chart 1.1 contains a partial list of the many duties that pharmacy technicians may be called upon to perform.

Chart 1.1

JOB DUTIES FOR PHARMACY TECHNICIANS

Prescription Preparation (under a Pharmacist's Supervision)

- Taking prescriptions in writing from patients, customers, or their representatives (In most states, prescriptions given by telephone must be taken by licensed pharmacists. While the technician may take a written prescription, it is expected that he or she will pass this along to the pharmacist.)
- Checking prescriptions for completeness and accuracy
- Preparing prescription labels
- Locating, counting, pouring, weighing, measuring, and mixing medications
- Reconstituting medications
- Selecting proper prescription containers
- Affixing labels to prescription containers

- Pricing prescriptions
- Filling prescriptions
- Establishing and maintaining patient profiles
- Repackaging and labeling medications
- Maintaining packaging and dispensing equipment
- Replenishing medications for nursing units, night cupboards, emergency boxes or trays, and cardiac arrest kits
- Preparing IVs and other solutions and admixtures using **aseptic** techniques
- Maintaining and cleaning equipment

Administrative Duties

- Preparing and reconciling **third-party billings** (those sent to carriers of prescription insurance), an activity that is known as third-party administration, or TPA
- Preparing receipts, invoices, letters, and memoranda
- Filing
- Generating and maintaining written or computerized patient medication records and medication reviews
- Maintaining drug information files
- Billing other departments for medication
- Basic bookkeeping/accounting
- Operating the cash register

Communication Duties

- Communicating with customers, physicians, and suppliers
- Referring questions related to prescriptions, drug information, poison information, and other health issues to the pharmacist
- Receiving and sending electronic communications via modem

Inventory Duties

- Monitoring stock levels
- Receiving and checking supplies purchased
- Issuing supplies
- Restocking medications and supplies
- Maintaining storage facilities
- Maintaining inventory records, including those for narcotics and other controlled substances
- Rotating stock and monitoring expiration dates
- Identifying and retrieving expired products for disposal, destruction, or return to manufacturer
- Repackaging of medications (including doing unit dose packaging)
- Delivering medications to wards

Chart 1.1
(cont.)

Duties Specific to Hospitals, Clinics, and Long-term Care Facilities

- Delivering medications to wards; maintaining nursing station medications
- Restocking of ward with narcotics and other controlled substances
- Preparing 24-hour supplies of medication for patients
- Collecting quality improvement data
- Delivering medications to patients' rooms
- Operating computerized or robotic dispensing machinery
- Maintaining files and statistics related to drug-information requests
- Maintaining the Drug Information Center's collection of literature
- Collating institutional data on adverse reactions and drug utilization

THE PHARMACY WORKPLACE: COMMUNITY AND HOSPITAL PHARMACIES

Community, or Retail, Pharmacies

Three-fifths of all pharmacists in the United States work in **community**, or **retail**, **pharmacies**. Some of these pharmacies are independently owned small businesses, while some are part of large retail chains, and still others are franchises. A **franchise** combines characteristics of an independent business and a large retail chain. Franchise agreements vary, but typically they involve a large retail company, the **franchiser**, that grants exclusive use of the company name and rights to sell company products to an owner/operator of a drugstore, the franchisee. An example of such a franchise operation is The Medicine Shoppe.® Most community pharmacies are divided into an R̲ area offering prescription merchandise and related items and a front area offering over-the-counter drugs, toiletries, cosmetics, cards, and so on. (The symbol R̲ means "take" and is commonly used in prescriptions.)

Typical duties of the pharmacy technician in a community pharmacy are to aid the pharmacist in the filling, labeling, and recording of prescriptions; to operate and be responsible for the pharmacy cash register; to stock and inventory prescription and **over-the-counter (OTC) medications** (those not needing a prescription); to maintain computerized or written patient records; to prepare insurance claim forms; and to order and maintain parts of the front-end stock. The last of these duties might involve interaction with a front-end manager responsible for the nonpharmacy area of the drugstore.

Hospital Pharmacies

A quarter of all pharmacists work in hospital settings. According to the American Hospital Association definition, a **hospital** is an institution that offers 24-hour healthcare service; that has six or more beds, a governing authority, and an organized medical staff; and that offers nursing and pharmacy services. Hospitals are classified by type of service into **general** and **specialized** hospitals; by length of stay into **short-term care** (under thirty days) and **long-term care** (thirty days or more) hospitals; and by ownership into **governmental** and **nongovernmental** hospitals, and into **for-profit** and **nonprofit** hospitals. In addition, hospitals are often described according to bed capacity. The functions of a hospital include the following:

- diagnosis and testing
- treatment and therapy
- patient processing (including admissions, record keeping, billing, and planning for postrelease patient care)
- public health education and promotion, done through a variety of programs, including smoking cessation programs, weight loss programs, support group programs, and screenings of community members (including mammographies and testing of blood pressure and cholesterol)
- teaching (training health professionals)
- research (carrying out programs that add to the sum of medical knowledge)

Traditionally, hospitals are run by a president who reports to a board of directors. Reporting to the president or to an executive vice president, in a typical hospital, are vice presidents in the following areas:

- ambulatory services
- community services
- fiscal services
- human and educational services
- management services
- medical services
- nursing services
- planning and program development
- professional services

The vice president for professional services usually oversees the departments responsible for anesthesiology, clinical services, laboratory testing, medical records, psychiatry, radiology, rehabilitation, respiratory care, social services, and pharmacy.

Similar to a community pharmacy, the hospital pharmacy carries out the functions of maintaining drug treatment records and ordering, stocking, compounding, repackaging, and dispensing medications and other supplies. It also prepares sterile intravenous medications (IVs), prepares 24-hour supplies of patients' medications, stocks nursing stations, and delivers medications to patients' rooms. The pharmacy technician in a hospital setting may take part in all of these functions. In addition, he or she may operate manual or computerized, robotic dispensing machinery.

In addition to the functions described in the preceding paragraph, a hospital pharmacy typically carries out numerous **clinical functions**, the purpose of which is dispensing not drugs but information. These clinical functions include providing drug information to healthcare professionals, monitoring drug therapy profiles, educating and counseling patients about their drug therapies, conducting drug usage evaluations, collecting and evaluating information about adverse drug reactions, participating in clinical drug investigations and research, providing in-service drug-related education, auditing for quality assurance, and providing expert consultation in such areas as **pediatric pharmacology** (the effects of drugs on babies and children) and **pharmacokinetics** (the absorption, distribution, and elimination of drugs by the body).

As part of their clinical functions, hospital pharmacies typically operate **Drug Information Centers**, the purpose of which is to collect and provide information and literature about drugs and their effects. The technician working in a Drug Information Center may be responsible for maintaining and filing correspondence and pharmacy-related literature, including abstracts, catalogs, correspondence, journals, microfilm, and newsletters; for logging information requests and compiling statistics about those requests; and for collating data on drug utilization and adverse reactions.

The staff of the hospital pharmacy may include administrators, **staff pharmacists** with BA degrees, **clinical pharmacists** with PharmD degrees, and pharmacy technicians. Hospital pharmacies and drugstore chains are more likely than community pharmacies to require that pharmacy technicians be certified. Some encourage people to become certified by paying for the certification exam and giving raises to people who pass it.

OTHER PHARMACY WORKPLACES

In addition to working in community and hospital pharmacies, both pharmacists and pharmacy technicians find employment with home healthcare services; nursing homes and other long-term care facilities; clinics; health maintenance organizations (HMOs); the federal government, including the military services; nuclear medicine pharmacies; mail-order prescription pharmacies; insurance companies; medical software developers; pharmaceutical manufacturers; drug wholesale companies; manufacturing companies in the food and beverage industries; and educational institutions offering training to pharmacists and pharmacy technicians.

Home Healthcare Systems

In recent years, spiraling hospitalization costs, regulatory changes, and advances in **parenteral therapies** (those involving the administration of nutrients and medications through subcutaneous and intravenous injection) have created an explosion in **home healthcare**, the delivery of medical, nursing, and pharmaceutical services to patients who remain at home. The home healthcare market grew from less than a billion dollars per year in the 1970s to over 30 billion per year in the late 1990s. Pharmacists and pharmacy technicians working in home healthcare—through a hospital, community pharmacy chain, HMO, or private home healthcare provider—provide educational materials, carry out traditional compounding and delivery functions, prepare and provide infusions and infusion equipment, and often must be available for emergencies on a 24-hour basis.

Long-term Care Facilities

Long-term care facilities provide institutional services to elderly patients and to others who cannot provide for themselves, including infants, children, and adults who suffer from severe birth defects, traumatic brain injuries, or **chronic** (long-lasting), debilitating illnesses. They also provide adult day-care services for persons with chronic psychiatric or medical disorders. Licensed pharmacists, who can be either employees of the facility or outside consultants, provide to long-term care facilities such services as establishing record-keeping systems related to controlled substances, reviewing the drug regimens of residents, reporting irregularities related to drug treatments or controlled substances, monitoring the on-site repackaging and storage of pharmaceuticals, ensuring that medications are uncontaminated and have not expired, calling attention to medication errors and possible adverse reactions or interactions, educating residents and sometimes their family members regarding drug therapies and self-medication, and providing medications to outpatients or residents on leave. In many of these areas, the pharmacist may play a crucial role in ensuring regulatory compliance by the long-term care facility, as long-term care is a highly regulated industry. For example, each patient profile in a long-term care facility must be checked monthly by a licensed pharmacist.

Under supervision by the pharmacist, the pharmacy technician in a long-term care facility may log prescriptions and refill orders via computer, prepare billings, maintain drug boxes or trays for emergencies, package and label medications, deliver medications to nursing stations, maintain records, retrieve patient charts and organize them for the pharmacist's review, conduct regularly scheduled inspections of drugs in inventory and in nursing stations to remove expired or recalled medications, and repackage drugs in **unit doses** labeled for each patient. **Unit dose systems** typically make use of a storage bin in a medication cart containing medication for a given resident for a 24-hour period. Some long-term care providers fill medication carts for longer periods—two, three, or five days.

chapter summary

The profession of pharmacy has ancient roots, dating to the use of drugs for magical and curative purposes before the beginning of civilization. Starting in the Middle Ages, pharmacy began to disengage itself from medicine and to become established as a distinct profession. Today, pharmacists are highly educated professionals who operate in a variety of settings, including community pharmacies, hospitals, home healthcare systems, and long-term care facilities. Pharmacy is primarily a knowledge-based profession. As such, it provides not only a dispensatory function, involving the ordering, preparation, and dispensing of medicines, but also a clinical function, involving the provision of information about drugs to patients and healthcare practitioners.

The pharmacy technician is a paraprofessional who, under the supervision of a pharmacist, carries out a wide range of duties related to prescription preparation, communication, and inventory control. The technician also typically has various clerical duties. At present, the job of the pharmacy technician is being redefined, moving away from lay clerical status to paraprofessional status involving education to the Associate degree level and, in many cases, professional registration and certification. Pharmacy technicians work in all the settings in which pharmacists are found, and the demand for competent technicians is expected to grow considerably in the near future.

chapter review

Knowledge Inventory

1. A list of drugs is known as a
   a. formulary
   b. dispensatory
   c. pharmacopeia
   d. all of the above

2. The humor associated with melancholy was
   a. blood
   b. phlegm
   c. yellow bile
   d. black bile

3. In days gone by, the pharmacist was commonly referred to as
   a. an apothecary
   b. a chemist
   c. a druggist
   d. all of the above

4. Knowledge of the medicinal functions of natural products of animal, plant, or mineral origin is known as
   a. pharmacognosy
   b. pharmacology
   c. Galenical pharmacy
   d. clinical pharmacy

5. The emergence of the pharmaceutical industry threatened to reduce the traditional role of the pharmacist to that of a
   a. compounder of medications
   b. pharmaceutical scientist
   c. drugstore operator
   d. toxicologist

6. The work that heralded the emergence of modern clinical pharmacy was the
   a. Code of Ethics of the American Pharmaceutical Association
   b. Millis Report
   c. Report of the President's Commission on Controlled Substances
   d. Kefauver-Harris Amendment to the Food, Drug, and Cosmetic Act of 1938

7. A technician who has completed the national certification examination is known as a
   a. PharmD
   b. CPhT
   c. RPhT
   d. PCT

8. Another name for a community pharmacy is a
   a. retail pharmacy
   b. long-term care facility
   c. home healthcare pharmacy
   d. health maintenance organization

9. The purpose of clinical pharmacy is to
   a. dispense medications
   b. compound medications
   c. report adverse reactions or interactions to medications
   d. provide information about medications

10. Licensing and general professional oversight of pharmacists and pharmacies is carried out by
    a. colleges of pharmacy
    b. the American Pharmaceutical Society
    c. the United States Pharmacopeial Convention
    d. state pharmacy boards

Pharmacy in Practice

1. Visit the site of the Pharmacy Technician Certification Board on the World Wide Web, at http://www.ptcb.org. Study the description given on the site of the content of the Pharmacy Technician Certification Examination and the sample questions provided. Take notes on these materials and then participate in a class discussion about the exam. The discussion should deal with the value of taking the exam, the structure of the exam, and the content covered by the exam. Consider this question: what influence might the creation of the national certification exam have had on elevating the status of the pharmacy technician in people's minds?

2. Do some library research to make a list of names, addresses, telephone numbers, and Web sites of pharmacy-related organizations in your state.

In class, compare your list with those prepared by other students and compile a complete list for future reference.

3. Go to the library and find a copy of the latest edition of the federal government's *Occupational Outlook Handbook.* Using information from the *Handbook,* prepare a short report on the work conditions, duties, training, salaries, and job outlook for one pharmacy-related profession.

4. Call some local drugstores and hospital pharmacies and arrange to interview two practicing pharmacy technicians about their job duties. Prepare an oral report for your class based on the interviews that you conduct.

5. Contact the admissions department of one college of pharmacy and ask them to send you information on admissions policies and degrees and programs offered at the school. Based upon the information that you receive, do a report on the various degrees and programs open to people in the pharmacy field.

Pharmacy Law, Standards, and Ethics for Technicians

2

The practice of pharmacy is controlled by a variety of mechanisms. These include common law—the system of precedents established by decisions in cases throughout legal history; statutory law—laws passed by legislative bodies at the federal, state, and local levels; regulatory law—the system of rules and regulations established by governmental bodies such as the FDA and state boards of pharmacy; professional standards—guidelines established by professional associations; and codes of ethics—rules for proper conduct, again established by professional associations. The complex system of interrelated laws, regulations, standards, and ethical guidelines helps to ensure that drug therapies and merchandising are carried out safely and in the public interest.

Learning Objectives

- Distinguish among common law, statutory law, regulatory or administrative law, ethics, and professional standards
- Explain the potential for tort actions under the common law related to negligence and other forms of malpractice
- List and describe the major effects on pharmacy of the major pieces of statutory federal drug law in the twentieth century
- Enumerate the major principles of the Code of Ethics for Pharmacists of the American Pharmaceutical Association and the Code of Ethics of the American Association of Pharmacy Technicians
- Enumerate the duties that may legally be performed by pharmacy technicians in most states

TERMS TO KNOW

Burden of proof In the law, the requirement to make a case, which in the United States generally falls upon the state or, in the case of a suit, on the person bringing the suit

Civil law That body of law that deals with noncriminal cases

Code of Federal Regulations, Title 21 The portion of the federal Code of Regulations that deals with the regulation of drugs

Common law That body of law that consists of precedents established by the history of decisions made by courts in individual cases

Compensatory damages A monetary award to a plaintiff made to redress an injury

Criminal law That body of law that deals with violations of statutes and/or regulations and with the penalties established for such violation

Ethics The subfield of philosophy that deals with the study of right action or the nature of good and evil

THE NEED FOR DRUG CONTROL

Not until 1951, with the passage of the Durham-Humphrey Amendment to the Food, Drug, and Cosmetic Act of 1938, was the distinction made under U.S. federal law between drugs that can and drugs that cannot be purchased without a prescription from a physician. In some countries yet today, any drug can be dispensed or sold by any person without legal restriction. To persons working in pharmacy in the United States today, such laxity of control over drugs seems astonishing, for pharmacy has become, in our time, one of the most highly proscribed professions. Contemporary pharmacy is subject to many kinds of control at the federal, state, and local levels (see Chart 2.1).

Why do all these levels of control exist? In the nineteenth century, the philosopher John Stuart Mill, in a book called *On Liberty,* expressed the opinion, sometimes referred to as **Mill's Doctrine**, that governments had the right to control people's behaviors only in those cases where the behaviors had a potential for bringing harm to others. Mill's Doctrine would seem to present a reasonable limit to arbitrary use of governmental authority, and it is the spirit of this doctrine that underlies the principle of **informed consent**, which allows people to accept or to reject treatment or medication after having received information about that treatment or medication. However, in practice, Mill's Doctrine presents difficulties. The drug addict, for example, may bring harm not only to himself but to others, and the patient who refuses, due to a psychiatric condition, to feed himself or herself may bring pain and suffering to relatives and friends. What is indisputable in Mill's Doctrine, however, is this: the social contract under which a legitimate government is established places a responsibility on that government to keep its citizens from bringing harm to others.

Because of the power of drugs to bring harm—directly through potency, toxicity, or contamination, or indirectly through lack of efficaciousness—most modern governments hold that they have a right and a duty to control the ways in which people develop, prescribe, store, and dispense drugs to and for others.

RULES OF THE PHARMACY PROFESSION: LAWS, STANDARDS, AND ETHICS

The controls exercised over drugs fall into three not entirely exclusive categories: laws, standards, and ethics. Laws are the rules established by governmental authority or court precedent. Often, violation of a law can result in criminal penalties, administrative sanctions such as license revocation, or lawsuits in which someone claims that the violation has caused him or her harm. Standards are guidelines for practice established by professional organizations. Violation of professional standards can lead to administrative sanctions even when the violation remains within the law. Ethics is the subfield of philosophy that deals with right and wrong action. An action might be within the law and might not be a violation of professional standards and yet still be unethical. For example, a pharmacist operating in an area with a high incidence of HIV infection might have an ethical responsibility to participate in local education programs involving the use of condoms and the sharing of needles, even though he or she is not required by law or by professional standards to do so. Of course, such ethical decisions are up to individuals, whereas compliance with the law and with professional standards is not.

Types of Law

A **law** is a rule established by legal precedent or by a governmental body, with or without mandated consequences for its violation. The three main kinds of law are: common law, statutory law, and regulatory or administrative law.

The **common law** is that body of law derived from the history of decisions made by courts in individual cases. Areas of common law include contracts, property law, domestic law, and **torts** (law related to personal injury). Because of the danger of injury from drugs, tort law is of particular relevance to the practice of pharmacy. Underlying the common law is the principle of *stare decisis,* meaning, literally, "to stand by things decided." Under the common law, when a particular matter is at issue in court, judges, attorneys, and juries make reference to **precedents**, decisions made by previous courts in similar cases. For example, it is a long-established principle in the common law that the physician is a learned intermediary between a drug product developer and a patient. Under the **learned intermediary doctrine**, a drug product developer has the responsibility to warn a physician of a potential **adverse reaction**, or negative consequence, of taking a drug, and the physician, in turn, has a responsibility to warn the patient. If the physician has been warned by the manufacturer of the adverse side effect, and if he or she knows that the patient runs a risk of substantive harm from this side effect and fails to warn the patient, then the physician, not the manufacturer, may

---

Law   The official rules of conduct established and enforced by the authority, legislation, or custom of a governmental body, including, in the United States system, common law, based on previous court decisions; statutory law, based on statues passed by legislative bodies; and regulatory law, based on rules and regulations promulgated by regulatory agencies

Learned intermediary doctrine   The legal principle that a physician acts as an intermediary between the drug manufacturer and the patient, with responsibility to pass on to the patient warnings by drug manufacturers about drugs given to him or her

Negligence   Failure to use a reasonable amount of care to prevent injury or damage to another

Precedent   A rule established by a court decision in a previous case

Prima facie **case**   The requirement that a plaintiff or the state demonstrate that there is sufficient reason for an action under the law

Punitive damages   Damages, often monetary, awarded by a court and meant not necessarily to compensate the victim but to punish the offender

Regulatory law   That body of law consisting of rules and regulations promulgated by agencies empowered by statute to issue said rules and regulations in order to enforce the statute

Standards of practice   Guidelines for professional practice, established by professional organizations, that are often referred by courts, especially in tort cases, as establishing minimum guidelines for the behaviors of professionals

Statutory law   That body of law which consists of laws passed by legislative bodies at the federal, state, and local level

Strict product liability   The legal principle by which a manufacturer is held liable for the sale of a dangerous product even if the product was developed and manufactured in good faith and according to the good manufacturing practices established by FDA regulations

Tort   Personal injury law

Chart 2.1

CONTROLS ON CONTEMPORARY PHARMACY

Controls on contemporary pharmacy are exercised by:

- State boards of pharmacy

- Courts

- Federal, state, and local legislative bodies such as the United States Congress, state legislatures, and municipal governing councils

- Federal and state regulatory agencies such as the **Food and Drug Administration (FDA)**, with general authority to regulate the manufacture and sale of drugs; the **Drug Enforcement Administration (DEA)**, with enforcement authority over controlled substances; the **Occupational Health and Safety Administration (OSHA)**, with authority over workplace safety; the **Federal Trade Commission (FTC)**, with authority over business practices; the **Health Care Financing Administration (HCFA)** of the **Department of Health and Human Services (DHHS)**, with authority over reimbursement under the Medicare and Medicaid programs; state health and welfare agencies; and **state boards of pharmacy**, with licensure and regulatory authority over pharmacy practice at the state level

- The private corporation known as the **United States Pharmacopeial Convention (USPC)**, which publishes the compendia setting standards for drug formulation and dosage forms

- Professional organizations such as the **American Pharmaceutical Association (APhA)**, the **American Association of Colleges of Pharmacy (AACP)**, the **National Association of Boards of Pharmacy (NABP)**, the **Joint Commission on Accreditation of Healthcare Organizations (JCAHO)**, and the **American Society of Health-System Pharmacists (ASHP)**

- Individual institutions such as community pharmacies, hospitals, long-term care facilities, and home healthcare organizations

be charged with **negligence**, or failure to use a reasonable amount of care to prevent injury or damage to another. In a case of negligence, the **burden of proof**, or requirement to make a case, falls on the **plaintiff**, or person bringing suit under the common law. He or she must first establish a *prima facie* case, showing sufficient reason for an action under the law. To establish a *prima facie* case for negligence, a plaintiff must demonstrate that

1. there was a duty owed,

2. the duty was breached,

3. this breach of duty caused substantive damages, and

4. these damages did occur.

To win the case, the plaintiff must prove each of these claims by a **preponderance of the evidence**, that is, he or she must show that most—more than 50 percent—of the evidence supports each of these claims. This standard of support by the preponderance of the evidence is less strict than the usual standard for criminal cases, that the culpability of the **defendant**, or person being charged, be established beyond a reasonable doubt. If convicted of negligence, the physician, or the physician's insurer, may be subject to paying **compensatory damages**, a monetary award to the plaintiff for redress of the injury. If the injury or negligence is severe, the pharmacist or technician may be subject to **punitive damages**, meant not to compensate the victim but to punish the offender. In most cases, the pharmacist who dispensed the medication cannot be held responsible as long as he or she filled the physician's prescription properly and otherwise abided by the law. However, the pharmacist also can be charged with negligence if he or she knows that a given customer or patient runs a particular risk in taking the medication and fails to warn the customer or patient of that risk. In some cases, pharmacists, or even technicians, are charged with **contributory negligence** (sharing in the negligence of the physician and/or manufacturer) or with **comparative negligence** (sharing in the negligence to some specified degree, say, 25 percent). A common defense against charges of negligence is the charge of contributory negligence on the part of the patient or customer. If a patient fails to heed the warnings of the manufacturer, physician, or pharmacist, this contributory negligence can be an absolute bar to recovery of damages.

When a patient has suffered injury as the result of taking of a drug, it can be because the drug was itself defective or because it was not prescribed, labeled, dispensed, or taken properly. Most tort cases brought against pharmacies, pharmacists, or pharmacy technicians involve one or more of the following failures of duty:

1. accidental substitution of another drug for the one prescribed

2. failure to warn, given knowledge (from a patient's record), of a substantive danger involved in taking the drug

3. improper compounding of the drug involving the wrong ingredients or quantities of ingredients

4. introduction into the drug of nonsterile, adulterated, or otherwise dangerous ingredients

5. failure to dispense the drug in the dosage form or amount prescribed

6. failure to label a drug properly

7. failure to package a drug properly

8. failure to interpret a drug order, prescription, or record properly

9. failure to fill a prescription or to do so in a timely fashion

10. dispensing of an expired or recalled drug or drug ingredients (An **expired drug** is one that has exceeded the federally mandated **expiration date**, or latest time for use, given on the labeling by the manufacturer. A **recalled drug** is one that has been discovered to involve excessive adverse reactions, or to have other problems and that is, on written notification, to be returned to the manufacturer. Loosely, people refer to a recall initiated by the manufacturer as a **voluntary recall** and to one required by the FDA as an **involuntary recall**.)

If the pharmacist or technician has taken an action that was in error, he or she is said to be guilty of **malfeasance**. If the pharmacist or technician has failed to take a necessary action required by law, regulation, or professional standards, he or she is said to be guilty of **nonfeasance**. Both malfeasance and nonfeasance are varieties of **malpractice**, the failure to perform properly the duties owed to the patient or customer under existing laws, regulations, and standards of practice. If the drug itself was defective, then the patient or customer may sue the manufacturer for damages on grounds of negligence, **breach of warranty** (claiming that the manufacturer violated an express or implied warranty that the product would not be harmful), or **strict product liability** (which holds the manufacturer strictly liable for the sale of a dangerous product even if the product was developed and manufactured in good faith and according to **good manufacturing practices (GMP)**, which are manufacturing practices for food and drug products established by FDA regulations).

Statutory law is the body of law created by the actions of legislatures. The laws thus created are known as **statutes**. The United States Constitution established a Congress, consisting of a House of Representatives and a Senate, empowered to pass laws in particular areas of legitimate government interest. The legislatures of the various states and commonwealths are similarly constitutionally enacted and empowered. Laws passed by federal or state legislatures must stand review by the courts and may be invalidated, in whole or in part, due to incompatibility with the Constitution. For example, a law may be struck down as unconstitutionally vague, or for not meeting the constitutional requirement that citizens be informed of the laws under which they are to abide. In the United States, when federal and state laws differ, *the stricter of the two laws generally applies*. For example, there is no federal law requiring the certification or registration of pharmacy technicians. However, a state law requiring such certification or registration would apply to a given case, being the stricter of the two.

Of primary importance in the statutory drug law of the United States are the Federal Food, Drug, and Cosmetic Act of 1938 and its subsequent amendments, and the Comprehensive Drug Abuse Prevention and Control Act of 1970, also known as the Controlled Substances Act (see "A Brief History of Statutory Pharmacy Law," p. 23). If, in the course of a negligent activity, a pharmacist violates a statute or regulation, then he or she may be charged with **negligence per se**. A finding of negligence per se might result, for example, if a pharmacist knowingly filled a forged prescription for a narcotic that then brought injury or death to the person receiving it. In such a case of negligence per se, the pharmacist's insurer could not be held accountable, and substantial **civil** (noncriminal) penalties likely to result would fall entirely on the pharmacist or on the pharmacist and his or her employing institution under the common law doctrine of *respondeat superior*, which allows a plaintiff to sue the employer of a negligent employee. Of course, having broken a law established by statute, the pharmacist would also be subject to separate criminal penalties as provided for under the statute.

Just as the Constitution establishes and empowers the Congressional bodies to create statutes, so statutes enacted by legislatures may establish and empower **regulatory agencies**, bodies that create rules, known as **regulations**, to carry out the intent of the statutes. Such **regulatory law**, created by agencies empowered by statutes, is an extremely important part of the law governing the profession of pharmacy. The Federal Food, Drug, and Cosmetic Act created the agency known as the **Food and Drug Administration (FDA)**. The **Drug Enforcement Administration (DEA)**, which enforces the Controlled Substances Act, was created in yet another way, by a presidential reorganization of agencies previously created by statute. Proposed and final versions of regulations created by these and other agencies are published daily in the **Federal Register (FR)**, and final versions are incorporated into an annual revision of the massive **Code of Federal Regulations, Title 21**. A court may overturn a regulation if it finds that the regulatory agency has exceeded its authority under its enabling statute.

We have already seen that pharmacists and technicians can be subject to civil actions, or lawsuits, under the common law if they cause injury to customers or patients. We have also seen that they can be subject to criminal actions if (and, in fact, only if) they violate a statute. Civil actions may lead to the payment of compensatory and punitive damages. If convicted of a criminal offense, the pharmacist or technician may be subject to a fine, imprisonment, or some combination thereof. Another kind of action that can be taken against an employing institution, such as a pharmacy or hospital, or against an individual pharmacist or technician is an **administrative action**, brought in a hearing conducted by a regulatory agency, such as the **state board of pharmacy** (the agency that typically, in each state, sets standards for the practice of pharmacy in the state and licenses pharmacies, pharmacists, and sometimes pharmacy technicians). An administrative action may result from violation of a statute, regulation, or of professional standards. Possible administrative actions include fines and, in order of severity, warnings, probation, license suspension, or license revocation. Technically, **standards** are statutes and regulations that bear upon how pharmacy operations are conducted. However, when making decisions regarding particular cases involving professionals, courts and regulatory agencies often consider not only specific statutes and regulations but also generally accepted professional practices as described in the **standards of practice** of professional organizations. For example, sloppiness in record keeping might not be subject to action under specific regulations, but in a given tort case, a court might view this violation of professional standards as an indication of breach of duty in an action charging negligence.

Standards of Practice

Examples of standards of practice include the "Practice Standards of the American Society of Hospital Pharmacists" and the "Competency Statements for Pharmacy Practice," jointly promulgated by the APhA, the AACP, and the NABP. Prospective pharmacy technicians are encouraged to secure copies of these documents and to study them. (Please note that professional standards, or standards of practice, differ from **drug standards**, which set requirements for the formulation of drug substances, ingredients, and dosage forms. These drug standards are contained in the **United States Pharmacopeia (USP)** and the **National Formulary (NF)**, published by the United States Pharmacopeial Convention.)

Codes of Ethics

Ethics, as a philosophical discipline, is the study of right action or of the nature of good and evil. Both pharmacists and technicians are expected to hold themselves to high ethical standards that both reinforce and go further than specific laws and standards of practice. Charts 2.2 and 2.3 present codes of ethics promulgated by the APhA and the American Association of Pharmacy Technicians (AAPT).

Chart 2.2

CODE OF ETHICS FOR PHARMACISTS OF THE AMERICAN PHARMACEUTICAL ASSOCIATION[1]

Preamble: Pharmacists are health professionals who assist individuals in making the best use of medications. This Code, prepared and supported by pharmacists, is intended to state publicly the principles that form the fundamental basis of the roles and responsibilities of pharmacists. These principles, based on moral obligations and virtues, are established to guide pharmacists in relationships with patients, health professionals, and society.

I. A pharmacist respects the covenantal relationship between the patient and pharmacist.

Considering the patient-pharmacist relationship as a covenant means that a pharmacist has moral obligations in response to the gift of trust received from society. In return for this gift, a pharmacist promises to help individuals achieve optimum benefit from their medications, to be committed to their welfare, and to maintain their trust.

II. A pharmacist promotes the good of every patient in a caring, compassionate, and confidential manner.

A pharmacist places concern for the well-being of the patient at the center of professional practice. In doing so, a pharmacist considers needs stated by the patient as well as those defined by health science. A pharmacist is dedicated to protecting the dignity of the patient. With a caring attitude and a compassionate spirit, a pharmacist focuses on serving the patient in a private and confidential manner.

III. A pharmacist respects the autonomy and dignity of each patient.

A pharmacist promotes the right of self-determination and recognizes individual self-worth by encouraging patients to participate in decisions about their health. A pharmacist communicates with patients in terms that are understandable. In all cases, a pharmacist respects personal and cultural differences among patients.

IV. A pharmacist acts with honesty and integrity in professional relationships.

A pharmacist has a duty to tell the truth and to act with conviction of conscience. A pharmacist avoids discriminatory practices, behavior or work conditions that impair professional judgment, and actions that compromise dedication to the best interests of patients.

V. A pharmacist maintains professional competence.

A pharmacist has a duty to maintain knowledge and abilities as new medications, devices, and technologies become available and as health information advances.

VI. A pharmacist respects the values and abilities of colleagues and other health professionals.

When appropriate, a pharmacist asks for the consultation of colleagues or other health professionals or refers the patient. A pharmacist acknowledges that colleagues and other health professionals may differ in the beliefs and values they apply to the care of the patient.

Chart 2.2
(cont.)

VII. A pharmacist serves individual, community, and societal needs.

The primary obligation of a pharmacist is to individual patients. However, the obligations of a pharmacist may at times extend beyond the individual to the community and society. In these situations, the pharmacist recognizes the responsibilities that accompany these obligations and acts accordingly.

VIII. A pharmacist seeks justice in the distribution of health resources.

When health resources are allocated, a pharmacist is fair and equitable, balancing the needs of patients and society.

Chart 2.3

CODE OF ETHICS OF THE AMERICAN ASSOCIATION OF PHARMACY TECHNICIANS[2]

Preamble: Pharmacy technicians are healthcare professionals who assist pharmacists in providing the best possible care for patients. The principles of this code which apply to pharmacy technicians working in all settings, are based on the application and support of the moral obligations that guide all in the pharmacy profession in relationships with patients, healthcare professionals, and society.

Principles: (1) A pharmacy technician's first consideration is to ensure the health and safety of the patient, and to use knowledge and skills most capably in serving others. (2) A pharmacy technician supports and promotes honesty and integrity in the profession, which includes a duty to observe the law, maintain the highest moral and ethical conduct at all times, and uphold the ethical principles of the profession. (3) A pharmacy technician assists and supports the pharmacist in the safe, efficacious, and cost-effective distribution of health services and healthcare resources. (4) A pharmacy technician respects and values the abilities of pharmacists, colleagues, and other healthcare professionals. (5) A pharmacy technician maintains competency in practice, and continually enhances professional knowledge and expertise. (6) A pharmacy technician respects and supports the patient's individuality, dignity, and confidentiality. (7) A pharmacy technician respects the confidentiality of a patient's records and discloses pertinent information only with proper authorization. (8) A pharmacy technician never assists in the dispensing, promoting, or distributing of medications or medical devices that are not of good quality or do not meet the standards required by law. (9) A pharmacy technician does not engage in any activity that will discredit the profession, and will expose, without fear or favor, illegal or unethical conduct in the profession. (10) A pharmacy technician associates and engages in the support of organizations that promote the profession of pharmacy through the use and enhancement of pharmacy technicians.

[2]Copyright by the American Association of Pharmacy Technicians. Reprinted with permission.

A BRIEF HISTORY OF STATUTORY PHARMACY LAW

Many people are familiar, from novels and movies, with the lawlessness that reigned during the nineteenth century with regard to medications. (An example of nineteenth-century dispensing practice is shown in Figure 2.1.) Consider the situation in John Irving's superbly researched novel *The Cider House Rules,* in which a character dies from taking a medication called French Lunar Solution, the label of which makes the following promises: "Restores Female Monthly Regularity! Stops Suppression!" and carries the warning: "Caution: Dangerous to Married Women! Almost Certainly Causes Miscarriages!" Suppression was a nineteenth-century euphemism for pregnancy, and the medication, a concentrated fluidextract of an extremely poisonous, or **toxic**, weed known as tansy, was meant as an aborticide. To combat real-life abuses of this kind—abuses in formulation and labeling—the United States Congress passed, in 1906, the first of a series of landmark twentieth-century laws to regulate the development, compounding, distribution, storage, and dispensing of drugs.

Figure 2.1 In the nineteenth century, the job of the pharmacist/ apothecary consisted largely of dispensing drugs and of compounding, or creating, drugs from plant and mineral materials such as those in this old-fashioned materia medica box on display at the History of Pharmacy Museum at the Arizona College of Pharmacy.
Used with permission from the University of Arizona College of Pharmacy.

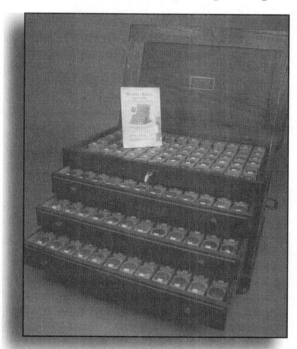

The Pure Food and Drug Act of 1906

The purpose of this act was to prohibit the interstate transportation or sale of adulterated and misbranded food and drugs. The act did not require that drugs be labeled, only that they not contain labels with false information about a drug's strength and purity. The act, though amended, proved unenforceable, and new legislation was required. In 1937, the need for new legislation was tragically demonstrated by 107 deaths resulting from the sale of a sulfa drug product that contained diethylene glycol, used today as an antifreeze for automobile radiators.

The Food, Drug, and Cosmetic Act (FDCA) of 1938

This act, the most important piece of legislation in pharmaceutical history, created the Food and Drug Administration and required pharmaceutical manufacturers to file a **New Drug Application** with the FDA. Under this act, manufacturers must, before marketing a drug product, prove to the FDA's satisfaction that the product is safe for use by humans. To do so, the manufacturer must conduct and submit the results of toxicological studies on animals followed by clinical trials with human beings. **Toxicological studies** are conducted to determine the degree of toxicity, or danger to living organisms, of a substance. **Clinical trials** are controlled experiments held to determine the effects of drugs on human subjects. The New Drug Application must detail the chemical composition of the drug and the processes used to manufacture it. The FDCA also extended and clarified the definitions of adulterated and misbranded drugs. It defined **adulterated drugs** as those

- consisting "in whole or in part of any filthy, putrid, or decomposed substance," ones "prepared, packed, or held under insanitary conditions"

- prepared in containers "composed, in whole or in part, of any poisonous or deleterious substance"

- containing unsafe color additives

- purporting to be or represented as drugs recognized "in an official compendium" but differing in strength, quality, or purity from said drugs

The relevant "official compendia" referred to are the *United States Pharmacopeia* and the *National Formulary*. The act defined **misbranded drugs**, in part, as those

- containing labeling that is "false or misleading in any particular"

- in packaging that does not bear "a label containing (1) the name and place of business of the manufacturer, packer, or distributor; and (2) an accurate statement of the quantity of the contents in terms of weight, measure, or numerical count"

- not conspicuously and clearly labeled with the information required by the act

- that are habit-forming but do not carry the label "Warning—May be habit forming"

- that do not contain a label that "bears (i) the established name of the drug, if any, and (ii) in case it contains two or more ingredients, the established name and quantity of each active ingredient, including the quantity, kind, and proportion of any alcohol, and also including, whether active or not, the established name and quantity" [of certain other substances listed in the act]

- that do not contain labeling with "adequate directions for use" and "adequate warnings against use in those pathological conditions or by children where its use may be dangerous to health, or against unsafe dosage or methods or duration of administration or application"

- that are "dangerous to health when used in the dosage or manner, or with the frequency or duration prescribed, recommended, or suggested in the labeling"

Under this act, the FDA has the power not only to approve or deny new drug applications but also to conduct inspections to ensure compliance. The Supreme Court later held that the act applied to interstate transactions as well as to intrastate transactions, including those within pharmacies. Unfortunately, the act required only that drugs be safe for human consumption, not that they be efficacious, or useful for the purpose for which they were sold.

The Durham-Humphrey Amendment of 1951

This amendment to the FDCA states that drug containers do not have to include "adequate directions for use" as long as they bear the legend "Caution: Federal law prohibits dispensing without a prescription." The dispensing of the drug by a pharmacist with a label giving directions from the prescriber meets the law's requirements. The amendment thus established the distinction between so-called **legend**, or prescription, drugs and **over-the counter (OTC)**, or nonprescription, drugs. It also authorized the taking of prescriptions verbally, rather than in writing, and the refilling of prescriptions. However, the refilling of prescriptions subject to abuse was limited. Under the amendment, prescriptions for such substances could not be refilled without the express consent of the prescriber.

The Kefauver-Harris Amendment of 1962

This amendment was passed in response to the birth, mostly in other countries, of thousands of infants with severe anatomical abnormalities to mothers who had taken the tranquilizer thalidomide. It extended the FDCA to require that drugs be not only safe for humans but also efficacious. The amendment requires drug manufacturers to file with the FDA, before clinical trials on humans, an **Investigational New Drug Application**. After extensive trials in which a product is proved both safe and effective, the manufacturer may then submit a New Drug Application that seeks approval to market the product.

The Comprehensive Drug Abuse Prevention and Control Act of 1970

This act, commonly referred to as the **Controlled Substances Act**, was created to combat and control drug abuse and to supersede previous federal drug abuse laws. The act classified drugs with potential for abuse into five categories, or **schedules**, from those with great potential for abuse to those with little such potential (see Table 2.1). The agency made primarily responsible under this act is the Drug Enforcement Administration (DEA), an arm of the Department of Justice. The DEA is charged with enforcement and prevention related to the abuse of controlled substances.

Table 2.1

DRUG SCHEDULES UNDER THE COMPREHENSIVE DRUG ABUSE AND CONTROL ACT OF 1970

Schedule I Drugs
Drugs with no accepted medical use, or other substances with a high potential for abuse (e.g., heroin, LSD, marijuana, mescaline, peyote, and psilocybin)

Schedule II Drugs
Drugs with accepted medical uses and a high potential for abuse which, if abused, may lead to severe psychological or physical dependence [e.g., amobarbital (Amytal), cocaine, codeine, Desoxyn, Dexedrine, hydromorphone (Dilaudid), meperidine hydrochloride (Demerol), methadone hydrochloride, morphine, opium, oxycodone hydrochloride (Percodan), oxymorphone (Numorphan), phenobarbital (Nembutal), Preludin, Ritalin, secobarbital (Seconal)]

Schedule III Drugs
Drugs with accepted medical uses and a potential for abuse less than those listed in Schedules I and II, which, if abused, may lead to moderate psychological or physical dependence [e.g., certain drugs compounded with small quantities of narcotics and other drugs with high potential for abuse (Tylenol with Codeine tablets), certain barbiturates, glutethimide (Doriden), methyprylon (Noludar), nalorphine (Nalline), paregoric]

Table **2.1**

(cont.)

Schedule IV Drugs

Drugs with accepted medical uses and low potential for abuse relative to those in Schedule III, which, if abused, may lead to limited physical dependence or psychological dependence relative to drugs in Schedule III [e.g., barbital, chloral hydrate (Noctec), chlordiazepoxide (Librium), clonazepam (Clonopin), diazepam (Valium), ethchlorvynol (Placidyl), lorazepam (Ativan), meprobamate (Equanil, Miltown), methohexital, oxazepam (Serax), paraldehyde, phenobarbital, propoxyphene hydrochloride (Darvon)]

Schedule V Drugs

Drugs with accepted medical uses and low potential for abuse relative to those in Schedule IV and which, if abused, may lead to limited physical dependence or psychological dependence relative to drugs in Schedule IV (e.g., Robitussin A-C syrup)

The Poison Prevention Act of 1970

This act, enforced by the Consumer Product Safety Commission, requires that most over-the-counter and legend drugs be packaged in child-resistant containers that cannot be opened by 80 percent of children under five but can be opened by 90 percent of adults. The law provides that on request by the prescriber or signed request by the patient/customer, the pharmacist may dispense a drug in a non-child-resistant container. The patient or customer, but not the prescriber, may make a blanket request that all drugs dispensed to him or her be in noncompliant containers. Other exceptions provided for by the law are detailed in Table 2.2.

Table **2.2**

EXCEPTIONS TO THE REQUIREMENT FOR CHILD-RESISTANT CONTAINERS PURSUANT TO THE POISON PREVENTION ACT OF 1970

1. Single-time dispensing of product in noncompliant container as ordered by prescriber

2. Single-time or blanket dispensing of product in noncompliant container as requested by the patient or customer in a signed statement

3. One noncompliant size of an over-the-counter product for elderly or handicapped users, provided that the label carry the warning "This Package for Households without Young Children" or, if the label is too small, "Package Not Child Resistant"

4. Drugs dispensed to institutionalized patients, provided that these are to be administered by employees of the institution

5. The following specific drugs:

   - Betamethasone tablets with no more than 12.6 mg per package

   - Erythromycin ethylsuccinate tablets in packages containing no more than 16 g

   - Inhalation aerosols

   - Mebendazole tablets with no more than 600 mg per package

   - Methylprednisolone tablets with no more than 85 mg per package

   - Oral contraceptives to be taken cyclically, in manufacturer's dispensing packages

   - Pancrelipase preparations

   - Potassium supplements in unit dose form, including unit dose vials of liquid potassium, effervescent tablets, and unit dose powdered potassium packets with no more than 830 mEq per unit dose

   - Powdered anhydrous cholestyramine

- Powdered colestipol up to 5 g per packet

- Prednisone tablets with no more than 105 mg per package

- Sodium fluoride products with not more than 264 mg of sodium fluoride per package

- Sublingual and chewable isosorbide dinitrate in strengths of 10 mg or less

- Sublingual nitroglycerin (tablets to be taken by dissolving beneath the tongue)

The Drug Listing Act of 1972

This act gives the FDA the authority to compile a list of currently marketed drugs. Under the act, each new drug is assigned a unique and permanent product code, known as a **National Drug Code**, or **NDC**, consisting of 10 characters that identify the manufacturer or distributor, the drug formulation, and the size and type of its packaging. The FDA asks, but does not require, that the NDC appear on all drug labels, including labels of prescription containers. Using this code, the FDA is able to maintain a database of drugs by use, manufacturer, and active ingredients and of newly marketed, discontinued, and remarketed drugs.

The Orphan Drug Act of 1983

An **orphan drug** is one that will be used by so few people that developing and marketing it is prohibitively expensive. This act encourages the development of orphan drugs by providing tax incentives and allowing manufacturers to be granted exclusive licenses to market such drugs.

Drug Price Competition and Patent-Term Restoration Act of 1984

A given drug typically has several names, including its chemical names and its official **generic** or **nonproprietary name** (e.g., ibuprofen), both of which are given in official compendia, and one or more **brand** or **proprietary names** (e.g., Advil, Motrin) given by manufacturers. A **generic drug** is one with the same chemical composition as a brand-name drug that can be substituted (under regulations now existing in every state) for the brand-name drug in prescriptions. The Drug Price Competition and Patent-Term Restoration Act encouraged the creation of both generic drugs and innovative new drugs by streamlining the process for generic drug approval and by extended patent licenses as a function of the time required for the drug application approval process.

Prescription Drug Marketing Act of 1987

Passed in response to concern over safety and competition issues raised by secondary markets for drugs, this act prohibits the reimportation of a drug into the United States by anyone except the manufacturer. It also prohibits the sale or trading of drug samples, the distribution of samples to persons other than those licensed to prescribe them, and the distribution of samples except by mail or by common carrier. In addition, it requires wholesalers who are not authorized distributors of the manufacturer to notify customers of the same prior to a sale.

The Omnibus Budget Reconciliation Act of 1990 (OBRA-90)

Embedded in this budget bill was legislation with a profound effect on how pharmacy is practiced. The act requires that, as a condition of participating in the Medicaid program, states must establish standards of practice for pharmacists requiring **drug use review (DUR)** by the pharmacist. Among other provisions, the act requires "a review of drug therapy before each prescription is filled or delivered to an individual receiving benefits under this subchapter, typically at the point-of-sale or point of distribution. The review shall include screening for potential drug therapy problems due to therapeutic duplication, drug-disease contraindications, drug-drug interactions (including serious interactions with non-prescription over over-the-counter drugs), incorrect drug dosage or duration of treatment, drug-allergy interactions, and clinical abuse/misuse."

Under the law, a pharmacist must make an offer to counsel the patient/customer, but this person may refuse such counseling. Matters discussed in the counseling should include, as necessary, the information described in Table 2.3.

Table 2.3

COUNSELING STANDARDS UNDER OBRA-90

The pharmacist must offer to discuss with the patient or the healthcare professional giving care all matters of significance, including

- Name and description of medication

- Dosage form

- Dosage

- Route of administration

- Duration of drug therapy

- Action to take following a missed dose

- Common severe side effects or adverse effects

- Interactions and therapeutic contraindications, ways to prevent the same, and actions to be taken if they occur

- Methods for self-monitoring of the drug therapy

- Prescription refill information

- Proper storage of the drug

- Special directions and precautions for preparation, administration, and use by patient

OBRA-90 uses the possibility of loss of Medicaid participation to enforce the clinical practices of screening prescriptions and counseling patients and caregivers. It also requires state boards of pharmacy or other state regulatory agencies to provide for the creation of DUR boards for prospective and retrospective review of drug therapies and educational programs for training physicians and pharmacists with regard to the use of medications. The law also requires that manufacturers rebate to state Medicaid programs the difference between the manufacturer's best price for a drug (typically the wholesale price) and average billed price.

LEGAL STATUS AND LEGALLY SANCTIONED DUTIES OF THE PHARMACY TECHNICIAN

As noted in chapter 1, definitions of the roles of the pharmacist and the pharmacy technician are in a state of flux. Increasingly, pharmacists are being called upon to perform clinical functions, counsel customers, monitor patient drug regimens, do prerelease and outpatient counseling, and participate in drug studies. As a result, increasing pressure has arisen for legal definition (or, in some cases, redefinition) of the role of the pharmacy technician, who, by assuming additional distribution, compounding, and dispensing responsibilities, could free the pharmacist to undertake his or her clinical duties. However, and this point is extremely important, **there is at the present time no statutory federal definition of the role of the pharmacy technician and no uniform definition from state to state.** Some states specifically authorize practice by technicians, detailing what duties they may perform. Others do not specifically recognize the technician in state laws and regulations but implicitly define what a technician may or may not do by detailing what the pharmacist must do.

By default, then, duties not required by law or regulation to be done by the pharmacist may be carried out by the technician. As a result of this situation, **it is important that a technician become familiar with the applicable statutes and regulations of the state in which he or she practices.** In some states, for example, technicians may compound solutions for intravenous infusion under the supervision of a pharmacist. In other states, such compounding may be done only by the pharmacist. In yet others, it may be done, as well, by nurses, but only for use by the nurse doing the compounding. The detailed analysis of state laws and regulations as they impact the practice of pharmacy technicians is beyond the scope of this book, but technicians in training are urged to contact knowledgeable professions in training institutions and/or state boards of pharmacy to learn about state-specific statutes and regulations, particularly those related to registration and/or certification by the state and to the specification of those duties that the technician may lawfully undertake. In most practice situations, a pharmacy **policies and procedures manual** will dictate the respective duties of the technician and the pharmacist.

Although statutes, regulations, and standards of practice vary from state to state, some rough generalizations can be made. Generally speaking, as a paraprofessional, the technician is expected to work under the supervision of the pharmacist, and his or her work, under all circumstances, is expected to be checked by the pharmacist. Table 2.4 lists duties that typically may be performed by technicians, while Table 2.5 lists duties that typically are performed by pharmacists, and may *not* be performed by technicians. Again, these vary from state to state, and a technician in training must learn how these duties do or do not differ in his or her locality.

Table 2.4	DUTIES TYPICALLY PERFORMED BY TECHNICIANS

Warning: The duties that technicians may or may not perform under the law differ from one locality to another, in accordance with state and local statutes and regulations. Allowable duties under established policies and procedures also differ from one community pharmacy or institution to another. Therefore, this table and Table 2.5 may or may not be completely accurate for a given practice site. In all practice locations, however, all duties listed in this table, if allowable, *must* be carried out under the direct supervision of a licensed pharmacist.

A. Dispensing, Record Keeping, and Pricing

Receiving written prescriptions and conveying them to the pharmacist

Answering telephone calls

Preparing records, including patient profiles and billing records

Table 2.4 (cont.)

B. Preparing Doses of Precompounded Medications

Retrieving medications from shelf or supply cabinet

Selecting containers

Preparing labels

Counting or pouring medications

Reconstituting prefabricated medications

Pricing prescriptions

C. Preparing Doses of Extemporaneously Compounded, Nonsterile Medications

Retrieving medications from shelf or supply cabinet

Selecting equipment for the compounding operation

Weighing and measuring

Compounding

Preparing labels

Selecting containers

Packaging

Maintaining and filing of records of extemporaneous compounding

Cleaning area and equipment

D. Preparing Doses of Extemporaneously Compounded, Sterile Medications

Retrieving medications from shelf or supply cabinet

Selecting equipment for the compounding operation

Using aseptic equipment and procedures

Weighing and measuring

Compounding

Preparing labels

Selecting containers

Packaging

Maintaining and filing records of extemporaneous compounding

Cleaning of area and equipment

E. Transporting Medications to and from Wards

Preparing cart, tray, or other means of conveyance

Delivering controlled drugs

Maintaining delivery records

Distributing medications to wards

Organizing medications for administration to patients

Retrieving, reconciling, and recording credit for unadministered medications

Returning unadministered medications to unit-dose bins and injectables to stock

F. Replenishing Floor Stocks

Replenishing stocks

Table 2.5

DUTIES TYPICALLY PERFORMED BY PHARMACISTS

A. Dispensing, Record Keeping, and Pricing

Receiving a verbal, or oral, prescription in person or by telephone

Preparing the written form of the verbal prescription

Interpreting and evaluating prescriptions

Reviewing patient profile (medication history, duplication of medications, allergies, drug interactions, etc.)

Verifying and certifying records

B. Preparing Doses of Precompounded Medications

Checking/verifying finished prescriptions

C. Preparing Doses of Extemporaneously Compounded, Nonsterile Medications

Checking/verifying that drugs were selected properly

Calculating weights and measures

Verifying that weighing and measuring was done properly

Verifying finished product

D. Preparing Doses of Extemporaneously Compounded, Sterile Medications

Verifying that drugs were selected properly

Calculating weights and measures

Verifying use of aseptic equipment and procedures

Verifying that weighing and measuring was done properly

Checking/verifying finished product

E. Transporting Medications to and from Wards

Checking/verifying delivery records

Examining returned medications for integrity and reusability

Emptying returned medications into stock containers

F. Replenishing Floor Stocks

Checking/verifying replenishment of stocks

Certifying/checking drug stations

Disposing of unused items and discontinued medications

chapter summary

In the modern era, it is generally recognized that governments and professional organizations have a right to exercise control over the manufacture, dispensing, and use of drugs in order to prevent harm to others due to the misuse or abuse of these potent substances. Controls over the use of drugs are embodied in laws, practice standards, drug standards, and ethical standards. All three kinds of law—common law, statutory law, and regulatory or administrative law—have important consequences for the pharmacy profession. In the area of common law, pharmacy is particularly affected by the potential for tort actions due to negligence or other forms of malpractice. In the area of statutory law, major acts passed by the United States Congress with effects on the pharmacy profession include The Food, Drug, and Cosmetic Act (FDCA), the enabling legislation for the major regulatory organization, the Food and Drug Administration; amendments to the FDCA, including the Durham-Humphrey Amendment and the Kefauver-Harris Amendment; the Comprehensive Drug Abuse Prevention Control Act, which established schedules for controlled substances; the Drug Listing Act; the Orphan Drug Act; the Drug Price Competition and Patent-Term Restoration Act; and the Prescription Drug Marketing Act.

In the area of regulatory law, important regulating agencies include the Food and Drug Administration, which approves or denies New Drug Applications and writes and enforces drug-related regulations, and state boards of pharmacy, which license pharmacies, pharmacists, and (sometimes) technicians; promulgate state regulations; and have the power to take administrative actions against people or organizations that violate laws, regulations, and standards. Standards for drugs are set by official compendia, the *United States Pharamacopeia* and the *National Formulary*. Standards for the practice of pharmacy are set by state boards of pharmacy and by various professional organizations. Several professional organizations, including the American Pharmaceutical Association and the American Association of Pharmacy Technicians also have codes of ethics by which their members are expected to abide. The legal status of pharmacy technicians and their allowable duties vary from state to state, but in all cases, technicians must act under the direct supervision of licensed pharmacists.

chapter review

Knowledge Inventory

1. The principle that governments have a right to control only those activities that involve a potential for harm to others was advanced by
   a. ex-Attorney General Dr. C. Everett Koop
   b. John Stuart Mill
   c. Galen
   d. Cornelius Agrippa

2. A rule promulgated by the FDA governing good manufacturing practice for the film-coating of tablets to be taken orally would be an example of a
   a. statute
   b. principle of the common law
   c. regulation
   d. administrative ruling

3. A particular over-the-counter antihistamine product has the side effect of causing drowsiness, an effect that is greatly increased by the ingestion of even a small amount of alcohol. A drug manufacturer has warned of this drug interaction in the labeling of its product and in its package insert. A physician prescribes the antihistamine to a patient whom he or she knows to be an alcoholic. The patient, while taking the medication, and after having had a glass of wine, has an automobile accident. The patient's attorney, at the law firm of Torts 'r Us, advises the patient that he may sue the physician but not the manufacturer under the legal principle known as
   a. *respondeat superior*
   b. *stare decisis*
   c. breach of warranty
   d. the learned intermediary doctrine

4. In the case of *Bemis vs. State of Indiana,* Bemis invited a woman to his apartment and gave her a bowl containing a dried mushroom. The woman ate the mushroom, left the apartment, and then began hallucinating. She was taken to a hospital by her son. On the following day, Bemis consented to a search of his apartment, where police officers discovered a container containing dried psilocybin mushrooms, several growing psilocybin mushrooms, and growing paraphernalia. Bemis was convicted of dealing and possession of a
   a. Schedule I controlled substance
   b. Schedule II controlled substance
   c. Schedule III controlled substance
   d. Schedule IV controlled substance

5. In a historic case, a sulfa drug marketed as an elixir caused a number of deaths because it was compounded with diethylene glycol. The drug was removed from the market because, as an elixir, it had to be compounded with alcohol. The grounds for removing the drug from the market were that it was
   a. adulterated
   b. misbranded
   c. unlabeled
   d. not in a child-resistant container

6. The legislation that requires drug packaging to bear a label giving an accurate statement of the quantity of the contents in terms of weight, measure, or numerical count is the
   a. Controlled Substances Act
   b. Drug Listing Act
   c. Pure Food, Drug, and Cosmetics Act
   d. Prescription Drug Marketing Act

7. Prior to human clinical trials, a manufacturer must submit
   a. a New Drug Application
   b. an Investigational New Drug Application
   c. a Human Toxicology Study
   d. an Adverse Effects Report

8. All states participate in the Medicaid program, and this fact makes it necessary for all states to meet the DUR requirements of
   a. the FDCA
   b. OBRA-90
   c. the Poison Prevention Control Act
   d. the Drug Price Competition and Patent-Term Restoration Act

9. Pursuant to OBRA-90, a state board of pharmacy might pass a regulation requiring that a
   a. pharmacist notify the local DEA office for instructions on disposal of medications containing controlled substances
   b. pharmacist advise a patient about what to do if he or she misses a dose if missing a dose might be significant
   c. manufacturer take precautions to avoid storage of drugs containing water solvents in places or under conditions that might lead to growth of bacteria
   d. manufacturer prepare a list of all its authorized wholesalers

10. A child-resistant container need not be used if
    a. for a refill, the prescriber has previously signed a blanket request for noncompliant containers
    b. for a refill, the customer has previously signed a blanket request for noncompliant containers
    c. the customer has made a verbal request for a noncompliant container
    d. the pharmacist determines that the customer or patient is of sufficient age to use a noncompliant container correctly

Pharmacy in Practice

1. Case: A pharmacy technician accidentally chooses the antidepressant drug Prozac instead of the prescribed medication, the antisecretory medication Prilosec, used for treatment of heartburn and gastroesophageal reflux disease. The pharmacist fails to check the medication, and the customer experiences no relief of the heartburn and a rare adverse reaction to the Prozac, rendering him temporarily impotent, a condition that causes the patient great psychological distress. The patient decides to sue the pharmacist and the pharmacy technician for negligence. To establish a *prima facie* case, what four claims must the patient prove and to what degree must he prove these? Given the facts as stated, what arguments and/or evidence can the patient put forward to support each of these four claims?

2. Case: In the case of *Baker vs. Arbor Drugs, Inc.,* which went to trial in 1966, the plaintiff, Baker, was taking the antidepressant drug tranylcypromine, under a prescription that he regularly filled at Arbor Drugs. The patient went to a physician with a cold, and the physician, despite having records indicating that the patient was taking tranylcypromine, prescribed phenylpropanolamine. When Baker came to Arbor Drugs to have his prescription filled, a pharmacy technician was warned by the pharmacy's

computer that a potential interaction existed between the new prescription and Baker's prescription for tranylcypromine that had been filled a few days earlier. The technician overrode the computer warning, and the pharmacist filled the prescription, unaware of the potential drug interaction. As a result of taking the phenylpropanolamine, Baker suffered a stroke. Baker brought suit, and on appeal, received a judgment against the pharmacy. Discuss this case with other students. Consider the following questions, given the facts as stated:

   a. Were both the pharmacist and the pharmacy technician guilty of negligence? Consider all four criteria for negligence.

   b. In what ways did the physician, the pharmacy technician, and the pharmacist fail to carry out their duties properly?

   c. What requirement, under OBRA-90, did the pharmacist fail to meet? What relevance does this case have to the expanded clinical role of the pharmacist?

   d. Under what legal principle might Baker sue the pharmacy for the actions of its employees, the pharmacist, and the technician?

   e. Under what legal principle could Baker not sue the manufacturer of the phenylpropanolamine product, given that the physician and the pharmacy had been warned of the dangerous drug interaction?

   f. What role do computers play, in contemporary pharmacy, in helping pharmacists and technicians to meet the counseling requirements of OBRA-90?

   g. Is this a case in which a court could conceivably make a finding of contributory negligence or comparative negligence? Explain.

   h. In what respect was the pharmacist guilty of nonfeasance? In what respect was the pharmacy technician guilty of malfeasance?

3. Case: In the course of his normal duties, a pharmacy technician employed by Hometown Drugs, Inc., discovers from a patient profile that the young man who is dating his daughter is taking a regular prescription for a powerful antipsychotic drug. The technician knows that his daughter and the young man are contemplating getting married. The technician tells his wife about this discovery, who then tells the daughter, who was unaware of her boyfriend's prescription for the drug. Has the pharmacy technician committed a breach of his ethical responsibilities? Explain in writing why you think this is or is not so.

4. Case: In the course of her normal duties, a pharmacy technician employed by Hometown Drugs, Inc., discovers from a patient profile that the young man who is dating her daughter is taking a regular prescription for a powerful antipsychotic drug. The technician keeps this information to herself but, in response to the information, attempts to dissuade her daughter from marrying the young man. Has the technician committed a breach of her ethical responsibilities? Explain in writing why you think this is or is not so.

5. Case: A pharmacist runs a community pharmacy in an area with a 30 percent Spanish-speaking population but does not himself speak Spanish nor employ anyone who speaks Spanish. Might this situation be a breach of the law? of professional ethics as defined by the "Code of Ethics for Pharmacists of the American Pharmaceutical Association"?

6. Case: A pharmacy technician discovers that her employer, Will Malpractice, regularly has been dispensing large amounts of a Schedule II amphetamine to

an obviously overweight individual. The prescription is allegedly for control of a rare hyperactivity disorder. However, the technician knows that both the prescribing doctor and her employer's business partner have a financial interest in a local weight loss clinic. The technician asks her employer about this and is told to mind her own business and get back to work. What legal and ethical obligations do you think that this situation might place on the technician? What is the technician's responsibility under the "Code of Ethics of the American Association of Pharmacy Technicians"? What risk does the technician run if she reports this matter to the state board of pharmacy? What would you do in this situation? Explain.

7. Contact your state board of pharmacy for information about the legal definition of the role of the pharmacy technician; licensure, registration, and/or certification requirements; and allowable duties of pharmacy technicians in your state. Write a report detailing these.

8. Explain what is done improperly in each of the following situations, citing relevant laws or regulations as explained in this chapter:
   a. A telephone call comes into the pharmacy, and the technician answers the phone. The pharmacist is very busy, and the pharmacy is understaffed. The technician takes the prescription, committing it to writing for review by the pharmacist.
   b. A pharmacy technician, working a long night shift in a hospital, takes a mild amphetamine from stock and ingests it in order to stay awake and to carry out his duties.
   c. A pharmacist takes a prescription over the telephone but fails to commit it to writing.
   d. A drug manufacturer sells capsules with labels that claim that the capsules contain phenobarbital 5 mg, but they actually contain phenobarbital 3 mg.
   e. A pharmacy dispenses 800 mg of Mebendazole tablets in a non-child-resistant container, with a specific request from the prescribing physician or the customer.
   f. A pharmacy technician weighs and measures the proper amounts of the ingredients of a powdered extemporaneous compound. The pharmacist then fills capsules with the powder, using the punch method.
   g. A hospital technician retrieves unused meds from a ward and then checks these to make sure that they are in good condition before returning them to stock.

9. In a group, choose either the "Practice Standards of the American Society of Hospital Pharmacists" or the "Competency Standards for Pharmacy Practice," review this document, and report to the class on its contents.

10. Pharmacists with alcohol or substance abuse problems sometimes fail to seek help for fear that a state board of pharmacy might take some disciplinary action should the problem become known. What might professional associations and state boards do, in your opinion, to combat this problem?

11. Amendments or new legislation are often passed in response to deficiencies in previous legislation. Give three examples from the text.

Pharmaceutical Terminology and Abbreviations

3

Like any profession, pharmacy has its own special language, or jargon. A pharmacy worker needs to be familiar with the wider jargon of health-related occupations in general and with the special abbreviations and symbols used to describe drugs, dosage forms, amounts, administration times, and other essential information on prescriptions and medication orders. Knowledge of these symbols and abbreviations, along with attention to sound-alike and look-alike drug names, can help ensure that medication errors do not occur.

Learning Objectives

- Identify common Greek and Latin roots used in medicine and pharmacy
- Define key terms used to describe drugs and their uses, including diagnosis, disease, trauma, disorder, acute, chronic, symptom, syndrome, mitigation, treatment, cure, prevention, generic name, and brand name
- List and describe a number of subfields within the field of pharmacy, including clinical pharmacy, pharmacology, clinical pharmacology, pharmacodynamics, pharmacokinetics, nuclear pharmacy, pharmacoeconomics, pharmacogenetics, and pharmacognosy
- Interpret abbreviations and symbols used in prescriptions and medication orders
- Identify common abbreviations and symbols used to describe weights and measures
- List some common sound-alike and look-alike names of drugs

TERMS TO KNOW

Acute Of short duration or especially severe, sharp, or immediate in impact

ADME The absorption, distribution, metabolism, and excretion of drugs over time

Brand name drug The proprietary name under which a manufacturer markets a drug or a particular dosage form of a drug

Chronic Of extended duration

Congenital Inborn

Cure The effective elimination of a diseased or disordered condition

Diagnosis The process by which a physician or other health-care professional determines the nature of a disease condition by examination of a patient's symptoms

THE NEED FOR SPECIAL TERMINOLOGY AND ABBREVIATIONS

Not so long ago, a dedicated student could go a long way toward mastering the available book-learning (if not the practical knowledge) of his or her culture. Today, all that has changed. Modern education and modern information technologies have created an explosion of knowledge. One consequence of the knowledge explosion is specialization. In the seventeenth century, a single person could comprehend the whole of biological science. In the nineteenth, that person's descendant could absorb the whole of, say, entomology, the study of insects. Today, as Harvard entomologist E.O. Wilson points out, several lifetimes is not enough time in which to learn all that is known about the behaviors of bees, wasps, termites, and other members of the single order of creatures known as Hymenoptera, which contains over a million known species.

To communicate precisely with other people involved in a particular field of endeavor, people find it necessary to invent new terminology, words, and phrases to describe the particular elements of their field. To communicate quickly as well as precisely, they create abbreviations and special symbols. Sometimes, the specialized words, phrases, abbreviations, and symbols used in a scientific field such as pharmacy or medicine can be intimidating. The name of a lung disease suffered by coal miners, for example, is

pneumonoultramicroscopicsilicovolcanokoniosis

and this is not even the longest of all technical words in chemistry, biology, and medicine! Do not let the foreign-sounding nature of scientific words intimidate you, however. With a little study and

Disease Any particular destructive physical process in an organ or organism with a specific cause, or causes, and characteristic symptoms

Disorder An ailment or abnormal functioning

Drug An agent intended for use in the diagnosis, mitigation, treatment, cure, or prevention of disease in man or animals

Generic drug The nonproprietary name of a drug

Medication order In a hospital or other institutional setting, an order for the administration of one or more medications to a patient

Mitigation The process of making something less painful, inconvenient, or otherwise severe

Prescription A direction for the preparation and use of medicine for a particular patient

Prevention The taking of steps before a disease or other abnormality occurs to ensure that it does not occur

Symptom Any condition accompanying or resulting from a disease, disorder, or other abnormality that provides evidence for the existence of the abnormality

Syndrome A set of symptoms that occurs together and that characterizes a particular disease or disorder

Therapy An extended treatment of a disease or disorder

Trauma A bodily wound, injury, or shock

Treatment The taking of action against a disease or disorder

practice in the field of pharmacy, you will soon master most of the specialized terms and abbreviations that you need to know. Most are far shorter and far clearer than the word given above.

GREEK AND LATIN ROOTS IN PHARMACY AND MEDICINE

At the beginning of the scientific revolution, in the Renaissance, most scholars in Western Europe were deeply learned in the Greek and Latin classics, and so it is not surprising that, when inventing new terms to describe their discoveries and observations, they borrowed bits and pieces of these ancient languages. Such coinage, based on Greek and Latin word parts, remains at the heart of scientific naming. Therefore, when you encounter in your practice as a pharmacy technician the names of procedures, parts of the body, drugs, chemicals, and so on, they will often look like this:

analgesia	from Greek *an*, "without," and *algos*, "pain"
diastolic	from Latin *dia*, "apart," and *stellein*, "to put"
streptomycin	from Greek *streptos*, "twisted," and *mykes*, "fungus"
sublingual	from Latin *sub*, "under, below," and *lingua*, "language, tongue"

Some common Greek and Latin roots encountered in medical and pharmaceutical terminology are listed in Table 3.1. You may wish to commit these to memory over a period of many weeks, learning a few at a time. Knowing these roots will be of considerable value in furthering your education about the effects, toxicity, and interactions of drugs.

Table **3.1**

COMMON GREEK AND LATIN ROOTS, PREFIXES, AND SUFFIXES USED IN MEDICAL AND PHARMACEUTICAL TERMINOLOGY

Note: A **root** is a word part that forms a major internal constituent of a word. A **prefix** is a word part added to the beginning of a word. A **suffix** is a word part added to the end of a word.

Root	Meaning	Example
aceto	vinegar, acid, sharp	acetaldehyde
acro	tip, end, sharpness	acromegaly
actin	ray, with radiated structure	actinomycin
acu	sharp, abrupt, sudden	acute
adeno	gland	adenoid, adenovirus
adipo	fat	adipose, adipoma
aero	air	aerogel, aerosol
aesth, esth	perception	anesthetic, anesthesia
agon	contest, struggle	agonist

Root	Meaning	Example
alb	white	albumin
algo, algia	pain	analgesia
allelo	one another, mutual	allergen
ambi/amph	both, two	amphoteric, ampicillin,
ambulo	walk	ambulatory
ameb, amoeb	constantly changing	antiamebic
amnio	membrane around the fetus	amniotic fluid
amylo	starch	amylase, amylolysis
andr, andro	male	androgen
angio	vessel	angiogram, angioplasty
anthrac	black	anthrax
aort	aorta (main artery of body)	aorta
aqu, aqua, aque	water	aqueous
argy	silver, shiny	arginase
artero	artery (as opposed to vein)	arterial
arthro	joint	arthritic
artic	little joint	articular
asthm	shortness of breath	asthma
atri	entry	atrium
aud	hear	auditory
aur	hear	aural
axilla	armpit	axillae
axo	center, axis	axial
azo	nitrogen	azotemia
bol	throw	bolus
blast	sprout	erythroblastosis
blephar, blepharo	eyelid	blepharoptosis
brachi	arm	brachial
brady	slow	bradycardia
bronch	bronchus (pathways from windpipe)	bronchoscope, bronchitis
bucc	inside of cheek	buccal membrane
burs	pouchlike cavity	bursa, bursitis
calc	calcium	hypocalcemia
canc	crab	cancer
cap, capi, capo	head, expansion	capillary
carbo	carbon	carbohydrate
carcin	crab, cancer	carcinogen
cardi	heart	cardiology
carp	wrist	carpal tunnel syndrome
caus	burn	causalgia
cele, -coele	tumor, hernia, cavity	cystocele
centesis	puncture	amniocentesis
centr	center	centrifuge
cephal	head, expansion	hydrocephalic
cereb, cerebr	brain	cerebellum
cervic	neck, cervix	cervicofacial, cervical
chemo	chemistry	chemotherapy

Table 3.1
(cont.)

Root	Meaning	Example
chir	hand	chiropractic
chlor	green	chlorocyte
chol, chole	bile	cholangiole, cholemia
chondr	cartilage; grain	enchondroma
chord, cord	cord, rope	spinal cord
chron	time, long	chronic
cili	eyelash, hair	cilia, penicillin
clino	bed	clinical
coagul	clot	anticoagulant
coccus	berry	staphylococcus
collo	glue	colloid
conios	dust	pneumoconiosis
core, coreo	pupil of eye	coreoplasty
corp	body	corpuscle
crani, cranio	cranium	craniotomy
crine	separation, secretion	endocrine
cule	small	molecule
cuta, cuti	skin	subcutaneous
cyan	blue	cyanosis
cycl	circle, wheel	tetracycline
cyst, cysti, cysto	bladder, cyst	cystic fibrosis
cyto	cell	cytologist
dacr	tear (crying)	dacryostenosis
dacty	finger	syndactylism
demos	people	pandemic, epidemic
dens, dent	tooth	dentifrice
derm	skin	epidermis, dermatology
diphth	leathery membrane	diphtheria
edem, edema	excess fluid in tissues	edema
emia	blood	hypoglycemia
encephal	brain	electroencephalogram
entero	intestine	parenteral, enteric
erythro	red	erythromycin, erythrocyte
esthesia	perception	anesthesia
fec	make, build, do, perform	infection
flat	blow	antiflatulent
galact	milk	galactopoietic
gangl	knot	ganglion
gastr	stomach	gastric acid
gen	become, beget, produce	antigen
genesis	origin	pathogenesis
ger	aged	gerontology
gest	produce	gestation
gli, glia, glio	glue	glial cells
glob	sphere, ball, round body	globule, hemoglobin
gloss	tongue	glossectomy
gluc, gluco	sugar	glucose
glute	buttocks	gluteal

Root	Meaning	Example
glyc, glyco	sugar	hyperglycemia
gnosis	know	prognosis
gonado	reproductive organ	gonadotropin
gram	record	sonogram
gran	grain	granule, granulocyte
graph	writing, record	sonograph
gynec	female	gynecological
haem, hem, hemo	blood	hemostat, hemorrhage
hepat	liver	hepatitis
hernia	rupture	hernia
hidr	sweat	hidradenoma
hippo	horse	hippocampus
hydro	water	hydrocephalus
hypno	sleep	hypnotic
hyster	uterus	hysterectomy
ichth	fishy, scaly	ichthyosis
immun, immuno	safe, safe from	immunologist, immune
insul	island	insulin
ject	throw	injection
jejun	jejunum, a section of the small intestine	jejunorrhaphy
kera, kerato	horned	cornea, keratolytic
kinesi, kinesio	motion	kinesiology
labio	lip	labia, labial
lachry	tear (from the eye)	lachrymal fluid
lacto	milk	lactose
lecith	egg yolk	lecithin
leuco	white	leukemia
liga, ligat	bind together, bandage	ligation
ling	tongue	sublingual
lith	stone	nephrolithiasis
lumb, lumbo	lower back, loin	lumbar, lumbodynia
lymph	water	lymphatic system
mal, mali	abnormal, bad	malpractice
malacia	soft	onychomalacia
mast, masto	breast	mastectomy
medi	middle	mediolateral
melano	black	melanoma
mening	membrane	meningitis
mens, menis	moon, month	menses
meter	measure	kilometer, thermometer
metro	uterus, womb	metrorrhea
mnem	memory	mnemonic
morb	sick	morbidity
morph, morpho	shape, dream	morphology, morphine
muscul	mouse, muscle	intramuscular
myc, myco	fungus	mycosis
myelo	soft, pith	myeloid

Table **3.1**
(cont.)

Root	Meaning	Example
myo	muscle	myocardial infarction
myxo, muco	slime	mucous membrane
narco	sleep	narcotic
naso	nose	nasal
nat, nata	birth	prenatal
necro	dead	necrosis
nephr	kidney	nephritis
neuro	nerve	neurotransmitter
nos, nox	unpleasant, sickening	noxious
ocul	eye	ocular, oculonasal
odont	tooth	orthodontics
odyn	pain	anodyne
olfact	smell	olfactory
oma	tumor, lump	steatoma, adipoma, carcinoma
onco	tumor, mass	oncology
onycho	nail	onychomalacia
ophthal	eye	ophthalmic
opi, opio	opium	opiate
optic	eye	optician
orchi, orchid	testes	orchiditis
oro	mouth	oral
ortho	straight	orthodontia
osmo, osmi	smell	anosmia
ost, osteo	bone	osteoporosis
ot, oto	ear	otic
ox, oxo, oxy	oxygen'	hypoxemia
paed, ped	child	pediatric
parit, part	have a baby	post–partum
patho	disease, misery	pathology
pect	chest	expectorant, angina pectoris
ped, pes	foot	orthopedic
pelvi	pelvis	pelvimetry
phac, phaco	lens of eye	phacocele
phage	eat	bacteriophage, dysphagia
pharmaco	sorcery, poison, drug	pharmacy
phasia	speech	aphasia
phero	carry, bear	pheromone
philo	like, love	hydrophilic
phleb	vein	phlebitis, phlebotomy
phleg	flame	phlegm
phone	voice	dysphonia
phori	carry, bear	iontophoresis
phos, phot	light	photosensitivity
phragm	divide into two, wall off	diaphragm
physi	nature, grow	physiological, diaphysis
phyte	plant, growth	osteophyte
pineo	pine cone	pineal

Root	Meaning	Example
plasm	molded	neoplasm
plegi	stroke, paralysis	paraplegic
pleur	rib, side	pleurisy
plex, plexy	braid, wind together	solar plexus
pneum, pneumat	breath	pneumonia
pod, podo	foot	podiatrist
poie, poiesis	making	erythropoiesis
prandial	meal	postprandial
procto	rectum	proctologist
pseud	false	pseudocyesis
psyche	spirit, mind	antipsychotic
pty, ptyalo	spit	hemoptysis
pulmo	lung	pulmonary
pyr, pyro	fever, fire	pyrogen
rach	spine	rachioplegia
radi, radio	radiation	radiography
ren, reni	kidney	renal
retin, retino	retina	retinopathy
rhea, rheo	flow	galactorrhea
rhino	nose	rhinovirus, rhinitis
rrha, rrhag	discharge, flow	hemorrhage
rub, rubr	red	rubella
sacch, sacchar	sugar	saccharine
sang, sangui	blood	consanguine
sarc, sarco	flesh	sarcoma
schis, schiz	split	schizophrenia, rachischisis
sclero	hard	atherosclerosis, sclerosing agent
scope	examine carefully	endoscopic, pharyngoscope
seb, sebo	fat, grease	sebum
sec, seg	cut	section
seps, sept	rot	antiseptic
sero	whey	serum
sial	saliva	sialolith
soma, somy	body	psychosomatic
spasmo	drawing tight	antispasmodic
spondylo	spine	spondylitis
sphygno	heartbeat, pulse	sphygmometer
spir	breathing	spirometer
staphyl	bunch of grapes	staphylococcus
stasis	standing up, being stable	homeostasis
stat	stop	bacteriostat
stern, sterno	breastbone	sternum
stigm	spot	stigmatism
stole	to pull, to draw	diastolic
stom, stoma , stomy	mouth	stomatitis
strepto	wavy	streptomycin
syring	pipe, tube, reed	syringe

Table **3.1**
(cont.)

Root	Meaning	Example
tachy	fast, swift	tachycardia
tact	touch	tactile
teno, tendo	stretch	tendonitis
thel	breast, covering	epithelium
thorac, thoraco	chest	pneumothorax, thoracic
thromb, thrombo	blood clot	thrombolysis
thym	thymus gland	thymectomy
thyro, thyro	thyroid	hypothyroidism
tom, tome	cut	lobotomy
tono	stretch	tonsils, tonsillotome
topo	place	topically
tox, toxo	poisonous	toxic, toxicology
troph, trop	growing, feeding	atrophy, somatotropin
tuber	knob, swelling, truffle	tuberculosis
tympan, tympano	membrane in ear	tympanocentesis
typho	smoky, fever	typhoid
uria, uro	urine	urology
uter, utero	uterus, womb	intrauterine
uvo	grape, iris, uvula	uvular, uvea
vacc	cow, vaccine	vaccinate
vago	nerve	vagotomy
vaso	blood vessel	vasodilation
velo	veil, cover	velamen
ven, veni, veno	vein (as opposed to artery)	ventricular
vener	sex	venereal
vert	turn	vertigo
viscero	internal organs	viscera, visceromegaly
xantho	yellow	xanthin
xero	dry	xeroderma
zema	boiled	eczema
zo	animals	zoomorphic
zygo	yoke	zygote
zyme	ferment	enzyme

Prefix	Meaning	Example
a-, ad-	towards	adsorbent, adsternal
a-, an-	without	amastia, anesthesia
ab-	from, away from	abaxial, abnormal, abscess
allo-	other, another	allopathy
ana-	up to, back, again,	anaplastic
ante-	before, forwards	antecubital
anti-	against, opposite	antitoxin, antiseptic
ap-, apo-	from, back, again	apoplectic
auto-	self	autoimmune
bi-, bis-	twice, double	biceps, bisulfite
bio-	life	biopsy, antibiotic
cata-	down	cataplectic

Prefix	Meaning	Example
circum-	around	circumoral
con-	together	congestion
contra-	against	contraindication
de-	from, away from, down from	decongestant
deca-	ten	dekaliter
di-, dis-	two	distillation
dia-	through, complete	diaphragm, dialysis
dipl-, diplo-	double	diplococci
dis-, dias-	separation	distended
dur-	hard, firm	epidural
dys-	bad, abnormal	dystrophy, dyspepsia
e-, ec-, ecto-	out, from out of	ectopic
em-	in	embolism
en-, endo-	into	endoarteritis, endometriosis
epi-	on, up, against, high	epidermis
eu-	well, normal, abundant	eupnea
ex-, exo-	out, from out of	exotropia
extra-	outside, beyond, in addition	extraoral
haplo-	single	haploid
hemi-	half	hemiplegia
hetero-	different	heterophilic
homo-	same	homeopathy, homeostasis
hyper-	above, excessive	hyperalimentation
hypo-	below, deficient	hypodermic
im-, in-	not	impotence
in-	into, not	invasive, insane
infra-	below, underneath	infracardiac
inter-	among, between	intercostal
intra-	within, inside, during	intravenous
iso-	equal, same	isomorphic
macro-	large	macrocytic
mal-	bad	malnutrition
medi-	middle	medial
mega-	large	megavitamin
megalo-	large	acromegaly
meso-	middle	mesoderm
meta-	change, between	metastasize, metacarpal
micro-	small	micron, microscope
mono	one	mononucleosis, monocyte
neo-	new	antineoplastic
non-	not	nontoxic
pan-	all, across, throughout	pandemic
para-	beside, to the side of, wrong	paranasal
path	disease of, suffering	pathology
per-	by, through, throughout	percutaneous
peri-	around	pericardia
poly	many	polymorphonuclear
post-	behind, after	postpartum

Table **3.1**
(cont.)

Prefix	Meaning	Example
pre-	before, in front	preoperative
primi-	first	primigravida
pro-	before, in front	prootic
pros-	besides, in addition	prosthetic
prox-	beside	proximal
pseudo-	false	pseudoplegia
quadri-	four	quadriplegia
re-, red-	back, again	reconstitute
retro-	backwards, behind	retrovirus
semi-	half	semiconscious
sub-	under, beneath	subcutaneous
super-	above, in addition, over, excessive	supersensitive
supra-	above, on upper side, excessive	suprarenal
syn-	together, with	synthetic
tachy-	rapid	tachycardia
tetra-	four	tetracycline
trans-	across, beyond, through	transocular
tri-	three	triceps
uni-	one	unicellular
ultra-	beyond, excess, more	ultrasound

Suffix	Meaning	Example
-ac	(makes an adjective)	cardiac
-al	(makes an adjective)	myocardial
-algesia	pain	analgesic
-algia	pain	synalgia
-ar	(makes an adjective)	lumbar
-arche	beginning	menarche
-ary	(makes an adjective)	salivary
-ase	enzyme (makes a noun)	amylase
-ate	(makes a verb)	expectorate
-cide	killer	spermicide
-clasis	break	osteoclasis
-desis	binding, fixation	arthrodesis
-dipsia	thirst	polydipsia
-ectomy	removal of, cut out	appendectomy
-emesis	vomiting	hematemesis, emetic
-gen	precursor	pyrogen
-ia	(makes a noun)	hernia
-iasis	condition	nephrolithiasis
-iatry	treatment	podiatry
-in	(makes a noun)	bacitracin
-ism	(makes a noun)	alcoholism
-ist	person	podiatrist
-itis	inflammation	colitis
-ity	(makes a noun)	alkalinity
-ium	(makes a noun)	Librium
-ize	(makes a verb)	immunize

Suffix	Meaning	Example
-lepsy	seizure	narcolepsy
-logy	study of, reasoning about	etiology
-oid	resembling	ovoid
-ol	alcohol	ethanol
-oma	tumor	melanoma
-opia	vision	myopia
-ose	carbohydrate	glucose
-osis	full of, condition	halitosis
-path, -pathy	disease, suffering	homeopathy
-pepsia	digestion	dyspepsia
-philia	attraction to, liking for	hydrophilia
-plasty	reshaping	rhinoplasty
-rhea	discharge, flow	diarrhea
-sis	process	diagnosis
-stomy	surgical opening	colostomy
-tomy	cut	nephrotomy
-tropia	turning	hypertropia
-ule	little, minute	venule

TERMS COMMONLY ENCOUNTERED IN PHARMACY PRACTICE

Drugs and Their Classification

The *United States Pharmacopeia* defines the term *drug* as "an agent intended for use in the diagnosis, mitigation, treatment, cure, or prevention of disease in man or animals." Let's examine this definition closely.

Diagnosis is the process by which a physician or other healthcare professional determines the nature of a disease condition by examination of a patient's symptoms.

If the definition in the *United States Pharmacopeia* is to cover all legitimate uses of drugs, then the term *disease* in the definition must be taken in its root sense of "not at ease," referring to any adverse condition. Ordinarily, however, people use the term with a more narrow meaning, to refer to any particular destructive physical process in an organ or organism with a specific cause, or causes, and characteristic symptoms. Of course, drugs are used to treat not only disease but also other abnormal or adverse conditions, including fractures, cuts, abrasions, wounds, and other such **traumas**, as well as various physical and mental **disorders**, which are **congenital** (inborn) or acquired abnormalities that are less than optimal, including physical disorders such as scoliosis, or curvature of the spine, and psychological disorders such as depression. Of course, the lines between diseases, traumas, and disorders is rarely clear-cut. A trauma can lead to an infection and thus the beginning of a disease process, a disease can cause a physical or psychological disorder, and a disorder, if it is destructive, may itself be considered a disease. A disease, trauma, or disorder is called **acute** if it is of short duration or is especially severe, sharp, or immediate in impact. This would be said, for example, of most traumas. A disease, trauma, or disorder is called

chronic if it is of extended duration. Chronic asthma, for example, is asthma with which the patient suffers over a long period of time.

In all cases, for the disease, trauma, or disorder to become known, it must present symptoms. A **symptom** is any condition accompanying or resulting from a disease, disorder, or other abnormality that provides evidence for its existence. Sometimes, symptoms are obvious upon examination and can lead to a ready **diagnosis**, or identification of the disease or disorder. At other times, extensive examination using special instruments or testing may be necessary to reveal the telltale symptoms of a given disease or disorder.

A set of symptoms that occurs together and characterizes a particular disease or disorder is known as a **syndrome**. It is usually the identification of a set of related symptoms that leads to a particular diagnosis.

Mitigation is the process of making something less severe or painful. An example of mitigation is the use of the drug morphine to relieve the pain of a cancer victim. Drugs can be used to mitigate symptoms without a particular diagnosis having been determined; however, in most cases, mitigation, treatment, and cure take place as a result of a plan of action based upon a particular diagnosis.

Treatment is the taking of action against a disease or other abnormality. Treatment may include a particular **therapy**, or extended treatment, such as physical therapy or drug therapy.

A **cure** is the effective elimination of a disease condition.

Prevention is taking steps before a disease or other abnormality occurs to keep it from occurring.

Drugs can be used to diagnose, mitigate, treat, cure, or prevent disease. To accomplish these purposes, a great variety of types of drugs, with particular kinds of effects, have been identified or created. Appendix A, at the back of this text, lists some of the most common categories of drugs, along with examples and specific purposes for which the drugs are used. Appendix B gives a list of commonly used drugs, with **generic** (nonproprietary) and **brand** (proprietary or trade) names for these drugs.

Pharmacy and Related Terms

As was noted in chapter 1, the word *pharmacy* derives from the Greek *pharmakon*, meaning "drug." As the term was used in the time of the Greek poet Homer, it meant, alternately, drug, poison, sorcerer's charm, or potion. Today, the same root has given us many terms related to pharmacy practice, as described in Chart 3.1.

ABBREVIATIONS IN PRESCRIPTIONS AND MEDICATION ORDERS

Under the law in most states, a pharmacist may not prescribe or engage in the manufacture of medications, although he or she can fill prescriptions and do small–scale **extemporaneous** (as needed) **compounding** (mixing and assembling) of medications in response to or in anticipation of prescriptions. In some states, registered pharmacists have been granted prescriptive authority. A **prescription**, or order for medication, must be written by a physician or by another licensed healthcare professional granted the right to prescribe under the applicable law (state, military, maritime, etc.). In a hospital, long–term care facility, or other institutional setting, a prescription is called a **medication order** or **physician's order**.

Chart 3.1

TERMS DERIVING FROM THE GREEK *PHARMAKON*

Pharmacy. As defined by the American Pharmaceutical Association, the word **pharmacy** *means "the health profession that concerns itself with the knowledge system that results in the discovery, development, and use of medications and medication information in the care of patients. It encompasses the clinical, scientific, economic, and educational aspects of the profession's knowledge base and its communication to others in the healthcare system." The word* pharmacy *also applies to the physical place where drugs are stored and dispensed, as a hospital pharmacy or community pharmacy.*

Clinical Pharmacology. Clinical pharmacology is that area of pharmacology (see below) that applies knowledge of pharmacological principles related to the effects of drugs on the body to particular drug therapies and to institutional practices and procedures, through counseling of customers, patients, or healthcare providers; through review of prescriptions, patient profiles, and drug therapies; through participation in drug use reviews; through establishment of **formularies**, or lists of drugs and dosage forms in stock; through monitoring of drug regimens; and through other means related to patient or customer care.

Clinical Pharmacy. Clinical pharmacy is that area of pharmacy that applies the pharmacist's knowledge and expertise to counseling related to drug therapies and to participating, as part of a total healthcare team, in the provision of clinical services to patients. See Clinical Pharmacology (above).

Nuclear Pharmacy. Nuclear pharmacy is that branch of the pharmacy profession that deals with the provisions of services related to radiopharmaceuticals.

Pharmaceutical. A **pharmaceutical** is any drug manufactured or compounded to be used for the mitigation, treatment, cure, or prevention of a disease or other abnormal condition.

Pharmacist. A **pharmacist** is a licensed professional, skilled in the procurement, compounding, and dispensing of drugs; knowledgeable in a wide range of areas related to drug formulation, dosage forms, use, and effects; skilled in the management of institutional or retail pharmacy operations; and dedicated to providing the service of dispensing drugs, drug information, and drug-related clinical services to customers, patients, and other healthcare professionals.

Pharmacodynamics. Pharmacodynamics is that branch of pharmacology (see below) that deals with the effects and reactions of drugs within the body, including their mechanisms of action.

Pharmacoeconomics is the study of the economic aspects of drugs. It includes study of the production, distribution, and consumption of drugs and of related costs and benefits. Aspects of pharmacoeconomics of particular interest include the following:

- Costs of drug development and therapy as weighed against therapeutic benefits
- The economic cost of drug abuse, misuse, diversion, misbranding, and adulteration

Chart **3.1**
(cont.)

- The economic forces and factors underlying drug distribution systems
- The effective control of drug costs at the development, federal, state, individual, institutional, wholesale, and retail levels
- The factors influencing the formulation, dosage forms, packaging, and marketing of drugs
- The management of pharmaceutical development, institutional pharmaceutical operations, and community or retail operations
- The study of drug utilization by consumers, within institutions, and by specific demographic groups by age, gender, race, and ethnicity
- The tensions among for-profit production, use of drugs, and societal needs

Pharmacogenetics. Pharmacogenetics is the study of genetic variation as revealed by reactions to drugs.

Pharmacognosy. Pharmacognosy is the science that deals with medicinal products of plant, animal, or mineral origin in their crude or unprepared state. The development of modern-day pharmaceuticals (see above) has, of course, dramatically decreased the importance of pharmacognosy to the practice of pharmacy.

Pharmacokinetics is that branch of pharmacology (see below) that deals with the scientific study of the absorption, distribution, metabolism, and excretion **(ADME)** of drugs over time. **Absorption** is the process by which a substance is taken up from the site of administration by the system. **Distribution** is the process of movement of the drug through the blood and transfer from the blood to other bodily fluids and tissues. **Metabolism** of a drug is the transformation of the drug by the physiological processes of the body into other forms, usually less potent or toxic than the original form, that can then be eliminated. **Excretion** is the elimination of the drug from the body, primarily through urination, defecation, perspiration, respiration, salivation, and, in lactating women, lactation.

Pharmacology. Pharmacology is the scientific study of the nature of drugs and of their interactions with food and drink, other drugs, and the biochemical processes of the body, including the therapeutic uses of drugs for treating conditions of disease or other abnormality, with special reference to the pharmacokinetics (see above) and toxicology, or adverse consequences, of drugs.

Pharmacopeia. A pharmacopeia is an authoritative reference containing a list and descriptions of drugs, pharmaceutical ingredients, and dosage forms, together with standards established under law for their production, dispensation, and use. The *United States Pharmacopeia (USP)*, published by the United States Pharmacopeial Convention, is the official pharmacopeia of the United States.

Pharmacy Fellowship. A pharmacy fellowship is a directed, highly individualized postgraduate program designed to prepare a graduate pharmacist to become an independent researcher in a scientific area related to pharmacy.

> **Pharmacy Residency.** A **pharmacy residency** is an organized, directed training program undertaken by a graduate of a pharmacy training program for the purpose of learning more about a defined area of practice.
>
> **Pharmacy Technician.** As defined by the AAPT, **pharmacy technicians** "are healthcare professionals who assist pharmacists in providing the best possible care for patients."

The forms of prescriptions and medication orders differ somewhat. Figure 3.1 shows a typical prescription. Figure 3.2 shows a typical institutional medication order. Sometimes a prescription or medication order calls for the pharmacist to dispense prefilled or prefabricated medications or dosage forms, such as a given number of capsules, tablets, patches, or prefabricated, prefilled syringes. At other times, the order requires that the pharmacist compound a medication, preparing a powder, for example, and filling capsules with it, or preparing a solution for intravenous infusion. The precise nature of these operations will be treated in subsequent chapters. The components listed in Chart 3.2 are generally found on a prescription.

Forms used by institutions for medication orders vary, but they typically include patient information (name, address, age, sex, etc.); the name of the physician; the patient's room number; and lines for physician's orders, including spaces for the date, time, and the orders themselves. Both prescriptions and medication orders are generally handwritten in ink on preprinted forms. Prescriptions typically make use of metric measurements, although other measurement systems are used (see chapter 7 for more information on pharmaceutical calculations and measurements). On a prescription form, decimal points used to express quantities and measurements may be replaced by handwritten or preprinted vertical lines, as follows:

1.94 mg = 1|94 mg

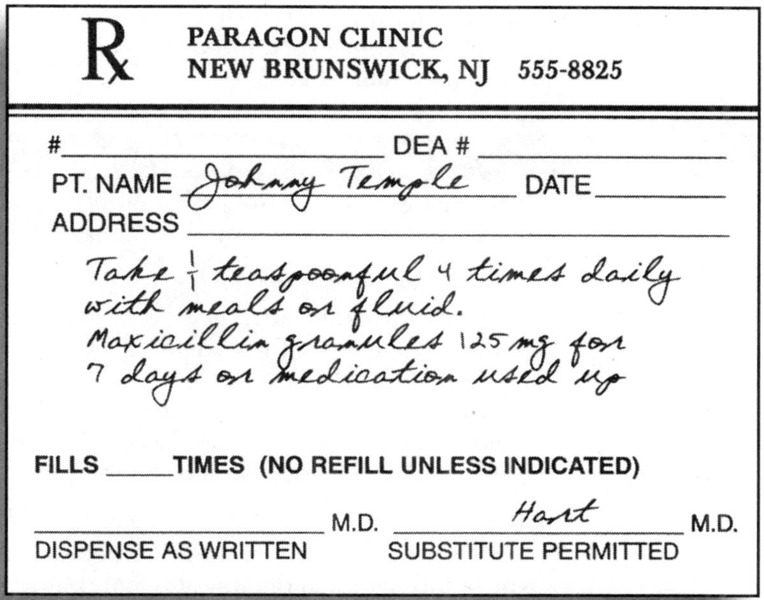

Figure 3.1 A typical prescription.

PARAGON CLINIC
NEW BRUNSWICK, NJ   555-8825

\#_____ DEA # _____
PT. NAME _Johnny Temple_____ DATE_____
ADDRESS _____

Take ½ teaspoonful 4 times daily
with meals or fluid.
Maxicillin granules 125 mg for
7 days or medication used up

FILLS _____TIMES (NO REFFILL UNLESS INDICATED)

_____ M.D.   _____ Hart _____ M.D.
DISPENSE AS WRITTEN   SUBSTITUTE PERMITTED

Figure 3.2
A typical institutional medication order.

PARAGON CLINIC PHARMACY

| Start Date Time: A.M. Here P. M. | Profiled by: | Filled by: | Checked by: | Patient name and ID. |

Give 275 mg oral Theraprofen tid

ALLERGIES:

PATIENT DIAGNOSIS

HEIGHT   WEIGHT

Patient: *Samay, Thelma*
Patient #
Admitted:
Physician:
Room:

PHYSICIAN'S ORDER

Prescriptions also make use of both **Arabic** (1, 2, 3, etc.) and **Roman** (i, ii, iii, etc.) **numerals**, as well as a great variety of special abbreviations and symbols. Information on Roman numerals is provided in chapter 7.

To the uninitiated, a prescription often reads like gobbledygook, and not just because of the famed illegibility of physicians' handwriting. Consider this example:

Sig: 1 cap p.o. c. aq. q.i.d. p.c. & h.s.

Translated, the example means, "Write on the label, 'Take one capsule by mouth, with water, four times daily, after meals and at bedtime.'" If these abbreviations and symbols seem at first like a foreign language, well, they are. For the most part, they are abbreviations of Latin terms. Chapter 8 deals in detail with receiving prescriptions and preparing orders based on them, but you can begin, now, to learn the abbreviations used in prescriptions and physicians' orders by studying the list given in Table 3.2.

Chart 3.2

PARTS OF A PRESCRIPTION

1. **Prescriber information:** The name, address, telephone number, and other information identifying the prescriber.

2. **Date:** The date on which the prescription was written.

3. **Patient information:** The name, address, and other pertinent information about the patient receiving the prescription. If the patient is an infant, a toddler, an elderly person, or someone else with special needs, the prescription may include such information as the age, weight, and **body surface area (BSA)** of the patient, information needed by the pharmacist in order to calculate appropriate dosages.

4. **R:** The symbol R, for the Latin word *recipe,* meaning "take."

5. **Inscription:** The medication or medications prescribed, including generic or brand names and amounts. States and most institutions have regulations and policies allowing pharmacists to substitute cheaper

generic equivalents of brand–name medications when appropriate. Lists of commonly prescribed medications and intravenous admixtures are given in Appendix B of this book.

6. **Subscription:** Instructions to the pharmacist on dispensing the medication, including such information as compounding or packaging instructions, labeling instructions, instructions on allowable refills, and, when a generic equivalent may not be substituted, instructions to that effect (e.g., "No substitutions" or "No substitutions allowed"). The abbreviation **PBO** means "Prescribe Brand Only." The abbreviation **DAW** means "Dispense as Written."

7. **Signa:** Directions for the patient to follow.

8. **Additional instructions:** Any additional instructions that the prescriber deems necessary.

9. **Signature:** The signature of the prescriber.

10. **DEA Number.** This number, identifying the prescriber as someone authorized to prescribe controlled substances, is required on all prescriptions for such substances.

Table 3.2

COMMON ABBREVIATIONS AND SYMBOLS IN PRESCRIPTIONS AND MEDICATION ORDERS

Note: Derivations given in this table are from Latin unless otherwise noted. Other symbols used are ME, Middle English, E, English, and GR, Greek. Individual prescriptions/medication orders will vary regarding whether abbreviations are given in uppercase or lowercase letters and with or without periods (e.g., gram = g., g, gm., gm, G., G, GM., GM). The most common forms in which abbreviations are written are given in the table. A complete list of abbreviations used in medical practice is beyond the scope of this book. See a standard reference work such as one of the following:

The Charles Press Handbook of Current Medical Abbreviations. Philadelphia: Charles Press, 1997.

Dorland, W. A. Newman. *Dorland's Medical Abbreviations.* Philadelphia: W.B. Saunders, 1992.

Mitchell–Hatton, Sarah Lu. *The Davis Book of Medical Abbreviations: A Deciphering Guide.* Philadelphia: F. A. Davis, 1991.

Stedman's Abbreviations, Acronyms, & Symbols. Ed. William R. Hensyl and Thomas Lathrop Stedman. Baltimore: Williams & Wilkins, 1992.

Stanaszek, Walter F., et al. *Understanding Medical Terms: A Guide for Pharmacy Practice.* Lancaster, PA: Technomic Publishing, 1992.

Amounts

Abbreviation*	Derivation	Definition
aa	ana	of each
ad	ad	up to, so as to make
C or C°	—	Celsius
C	congius	gallon
cc	—	cubic centimeter (mL)
d.t.d.	datur talis dosis	give such doses
g or gm	gramma	gram

*Some healthcare professionals write the Latin abbreviations *without* the periods.

Table **3.2**

(cont.)

Abbreviation*	Derivation	Definition
gr	granum	grain
GT	—	gastrostomy tube
gt.	gutta (ME)	drop
gtt.	guttae (ME)	drops
h. or hr.	hora	hour
IU	—	International Unit
lb.	libra	pound
m^2	—	square meter
mcg, μg	—	microgram
mEq	—	milliequivalent
mg	—	milligram
mg/kg	—	milligrams of drug per kilogram of body weight
mg/m^2	—	milligrams of drug per square meter of body surface area
♏	—	minim
ml, mL	—	milliliter
ml/h	—	milliliters of drug administered per hour
mOs or mOsm	—	milliosmole
NMT	—	not more than
no. or No.	numerus	number
O	octarius	pint
q.p.	quantum placeat	as much as you please
q.s.	quantum sufficiat	a sufficient quantity
q.s.ad	quantum sufficiat ad	a sufficient quantity to make
ss	semis	one-half
stat.	statim	immediately
t.	talis	of such
T	—	temperature
tal.	talis	of such
tal. dos.	talis dosis	of such doses
tbs or tbsp.	—	tablespoon
tsp.	—	teaspoon
U	unitas	unit
u	unitas	unit
w/v	—	weight to volume ratio
&	—	and
+	—	and

Bodily Functions or Conditions

Abbreviation	Derivation	Definition
BM	—	bowel movement
BP	—	blood pressure
BS	—	blood sugar

*Some healthcare professionals write the Latin abbreviations *without* the periods.

Abbreviation	Derivation	Definition
CHF	—	congestive heart failure
DT	—	delirium tremens
HA	—	headache
HBP	—	high blood pressure
HT or HTN	—	hypertension
N&V	—	nausea and vomiting
SCT	—	sickle-cell trait
SOB	—	shortness of breath
URI	—	upper respiratory infection,
UTI	—	urinary tract infection
VS	—	vital signs
WBC	—	white blood cell (count)

Dosage Forms, Solutions, and Delivery Systems

Abbreviation	Derivation	Definition
amp	ampulla	ampule
aq.	aqua	water
cap	capsula	capsule
chart.	carta	divided powders
D5LR or D_5LR	—	5% dextrose in lactated Ringer's solution
D5NSS or D_5NSS	—	5% dextrose in normal saline solution
DT	—	dispensing tablet
DW	—	distilled water
D5W or D_5W	—	5% dextrose in water
D10W or $D_{10}W$	—	10% dextrose in water
ECT	—	enteric-coated tablet
elix.	elixir	elixir
ex aq.	ex aquam	out of water
ext or ext.	extractum	extract
FCT	—	film-coated tablet
fl, fl., or fld.	fluidus	fluid
fl. oz.	—	fluid ounce
H	hypo + derma (GR)	hypodermic
inj.	injectio	injection
IV	intra venosus	intravenous
IVP	—	intravenous push
IVPB	—	intravenous piggyback
LCD	liquor carbonis detergens	coal tar solution
NS	—	normal saline (0.9% sodium chloride)
1/2 NS	—	half-strength normal saline
NTG	—	nitroglycerin
oint.	—	ointment

Table **3.2**

(cont.)

Abbreviation	Derivation	Definition
O/W	—	oil-in-water
pulv.	pulvis	powder
RL, R/L	—	Ringer's lactate (solution)
SCT	—	sugar-coated tablet
sol.	solutio	solution
supp.	suppositorium	suppository
susp	suspensus	suspension
syr.	syrupus	syrup
tab.	tabella	tablet
TDS	—	transdermal delivery system
TPN	—	total parenteral nutrition
Tr., tinct.	tinctura	tincture
TT	—	tablet triturate
ung.	unguentum	ointment
W/O	—	water in oil

Drugs and Drug References

Abbreviation	Derivation	Definition
ASA	acetylsalicylic acid (E)	aspirin
HC	—	hydrocortisone
LCD	liquor carbonis detergens	coal tar solution
MS	—	morphine sulfate
NF	—	*National Formulary*
NTG	—	nitroglycerin
USP	—	*United States Pharmacopeia*
ZnO	—	zinc oxide

Time/Time of Administration

Abbreviation	Derivation	Definition
ā	ante	before
a.c.	ante cibum	before meals
ad lib.	ad libitum	at pleasure, freely
a.m.	ante meridian	morning, before noon
ATC	—	around the clock
b.i.d.	bis in die	twice a day
h.s.	hora somni	at bedtime
noct.	nocte	at night
p	post	after
p.c.	post cibum	after meals
p.m.	post meridiem	after noon
post-op	—	postoperative
pp	postprandial	after meals
p.r.n.	pro re nata	as needed
q.	quaque	each, every
q.d.	quaque die	every day

Abbreviation	Derivation	Definition
q.h.	quaque hora	every hour
q.3h.	quaque 3 hora	every three hours
q.i.d.	quater in die	four times a day
t.i.d.	ter in die	three times a day
tiw	—	three times a week
wk.	—	week

Sites of Administration/Parts of the Body

Abbreviation	Derivation	Definition
A.D.	auris dextra	right ear
A.S.	auris sinistra	left ear
A.U.	auris uterque	each ear
BSA	—	body surface area
GI	—	gastrointestinal
GU	—	genitourinary
IA	—	intra-arterial
ID	—	intradermal
IM	—	intramuscular
IT	—	intrathecal
NPO, n.p.o.	non per os	nothing by mouth
O.D.	oculus dexter	right eye
O.S.	oculus sinister	left eye
O.U.	oculus uterque	each eye
p.o.	per os	by mouth
R	rectum	rectal
SC, SQ, or subq.	sub cutis	subcutaneous
SL	sub lingua	sublingual
top	topikos	topical

Other Instructions

Abbreviation	Derivation	Definition
c., c̄	cum	with
comp.	compositus	compound
d.	dentur	give
D/C	discontinuare	discontinue, discharge
dil.	diluere	dilute, dissolve
disc.	discontinuare	discontinue
disp, disp.	dispensare	dispense
div.	dividere	divide
DT	—	discharge tomorrow
ECT	—	electroconvulsive therapy
Emp.	ex modo praescripto	as directed, in the manner prescribed
et	et	and
f., ft.	fac, fiat, fiant	make
m	misce	mix

Table 3.2
(cont.)

Abbreviation	Derivation	Definition
m.	mitte	send
m. ft.	misce et fiat	mix and make
m.t.	mitte talis	send like this
non rep.	non repetatur	do not repeat
NR	non repetatur	do not repeat
O_2	—	oxygen
Rx	recipe	take
s̄	sine	without
sig.	signa, signetur	write on label
s.o.s.	si opus sit	if there is need
TAb	—	therapeutic abortion
TT	—	thrombin time
u.d.	ut dictum	as directed
ut dict.	ut dictum	as directed
w/	—	with
w/o	—	without
YO, y/o	—	years old

COMMON APOTHECARY SYMBOLS

Occasionally, prescriptions and medication orders make use of older systems of measurement such as the **apothecary** and **avoirdupois systems**. These systems are treated in chapter 7. The related symbols are described in Table 3.3.

Table 3.3

COMMON SYMBOLS FROM THE APOTHECARY AND AVOIRDUPOIS MEASUREMENT SYSTEMS

FLUID MEASURE

Symbol	Name	Equivalent in Metric System
ℳ	minim (apoth)	0.06 mL
f℥	fluiddrachm, fluidram (apoth)	3.69 mL
f℥	fluidounce (apoth)	29.57 mL
pt	pint (apoth)	473 mL
qt	quart (apoth)	946 mL
gal	gallon (apoth)	3785 mL

DRY MEASURE

Symbol	Name	Equivalent in Metric System
gr	grain (apoth and avoir)	65 mg
℈	scruple (apoth)	1.3 g
ℨ	drachm, dram (apoth)	3.9 g

Symbol	Name	Equivalent in Metric System
℥	ounce (apoth)	31.2 g
#	pound (apoth)	374.4 g
℥	ounce (avoir)	437.5 gr

COMMONLY CONFUSED NAMES OF MEDICATIONS

One of the most serious events that can occur in pharmacy practice is the accidental substitution of one drug or pharmaceutical ingredient for another. At all times, great caution must be taken to make sure that such substitution does not occur. In one infamous case, *Toppi v. Scarf, 1971,* a pharmacist accidentally dispensed Nardil, an antidepressant, instead of Norinyl, a contraceptive. The woman who received the wrong drug gave birth to a child, and the Michigan Court of Appeals held the pharmacist liable not only for the medical expenses incurred in the woman's pregnancy but also for the costs of raising the child. Given the potency and potential toxicology of drugs and the danger of not receiving the drug prescribed for treatment or prevention, one must be extremely careful not to substitute drugs that have similar names. Table 3.4 lists the names of some drugs that are near **homonyms** (words that sound alike) or **homographs** (words that are similar in spelling).

Table 3.4

NEAR HOMONYMS AND HOMOGRAPHS AMONG DRUG NAMES

Note: This is by no means a complete list of names of drugs that sound and/or look alike. The highest degree of caution must be exercised at all times to avoid accidental substitution of one drug or pharmaceutical product for another.

acetazolamide	acetohexamide	enalapril	Anafranil
albuterol	atenolol	Fioricet	Fiorinal
Aldomet	Aldoril	glipizide	glyburide
alprazolam	lorazepam	hydralazine	hydroxyzine
amitriptyline	imipramine	Inderal	Isordil
amitriptyline	nortriptyline	lamotrigine	lamivudine
Amoxil	Amcill	Lanoxin	Levoxyl
Apresazide	Apresoline	Lioresal	lisinopril
Catapres	Captopril	Lithotabs	Lithobid
Catapres	Combipres	Levoxine	Lanoxin
chlorpromazine	chlorpropamide	Norvasc	Navane
chlorpromazine	promethazine	Orinase	Ornade
clonidine	Klonopin	prednisolone	prednisone
Cytotec	Cytomel	Prilosec	Prozac
Cytotec	Cytovene	quinine	quinidine
Darvocet–N	Darvon–N	Seldane	Feldene
desipramine	diphenhydramine	Sinequan	saquinavir
desipramine	imipramine	tolazamide	tolbutamide
digitoxin	digoxin	Xanax	Zantac
diphenhydramine	dimenhydrinate		

chapter summary

In order to communicate precisely with other professionals, specialists in various fields of endeavor, including pharmacists, create unique terminology, abbreviations, and symbols to describe the elements of their disciplines. Medical terminology commonly encountered in the practice of pharmacy makes extensive use of Greek and Latin roots, prefixes, and suffixes, as illustrated by words such as analgesia, diastolic, streptomycin, and sublingual. Pharmacy, of course, is the practice of dispensing drugs and information about drugs. A clear understanding of what, exactly, a drug is involves an understanding of its uses and of terms related to drug uses, including diagnosis, disease, trauma, disorder, acute, chronic, symptom, syndrome, mitigation, treatment, cure, prevention, generic name, and brand name. A wide variety of drugs is currently used, from absorbents to take up toxic chemicals in the body to vitamins to aid metabolism.

The Greek word from which the word *pharmacy* derives also provides the root of words to describe many fields of study and activity within pharmacy, including clinical pharmacy, pharmacology, clinical pharmacology, pharmacodynamics, pharmacokinetics, nuclear pharmacy, pharmacoeconomics, pharmacogenetics, and pharmacognosy. Persons practicing pharmacy must be familiar with a great many abbreviations used on prescriptions and medication orders, including ones used to name amounts, bodily functions and conditions, dosage forms and delivery systems, drugs, drug references, time, time of administration, sites of administration, and parts of the body. A pharmacist or pharmacy technician must also be familiar with common symbols for weights and measures and with sound–alike and look–alike names of drugs which have the potential for leading to severe medication errors.

chapter review

Knowledge Inventory

Choose the best answer from those provided.

1. The word part *sub* is a
   a. suffix meaning "above"
   b. prefix meaning "above"
   c. suffix meaning "below"
   d. prefix meaning "below"

2. The determination of the nature of a disease condition by examining a patient's symptoms is known as a
   a. disease
   b. disorder
   c. syndrome
   d. diagnosis

3. An abnormality with which a person is born (that is, one that is not caused by environmental factors after birth), such as a cleft palate, is described as
   a. acute
   b. congenital
   c. mitigated
   d. traumatic

4. A group of symptoms that together characterize a particular abnormal condition is known as a
   a. disorder
   b. disease
   c. syndrome
   d. treatment

5. Bayer Aspirin is a
   a. generic drug name
   b. nonproprietary drug name
   c. brand name
   d. chemical name

6. The practice of counseling people about drug therapies and participating, as part of a total healthcare team, in the provision of services to patients is known as
   a. pharmacology
   b. clinical pharmacy
   c. pharmacokinetics
   d. pharmacodynamics

7. Drugs may be eliminated from the body via
   a. urination
   b. perspiration
   c. respiration
   d. all of the above

8. The equivalent of a prescription, in a hospital or other institutional setting, is the
   a. medication order
   b. drug list, or formulary
   c. dispensatory
   d. materia medica

9. An abbreviation that does *not* describe an amount of a medication to be taken is
   a. g
   b. mL
   c. N&V
   d. ss

10. In the case of *Toppi vs. Scarf,* a pharmacist accidentally substituted Nardil, an antidepressant, for Norinyl,
    a. an antiemetic
    b. a contraceptive
    c. an antipsychotic
    d. a vasoconstrictor

Pharmacy in Practice

1. Rewrite each of the following prescriptions or medication orders in standard English:

MT. HOPE MEDICAL PARK
MY TOWN, USA 822-3591

\# _____ DEA # _MJ/564293_

PT. NAME _Nancy Crutch_ DATE _____

ADDRESS _314 Crutch Way_

My Town

℞ Demerol 50 mg
Take ī PO daily prn AM pain
#30

REFILLS ___ TIMES (NO REFILL UNLESS INDICATED)

_____ M.D. _M Johnson_ M.D.
DISPENSE AS WRITTEN   SUBSTITUTE PERMITTED

a.

MT. HOPE MEDICAL PARK
MY TOWN, USA 822-3591

\# _____ DEA # _____

PT. NAME _Debbie White_ DATE _____

ADDRESS _____

_____

℞ Trimox Suspension 125 mg
Take ī tsp tid c̄ meals and fl
50 ml

REFILLS ___ TIMES (NO REFILL UNLESS INDICATED)

_____ M.D. _____ M.D.
DISPENSE AS WRITTEN   SUBSTITUTE PERMITTED

b.

MT. HOPE MEDICAL PARK
MY TOWN, USA 822-3591

\# _____ DEA # _____

PT. NAME _Larry Walkover_ DATE _____

ADDRESS _____

℞ Timolol 0.25% Solution
ī gtt AM o.d.
ī gtt Bid PM & HS O.U.

REFILLS _2_ TIMES (NO REFILL UNLESS INDICATED)

M. Johnson M.D. _____ M.D.
DISPENSE AS WRITTEN   SUBSTITUTE PERMITTED

c.

MT. HOPE MEDICAL PARK
MY TOWN, USA 822-3591

\# _____ DEA \# _____

PT. NAME _David Morrell_ DATE _____

ADDRESS _____

_____

℞ Zantac 150
Take ɉ tab Bid 30min Ac
and HS   \#60

REFILLS _/_ TIMES (NO REFILL UNLESS INDICATED)

_____ M.D. _M.D. Anderson_ ___ M.D.

DISPENSE AS WRITTEN   SUBSTITUTE PERMITTED

d.

e.

PHYSICIAN'S ORDERS

A GENERICALLY EQUIVALENT DRUG MAY BE
ADMINISTERED UNLESS CHECKED HERE.

(ADDRESSOGRAPH)

(✓)	START HERE →	DATE 3-6-94	TIME 0540	A.M. P.M.		(1)

Admit to 7E or 7W

Dx 2° burns to hands, arms, face

All- NKA

whirlpool in am

Silvadene cream Bid to wounds

D5½ NS w/ 20 kcl/L at 125 cc/hr

Zantac 50mg IV Q8°

MsO4 2-4mg IV Q2° prn pain

Ampicillin 1gm IV Q6°

Gentamicin 85mg IV Q8°   Dr. P. Brown

Ruff, Mary
748-1
7942153

(✓)	START HERE →	DATE	TIME	A.M. P.M.		(2)

Procardia 10mg Bite + swallow prn syst > 150
                                    diast > 110

MVI ɉ PO QD

Zinc 200mg po QD

reg diet

when taking po Percocet Q4-6 prn

f.

PHYSICIAN'S ORDERS

A GENERICALLY EQUIVALENT DRUG MAY BE
ADMINISTERED UNLESS CHECKED HERE.

(ADDRESSOGRAPH)

(✓)	START HERE	DATE	TIME	A.M. P.M.		(1)

Admit Dr. Cook
RO MI
Allerg - codeine

Nitrol 2% ½" Q6° off 12M-6A
Nitro 0.4mg SL prn CP
Nifedipine 10mg SL SBP >170; DBP >100
tylenol gr X po Q4° prn
MOM 30ml prn
⊘ ½ NS w/ 20meq KCl/L at 50ml/hr   Dr. Cook

Johnson, St.

g.

PHYSICIAN'S ORDERS

A GENERICALLY EQUIVALENT DRUG MAY BE
ADMINISTERED UNLESS CHECKED HERE.

(ADDRESSOGRAPH)

(✓)	START HERE	DATE 3-4-94	TIME	A.M. P.M.		(1)

Admit
RO Pneumonia

Claforan 1gram IV Q8°
Erythromycin 500mg IV Q6°
D5 ½ NS at 125cc/hr
Tylenol 650mg Q4° prn pain or temp >101
                          J. Roger, MD

Spokis, Tom
1049

(✓)	START HERE	DATE 3-4-94	TIME	A.M. P.M.		(2)

Continue home meds:
Digoxin 0.125mg Qday
Hydralazine 75mg po tid
Zantac 150mg BID
ASA EC Qday
Maalox 30cc Q4° prn indigestion
                          J. Rogers MD

h.

PHYSICIAN'S ORDERS

↓ A GENERICALLY EQUIVALENT DRUG MAY BE
ADMINISTERED UNLESS CHECKED HERE.

(ADDRESSOGRAPH)

(✓)	START → HERE	DATE	TIME	A.M. P.M.		(1)

Admit to Dr. Cook

Solumedrol 125mg IVPB Q8° x4 doses

Albumin 25gm IVPB yellow w/ 40mg IV lasix

Biaxin 500mg po Q12h

Rocephin 1gm IVPB Qday

Albuterol Aerosol Q4° WA

D5 ½ NS at 100cc/hr x4 then 60cc/hr

Tylenol gr X po Q4° T° > 101 or mild pain

Restoril 15mg Q HS

Zantac 150mg BID 30min AC + HS   J. Cook MD

(✓)	START → HERE	DATE	TIME	A.M. P.M.		(2)

K+omeq Ti po QAM

J Cook MD

Taylor, Mark
649-1
7942197

2. The following is a passage from a package insert included with Albuterol, USP Inhalation Aerosol. Read the passage and locate five medical terms used in it for which you can find prefixes, suffixes, and/or roots from the list given in this chapter. List the terms and their prefixes, suffixes, and/or root(s). Then look up each term in a medical dictionary and write its definition.

PRECAUTIONS General: Albuterol, as with all sympathomimetic amines, should be used with caution in patients with cardiovascular disorders, especially coronary insufficiency, cardiac arrhythmias, and hypertension; in patients with convulsive disorders, hyperthyroidism, or diabetes mellitus; and in patients who are unusually responsive to sympathomimetic amines.

Large doses of intravenous albuterol have been reported to aggravate preexisting diabetes and ketoacidosis. Additionally, beta–agonists, including albuterol, when given intravenously may cause a decrease in serum potassium, possibly through intracellular shunting. The relevance of this observation to the use of Albuterol Inhalation Aerosol is unknown, since the aerosol dose is much lower than the doses given intravenously.

Although there have been no reports concerning the use of Albuterol Inhalation Aerosol during labor and delivery, it has been reported that high doses of albuterol administered intravenously inhibit uterine contractions. Although this effect is extremely unlikely as a consequence of aerosol use, it should be kept in mind. . . .

ADVERSE REACTIONS The adverse reactions of albuterol are similar in nature to those of other sympathomimetic agents, although the incidence of certain cardiovascular effects is less with albuterol. A 13–week double–blind study compared albuterol and isoproterenol aerosols in 147 asthmatic patients. The results of this study showed that the incidence of cardiovascular effects was: palpitations, less than 10 per 100 with albuterol and less than 15 per 100 with isoproterenol; tachycardia, 10 per 100 with both albuterol and isoproterenol; and increased blood pressure, less than 5 per 100 with both albuterol and isoproterenol. In the same study, both drugs caused tremor or nausea in less than 15 patients per 100; dizziness or heartburn in less than 5 per 100 patients. Nervousness occurred in less than 10 per 100 patients receiving albuterol and in less than 15 per 100 patients receiving isoterenol.

Rare cases of urticaria, angioedema, rash, bronchospasm, and oropharyngeal edema have been reported after the use of inhaled albuterol.

In addition, albuterol, like other sympathemimetic agents, can cause adverse reactions such as hypertension, angina, vomiting, vertigo, central nervous system stimulation, insomnia, headache, unusual taste, and drying or irritation of the oropharynx.

3. Use the Merck Manual online, at

   http://www.merck.com/!!qpRmU0yhYqpRmU2PGT/pubs/mmanual

   to look up a disease condition or disorder in which you are interested. Explain whether the condition is an acute or chronic condition. List its symptoms and describe its normal treatment.

4. Choose one of the following subfields of pharmacy in which you are particularly interested, do some research on it, and prepare a written or oral report explaining to other pharmacy technician students the subjects of interest to practitioners in this field.

   Clinical Pharmacy
   Pharmacology
   Clinical Pharmacology
   Pharmacodynamics
   Pharmacokinetics
   Nuclear Pharmacy
   Pharmacoeconomics
   Pharmacogenetics
   Pharmacognosy

5. Choose four of the pairs of drugs listed in Table 3.4. Do some research on each drug by looking it up in the *Physician's Desk Reference* or another standard reference work. (See chapter 6, "Sources of Information.") Explain the purpose or purposes for which each drug is used.

Drugs, Dosage Forms, and Delivery Systems

4

In no area of modern life, with the possible exception of computing, has technology so transformed everyday lives as in the area of pharmaceuticals. Modern pharmaceutical science has given us a vast array of medicines used for a wide variety of purposes and administered in an equally wide variety of forms. In this chapter, you will learn the uses of the modern pharmaceutical arsenal and about the many different forms—the dosage forms and delivery systems—that pharmaceutical scientists have created.

Learning Objectives

- Define the term *drug*
- Distinguish between over-the-counter and legend drugs
- Explain the parts of a National Drug Code number
- Categorize drugs by source as natural, synthetic, synthesized, or semisynthetic
- Explain the uses of drugs as therapeutic, phamacodynamic, diagnostic, prophylactic, and destructive agents
- Define and differentiate between the terms *dosage form* and *delivery system*
- Enumerate and explain the properties of the major dosage forms and delivery systems for drugs

TERMS TO KNOW

Capsule A solid dosage form consisting of a drug enclosed within a conical gelatin shell

Dispersion A liquid dosage form in which undissolved ingredients are dispersed, or scattered, throughout a liquid vehicle

Dosage form The physical manifestation of a drug as a solid, liquid, or gas that can be used in a particular way; the form of a drug, as for example, a tablet, cream, solution, injection, or aerosol

Drug Any substance taken into or applied to the body with the purpose of altering the body's biochemical functions and thus its physiological processes

Emulsion A dispersion in which one liquid is dispersed, or scattered about, within another, immiscible liquid

Legend drug A drug that can be sold only by prescription and that must bear a federally mandated warning, or legend

Lotion A liquid for topical application containing insoluble dispersed solids or immiscible liquids

DEFINING THE TERM *DRUG*

A *drug* is any substance taken into or applied to the body with the purpose of altering the body's biochemical functions and thus its physiological processes. The biochemically reactive component or components of a drug, the **active ingredient** or **ingredients**, are rarely given in pure (that is, in undiluted or uncut) form. Instead, one or more active ingredients are combined with one or more **inert ingredients**, which have little or no physiological consequences. Most drugs contain one or more active ingredients commingled, dispersed, or in solution or suspension within an inert primary **base**, or **vehicle**, that may contain other ingredients, such as antimicrobial preservatives, colorings, and flavorings (see Figure 4.1).

References for Definition and Description of Particular Drugs

Two reference works published by the United States Pharmacopeial Convention establish the official legal standards for drugs in the United States: the *United States Pharmacopeia (USP)* and the *National Formulary (NF)*. The *USP* describes drug substances and dosage forms. The *NF* describes pharmaceutical ingredients. Both are revised every five years, and supplements are published in the interim between revisions. Useful to practitioners is the three-volume work *USP Drug Information (USP DI),* available in print and computer database form, which includes *Drug Information for the Health Care Professional* (Vol. 1), *Advice for the Patient* (Vol. 2), and *Approved Drug Products and Legal Requirements* (Vol. 3). Also useful is the *Physician's Desk Reference,* published annually, a reference work that contains package inserts for commonly used drugs. (For more information on drug literature, see chapter 6.) Under the Drug Listing Act of 1972, a unique **National Drug Code (NDC)** number appears on all drug labels, including labels of prescription containers. The 10-character NDC includes a 4-number **Labeler Code**, identifying the manufacturer or distributor of the drug; a 3- or 4-number **Product Code**, identifying the drug; and a 2- or 3-number **Package Code**, identifying the packaging size and type, as follows:

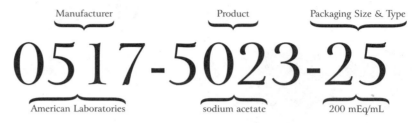

Manufacturer   Product   Packaging Size & Type

0517-5023-25

American Laboratories   sodium acetate   200 mEq/mL

Classes of Drugs

Drugs are classified as over-the-counter (OTC) or legend. An **over-the-counter drug** is one that can be dispensed without a prescription. A **legend drug** can be dispensed only with a prescription and must bear on its label the legend "Caution: Federal Law Prohibits Dispensing Without Prescription" (see Figure 4.2). Drugs with potential for abuse are classified, under the Comprehensive Drug Abuse Prevention and Control Act of 1970, according to five **drug schedules**, from Schedule I drugs with no accepted medical use and a high potential for abuse to Schedule V drugs with accepted medical uses, low potential for abuse, and limited potential for creating physical or psychological dependence. (For more information on drug schedules, see chapter 2.)

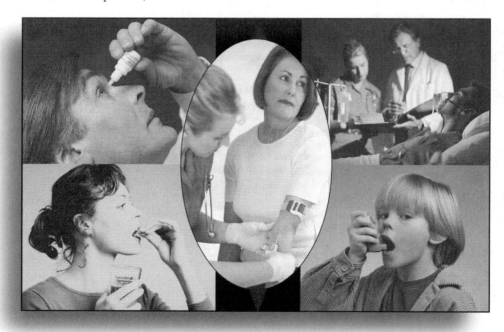

Figure 4.1 Modern development and manufacturing processes have made available thousands of drugs and hundreds of drug delivery systems and dosage forms.

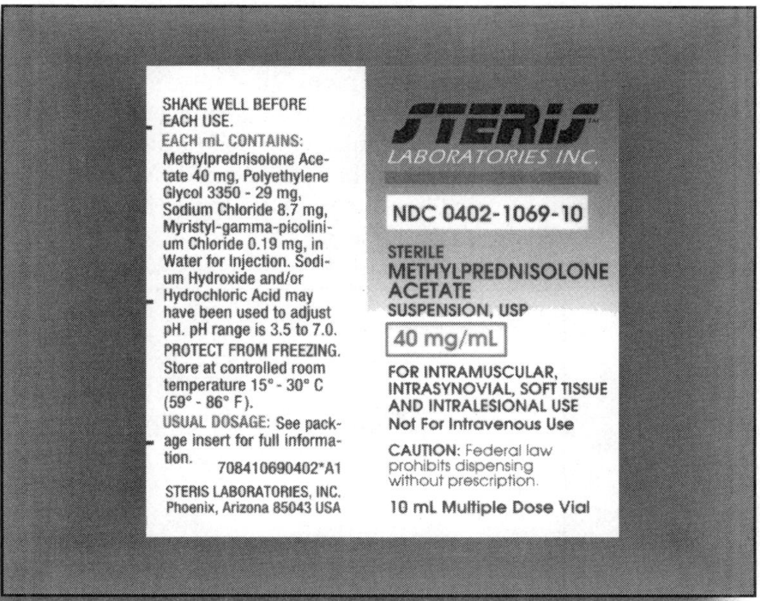

Figure 4.2 Federal law requires that prescription drugs bear the legend "Caution: Federal Law Prohibits Dispensing Without Prescription." Therefore, such drugs are known as legend drugs.

SOURCES OF DRUGS

Drugs come from various sources and can be classified as **natural** (taken from prokaryotic, eukaryotic, animal, plant, fungal, or mineral sources), **synthetic** (created artificially), **synthesized** (created artificially but in imitation of naturally occurring substances), and **semisynthetic** (containing both natural and synthetic components).

Drugs from Natural Sources

Some drugs are naturally occurring biological products, made or taken from single-celled organisms, plants, animals, people, or fungi. Both Vitamin B_{12} and the antibiotic streptomycin are produced from cultures of the bacterium *Streptomyces griseus*. Opium, the narcotic, comes from poppies; quinine, used to treat malaria, comes from cinchona bark. Thousands of years ago, people learned that they could combat pain by drinking teas made from white willow leaves. Today, we know that these leaves contain salicylic acid, which, in the form of acetylsalicylic acid, we know as aspirin. Insulin for the treatment of diabetes mellitus can be extracted from the pancreas of sheep or oxen. The human growth hormone somatotropin comes, as its name suggests, from human bodies, where it is produced by the anterior pituitary. As most everyone knows, naturally occurring forms of the antibiotic penicillin are extracted from certain molds. Some drugs are minerals. One example is magnesia (magnesium oxide or hydrated magnesium carbonate), which is used as an antacid and laxative.

Synthetic, Synthesized, and Semisynthetic Drugs

In the modern era, many naturally occurring chemicals, such as adrenaline, have been synthesized, or artificially created by humans, and used as drugs. Other drugs, such as barbiturates, are completely synthetic. Still others are semisynthetic, and contain both natural and synthetic molecules; an example would be some forms of penicillin. This widely used antibiotic, derived from the molds *P. notatum* and *P. chrysogenum,* was discovered by Alexander Fleming in 1928. Today, natural penicillins are still manufactured from molds, but new semisynthetic penicillins have also been developed. These penicillins combine artificially created molecules with naturally occurring ones, and are effective against bacteria that have developed resistance to the natural penicillins. Like the natural penicillins, the semisynthetics are administered by hypodermic injection (see Figure 4.3).

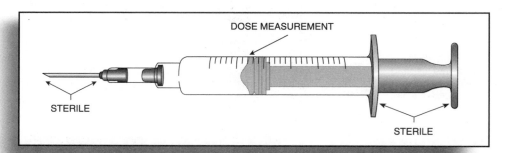

Figure 4.3 A hypodermic syringe, used in the administration of medication beneath the skin.

Synthetic drugs can be created by means of the recombinant DNA techniques of genetic engineering. **DNA**, or **deoxyribonucleic acid**, is the complex, helically shaped molecule that carries the genetic code (see Figure 4.4). This molecule contains the instructions, or recipe, for creating **messenger RNA**, or **ribonucleic acid,** which in turn contains the recipe for creating **amino acids**, the building blocks of proteins and thus of the bodies of organisms. **Recombinant DNA** is DNA constructed of segments taken from different sources, as, for example, from a human being and a sheep. By transferring a segment of recombined DNA into a host cell, scientists can change what proteins the cell produces, in effect converting the cell into a small-scale protein factory. By this means, for example, the bacterium *E. coli*—the microbiologists' and geneticists' experimental subject of choice—can be induced to produce human insulin or human growth hormone.

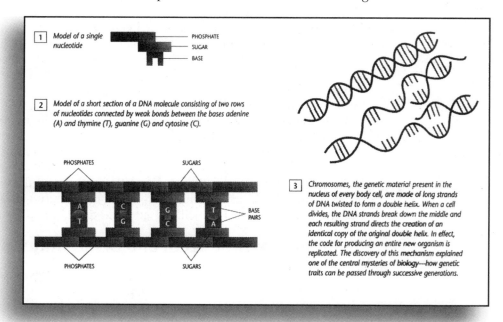

Figure 4.4 By making alterations in the DNA of an organism, which carries the organism's genetic code, scientists can create genetic instructions that lead the organism to produce chemical substances that can be used in drugs.

Another biotechnological method of drug production is the use of cells from inoculated animals to produce, in the laboratory, hybrid cells that create what are known as **monoclonal antibodies**. **Antibodies** are created by the immune system in response to foreign substances in the body known as **antigens**. Laboratory-produced monoclonal antibodies can be used to attack tumors and to diagnose a great variety of conditions, from pregnancy to anemia to syphilis. Genetic engineering, the hybridization techniques for creating monoclonal antibodies, and other biotechnologies are already used to create a great variety of drugs, such as clotting factors used to treat hemophiliacs and interferons for combating viral infection. Such technologies promise to bring many new drugs to the market and to decrease the difficulty and cost of producing drugs already known.

USES OF DRUGS

Some common uses of drugs are as noted in Chart 4.1.

Chart 4.1

COMMON USES OF DRUGS

1. **As Therapeutic Agents.** A **therapeutic agent** helps to maintain health, relieve symptoms, combat illness, and reverse disease processes. Examples of such drugs include vitamins to regulate metabolism and otherwise contribute to the normal growth and functioning of the body, electrolytes, enzymes, hormones, anti-inflammatories, antibiotics, sulfa drugs, laxatives, painkillers, antidepressants, insulin, and antiviral or antifungal agents.

2. **As Pharmacodynamic Agents.** A **pharmacodynamic agent** alters bodily functioning in a desired way. Drugs can be used, for example, to stimulate or relax muscles, to dilate or constrict pupils, or to make blood more or less coagulable. Examples of pharmacodynamic agents include caffeine to forestall sleep, oral contraceptives to prevent pregnancy, expectorants to increase fluid in the respiratory tract, anesthetics to cause numbness or loss of consciousness, and digitalis to increase heart muscle contraction.

3. **As Diagnostic Agents.** A **diagnostic agent** facilitates an examination, usually one conducted in order to arrive at a diagnosis, or conclusion as to the nature or extent of a disease condition. Examples of diagnostic agents include barium meals or enemas given to facilitate X-ray observation of the gastrointestinal tract and the radiopharmaceutical thallous chloride given to facilitate a SPECT (Single Photon Emission Computed Tomography) scan (see "Radiopharmaceuticals," p. 90).

4. **As Prophylactic Agents.** A **prophylactic agent** prevents illness or disease from occurring. Examples of prophylactic agents include the antiseptic and germicidal liquid iodine used for prevention of infection, emetics given to induce vomiting of previously ingested toxic substances, smallpox vaccine, and the Salk and Sabin vaccines used to prevent the disease poliomyelitis.

5. **As Destructive Agents.** A **destructive agent**, as the name suggests, destroys. Examples of destructive agents are antiseptics for killing bacteria and antineoplastic (literally "anti-new-formation") drugs used in chemotherapy to destroy malignant tumors. Another example is radioiodine, which is used to destroy the thyroid gland in patients suffering from hyperthyroidism or thyroid cancer prior to placing these patients on natural or synthetic thyroid hormone medication.

Of course, Chart 4.1 does not present mutually exclusive categories. In the eighteenth century, William Withering discovered the effective ingredient in certain folk concoctions for treating people with heart conditions to be leaves of the foxglove plant. We now know the active ingredient in foxglove as the drug digitalis. Digitalis is pharmacodynamic in that it increases heart muscle contractions. It is therapeutic in that it can be used to treat congestive heart failure and irregular heartbeat. A bactericidal ointment is both a destructive agent that kills bacteria and a prophylactic agent that prevents infection. Radioiodine is a diagnostic agent when it is used in imaging and both a destructive and therapeutic agent when used to treat hyperthyroidism.

DEFINING THE TERMS *DOSAGE FORM* AND *DELIVERY SYSTEM*

The term ***dosage form*** refers to the physical manifestation of a drug as a solid, liquid, or gas that can be used in a particular way. Examples of dosage forms include tablets, creams, solutions, injections, and aerosols (see Figure 4.5). The term ***delivery system*** encompasses the drug in its particular solid, liquid, or gaseous form; any mechanism used to deliver the drug (such as a teaspoon, hypodermic, IV, or osmotic pump); and any design feature of the dosage form that affects the delivery of the drug (such as the coating on some capsules that resists breakdown by the gastric fluids in the stomach so that the capsule will release medication, instead, into the intestines). Health practitioners use the term *delivery system* when they wish to refer to a means for delivering a particular amount of a drug at a certain rate to the particular site or sites of action of the drug within the body.

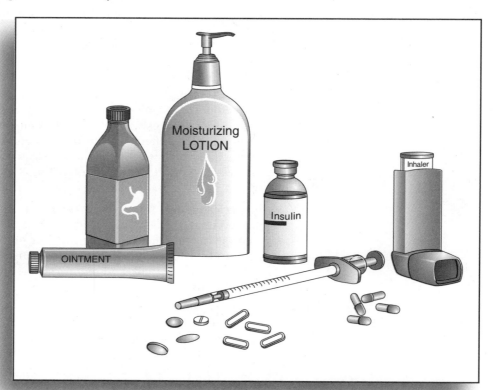

Figure 4.5 Drugs come in many dosage forms that vary in unit volume, active ingredient(s) per unit volume, rate of action, site(s) of action, and deliverable quantity to the site(s) of action. Different dosage forms and their associated apparatus and designs act as unique delivery systems, providing active ingredients to their effective sites in differing ways.

Delivery systems differ in their **pharmacological** properties, that is, in their sites of action, rate of delivery, and quantities of active ingredient delivered. Consider, for example, the drug nitroglycerin, commonly used to treat **angina pectoris** (pain in the chest and left arm associated with a sudden decrease in blood supply to the heart). Nitroglycerin dilates blood vessels, thus increasing blood supply to the heart and decreasing blood pressure. Two common delivery systems for nitroglycerin are sublingual tablets, placed under the tongue, and transdermal patches, worn on the skin. Sublingual nitroglycerin tablets are fast-acting but deliver their active ingredient for only a short period of time, about 30 minutes. Transdermal patches, in contrast, act slowly, with a delivery onset of about 30 minutes, but can deliver a steady amount of the drug for up to 24 hours. Another example of differing delivery systems is the use of acetylsalicylic acid (aspirin) in tablet form taken **orally** (by mouth) for relief of minor aches and pains as opposed to salicylic acid applied **topically** (locally) in a liquid solvent mixture to remove a corn on the foot. Obviously, the choice of delivery system depends upon many factors, including

- what active ingredient is to be delivered
- how much of the active ingredient is to be delivered
- by what means or by what route the ingredient is to be delivered
- to what sites
- at what rate
- over what period of time
- and for what purpose

Classification of Dosage Forms and Delivery Systems

Today, drugs are administered in a wide variety of dosage forms that are part of an even wider variety of delivery systems. Because of the variety and overlap of dosage forms and delivery systems, is impossible to create a rigid, mutually exclusive taxonomy or classification of them. However, for ease of learning, the next three sections of this chapter will present these forms and systems under the rough categories of solids, liquids, and "other." Various semisolid, semiliquid, and semigaseous dosage forms and specialized delivery systems will be considered under the "other" category.

SOLID DOSAGE FORMS

Capsules

The **capsule** is a solid dosage form consisting of a gelatin shell that encloses the drug. **Gelatin** is a protein substance obtained from vegetable matter and from the skin, white connective tissue, and bones of animals. A capsule may be a **placebo**, containing no active ingredients. (Placebos in encapsulated or other dosage forms are commonly given to people as controls in drug tests and experiments.) Generally, however, the capsule contains powder, granules, liquids, or some combination thereof with one or more active ingredients. In most cases, the powder, granules, or liquids in the capsule also contain one or more pharmacologically inert filler substances, or **diluents**. The capsule may also contain **disintegrants** (which help to break up the ingredients), **solubilizers** (which maintain the ingredients in solution or help the ingredients to pass into solution in the body), **preservatives** (to maintain the integrity of the ingredients), colorings, and other materials. Because a capsule is enclosed, flavorings are not common for this dosage form. The gelatin shell of a capsule, which can be hard or soft, may be transparent, semitransparent, or opaque and may be colored or marked with a code to facilitate identification. In most cases, the capsule is meant to be swallowed whole. Examples of drugs available in capsule form include amoxicillin 250 and 500 mg, indomethacin 25 and 50 mg, and secobarbital sodium 30 mg (see Figure 4.6).

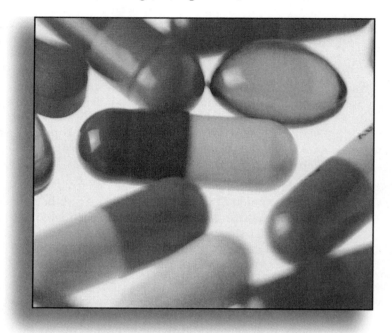

Figure 4.6 Capsules come with both hard and soft shells.

Hard gelatin shells consist of two parts: the **body**, which is the longer and narrower part, and the **cap**, which is shorter and fits over the body. In some cases, capsules have a **snap-fit design**, with grooves on the cap and the body that fit into one another to ensure proper closure (see Figure 4.7). Hard gelatin shells are made of gelatin, sugar, and water. Such shells commonly contain powders or granules and are used for **extemporaneous** (to order) hand-filling operations and

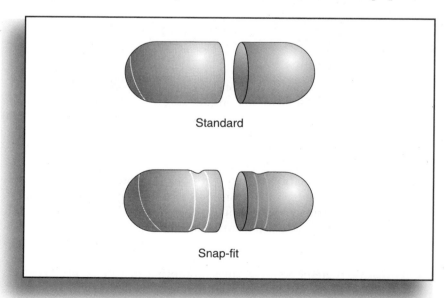

Standard

Snap-fit

Figure 4.7 Hard-shell capsules come in regular and snap-fit designs.

for commercial manufacturing. In commercial manufacturing, the body and the cap may be sealed to protect the integrity of the drug within (a practice that has increased since the 1980s, when highly publicized incidents of capsule tampering occurred). Hard-shell capsules come in standard sizes indicated by the numbers 000, 00, 0, 1, 2, 3, 4, 5 (from largest to smallest). The largest capsule, size 000, can contain about 1040 mg of aspirin; the smallest, size 5, about 97 mg (see Figure 4.8).

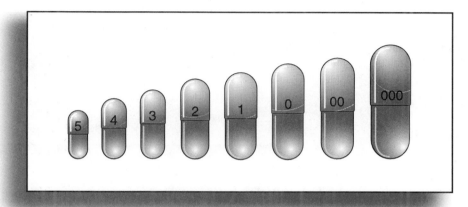

Figure 4.8 The sizes in which hard-shell capsules are available range from 5, the smallest, to 000, the largest.

Most hard-shell capsules are meant to be swallowed whole, but a few are meant only as conveyances for granules or powders to be sprinkled on food or in drink. Capsules should not be used in this latter fashion, however, except when specifically intended for this purpose, because opening the capsule can defeat the capsule's **controlled-release** properties. A controlled-release dosage form may be used to deliver a drug over a particular period of time **(sustained release)** or at a particular site **(delayed action)**. Some capsules and tablets, for example, have an **enteric coating** allowing the dosage form to pass through the gastric fluids of the stomach relatively undisturbed and to then dissolve and release the medication into the intestines. Others are designed to disintegrate at a particular rate, matching that of the metabolism of the drug by the body and so providing a steady replenishment of the medication, over time, in a more or less precise amount. The design of a wide variety of controlled-release tablets, capsules, granules, and other dosage forms has proved to be a fertile field for the imaginations of pharmaceutical developers, and the naming of these varieties has provided much diversion to these developers' marketing personnel. A few of the names by which controlled-release dosage forms are called include *constant release, continuous action, continuous release, controlled release, delayed absorption, depot, extended action, extended release, gradual release, long acting, long lasting, long-term release, programmed release, prolonged action, prolonged release, protracted release, rate controlled, repository, retard, slow acting, slow release, sustained action, sustained release, sustained release depot, timed coat, timed disintegration,* and *timed release.*

When hand-filling a capsule with powder, a pharmacist or technician generally uses the **punch method**. First, the number of capsules to be filled is counted out. Then, the powder is placed on a clean surface of paper, porcelain, or glass and formed into a cake with a spatula. The cake should be approximately 1/4 to 1/3 the height of the capsule body. The body of the capsule is then punched into the cake repeatedly until the capsule is full (see Figure 4.9). The cap is then placed snugly over the body. Granules are generally poured into the capsule body from a piece of paper. Sometimes, hand-operated capsule filling machines are used.

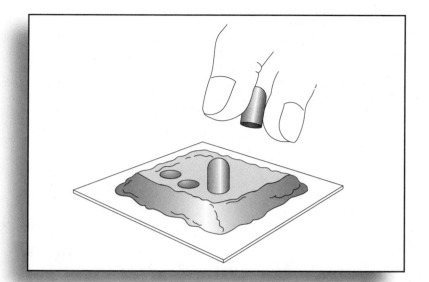

Figure 4.9 The punch method is used for extemporaneous filling of capsules.

Soft gelatin shells are spherical, oblong, ovoid, or elliptical dosage forms of sealed, one-piece construction that come prefilled from commercial manufacturers with powders or, more commonly, with liquids, suspensions, pastes, or other materials that could leak from capsules having a two-part, hard shell construction. Soft-shell capsules are particularly suited to **volatile** preparations, which vaporize or evaporate rapidly in air, and to preparations otherwise subject to deterioration on exposure. Soft capsule shells are made of gelatin and added substances, such as glycerin or sorbital, that give the gelatin its softness, or plasticity. They generally contain from 1 to 480 minims (from .0616 to about 30 mL).

Effervescent Salts

Effervescent salts are granules or coarse powders containing one or more medicinal agents (such as an analgesic), as well as some combination of sodium bicarbonate with citric acid, tartaric acid, or sodium biphosphate. When dissolved in water or some other liquid, effervescent salts release carbon dioxide gas, causing a distinctive bubbling. A common example of an effervescent salt is effervescent sodium phosphate, used as a **cathartic**, or purgative (a medicine for stimulating evacuation of the bowels).

Implants/Pellets

Implants, or **pellets**, are dosage forms that are placed under the skin by means of minor surgery and/or special injectors. They are used for long-term, controlled release of medications, especially hormones. An example of an implant is Norplant, which contains levonorgestrel to prevent pregnancy.

Lozenges/Troches/Pastilles

Lozenges, also known as **troches** or **pastilles**, are dosage forms containing active ingredients and flavorings, such as sweeteners, that are administered **buccally** (dissolved in the mouth). They generally have local effects. Commercial over-the-counter lozenges for relief of sore throat are quite common, although many other drugs, including such prescription drugs as nystatin or clotrimazole, are also available in lozenge form.

Pills

The small, almost perfectly spherical dosage form known as the **pill**, once very common in pharmacy, has now largely been replaced by tablets and capsules.

Plasters

Plasters are solid or semisolid, medicated or nonmedicated preparations that adhere to the body and contain a backing material such as paper, cotton, linen, silk, moleskin or plastic. An example is salicylic acid plaster used to remove corns.

Powders and Granules

To a layperson, a powder is any finely ground substance. To a pharmacist, a **powder** is a finely divided combination, or admixture, of drugs and/or chemicals ranging in size from extremely fine (1 micron or less) to very coarse (about 10 mm). Official definitions of powder size include very coarse (No. 8 powder), coarse (No. 20 powder), moderately coarse (No. 40 powder), fine (No. 60 powder), or very fine (No. 80 powder), according to the amount of the powder that can pass through mechanical sieves made of wire cloth of various dimensions (No. 8 sieves, No. 20 sieves, and so on). In the past, it was common for the pharmacist/apothecary to prepare medicines in the form of powders. However, powders dispensed in bulk amounts had the disadvantage of leading to inaccuracy in the dosage taken by the patient. Commonly dispensed bulk powders include antacids, brewer's yeast, laxatives, douche powders, dentifrices and dental adhesives, and powders for external application to the skin. In the past, pharmacists often dispensed **divided powders**, or **charts**, that were prepared, measured, mixed, divided into separate units, and placed upon pieces of paper that were then folded. Today, dispensing of medicines in the divided powder dosage form is rare, although powders are very widely used as components of such commercially prepared dosage forms as capsules and tablets.

Powders are combined and mixed by a variety of means, including **spatulation** (blending with a pharmaceutical spatula), **trituration** (grinding or pulverizing, as with a mortar and pestle), **sifting**, and **tumbling** in a container or blending machine. They may also be **levigated**, or formed into a paste employing a small amount of liquid, in preparation for being added to an ointment base. In large-scale commercial manufacturing, powders are milled and pulverized by machines. An example of a medication in the powder dosage form is polymyxin b sulfate and bacitracin zinc topical powder, which is used to prevent infection.

Granules are larger than powders and are formed by adding very small amounts of liquid to powders and then passing these through a screen or a granulating device (see Figure 4.10). Granules are generally of irregular shape, have excellent flow characteristics, are more stable than powders, and are generally better suited than powders for use in solutions because they are not as likely simply to float on the surface of a liquid. Tablets are often prepared by compressing granules, and capsules are often filled with granules. Granules may contain colorings, flavorings, and coatings and may have controlled release characteristics. Some drug products in granular form are combined by the pharmacist with water before dispensing. Some are dispensed as granules and measured, for prescription and dosage, by the teaspoonful or tablespoonful.

Suppositories

Suppositories are solid dosage forms designed for insertion into bodily orifices, generally the rectum or the vagina or, less commonly, the urethra (see Figure

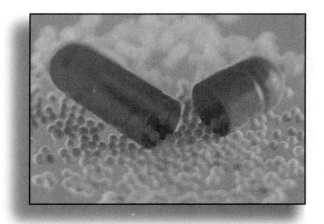

Figure 4.10 Both granules (in photo) and powders are commonly used in capsules.

4.11). Suppositories vary in size and shape, depending on their site of administration and the age and gender of the patient for whom they are designed. Some are meant for local action. Rectal suppositories, however, are often used as vehicles for systemic drugs because the large numbers of blood and lymphatic vessels in the rectum provide for exceptional absorption. A variety of bases are used in suppositories, including cocoa butter, hydrogenated vegetable oils, and glycerinated gelatin. Suppositories are produced by molding and by compression.

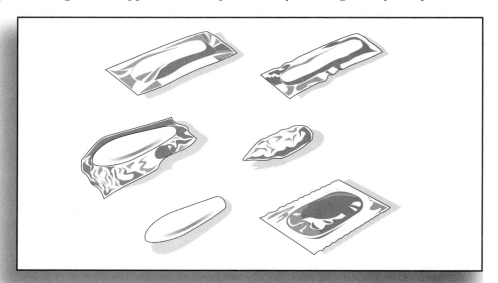

Figure 4.11 The size and shape of a suppository are determined by its site of administration.

Tablets

The **tablet** is a solid dosage form produced by compression (or, in the past, by molding) and containing, as capsules do, one or more active ingredients and, commonly, other pharmacological ingredients, including diluents, **binders** (to promote adhesion of the materials in the tablet), **lubricating agents** (to give the tablet a sheen and to aid in the manufacturing process), disintegrants, solubilizers, colorings, and coatings (see Figure 4.12). For obvious reasons, tablets also commonly contain flavorings. Coatings can be used to protect the stability of the ingredients in tablets; to improve appearance, flavor, or ease of swallowing; or to provide for controlled (sustained or delayed) release of medication. Tablets are

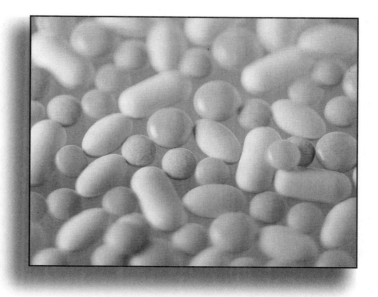

Figure 4.12 Tablets come in a wide variety of shapes, sizes, and colors, with a wide variety of external markings.

available in a wide variety of shapes and sizes, with a wide variety of surface markings. They are extremely convenient because of the ease with which various doses can be delivered. A patient can take one tablet, several tablets, or a portion of a tablet, as required. Some tablets are scored to facilitate breaking into portions (see Figure 4.13). Several routes of administration are possible for tablets. Most tablets are meant to be swallowed whole and to dissolve in the gastrointestinal tract. However, some tablets are designed to be chewed or to be dissolved in liquid, in the mouth, under the tongue, or in the vagina. Examples of drugs available in tablet form include digoxin 0.125, 0.25, and 0.5 mg; ibuprofen 300, 400, 600, and 800 mg; nitroglycerin 0.15, 0.3, 0.4, and 0.6 mg; and penicillin v potassium 250 and 500 mg. Types of tablets include those described in Chart 4.2.

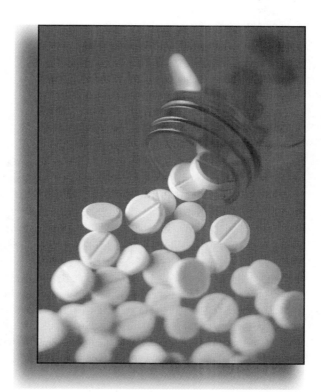

Figure 4.13 Tablets are often scored to facilitate breaking into smaller dosage forms.

Chart 4.2

TYPES OF TABLETS

Note: In this chart, common pharmaceutical abbreviations for tablet dosage forms are given in parentheses where applicable.

Single Compression Tablets (CT). Almost all tablets produced today are created by punch and die machines that compress the ingredients of each tablet in a single stroke.

Multiple Compression Tablets (MCT). Some tablets are produced by multiple compressions and are, in effect, either tablets on top of tablets or tablets within tablets. A multiple compression tablet may contain a core and one or two outer shells or two or three different layers, each containing a different medication and colored differently. Multiple compression tablets are created for appearance alone, to combine incompatible substances into a single medication, or to provide for controlled release in successive events, or **stages** (see Figure 4.14).

Figure 4.14 A multiple compression tablet may contain more than one medication in a core and one or two outer shells (left) or in two or three layers (right).

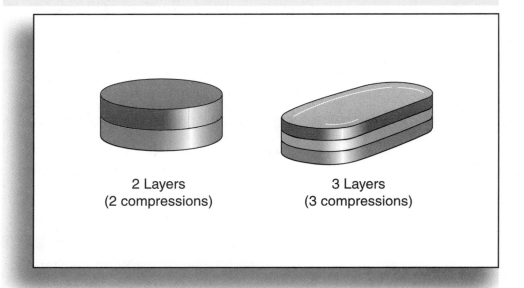

2 Layers
(2 compressions)

3 Layers
(3 compressions)

Molded Tablets. Trituration is the process of rubbing, grinding, or pulverizing a substance into fine particles or powder. In the past, tablets were created by placing moist, triturated ingredients into a mold. Today, however, such **molded tablets** have been almost entirely replaced by ones produced by the compression methods described above (see the next page, however, for information on tablet triturates).

Coated Tablets. Tablets can be **coated**, containing a special outside layer that dissolves or ruptures at the site of application, or **uncoated**, not containing such a layer. **Sugar-coated tablets (SCT)** contain an outside layer of sugar that provides protection for the medication and improves both appearance and flavor. If a drug is particularly foul tasting, then sugar coating and other flavoring may be necessary. Of course, in pharmacy, as in life, sugar-coating tends to improve **compliance**, which pharmacy personnel define as the taking of medication in the prescribed amount and at the prescribed times. Unfortunately, sugar-coating, both in pharmacy and in life, has disadvantages as well. The sugar-coating of tablets makes them much larger and heavier. **Film-coated tablets (FCT)** contain a thin outer layer of a **polymer** (a substance containing very large molecules) that can be either soluble or insoluble in water. Film coatings are thinner, lighter in weight, and cheaper to manufacture than sugar coatings and are colored to provide an attractive appearance. **Enteric-coated tablets (ECT)** are used for drugs that are destroyed by gastric acid, that might irritate the esophageal tract or stomach, or that are better absorbed by the intestines if they bypass the stomach. The enteric coating is designed to resist destruction by gastric fluids and to break down once the tablet reaches the intestines.

Chewable Tablets. Containing a base of flavored and/or colored **mannitol** (a sugar alcohol), **chewable tablets** are designed to be masticated and are a preferred dosage form for antacids, antiflatulents, commercial vitamins, and tablets for children.

Effervescent Tablets. **Effervescent tablets** are made with granular effervescent salts or other materials that release gas and so dispense active ingredients into solution when placed in water. Most people are familiar with such tablets in the form of commercial analgesics. (An **analgesic** reduces pain without affecting consciousness.)

Buccal Tablets. **Buccal tablets**, such as those used to deliver progesterone, are meant to be placed in the **buccal pouches** (between the cheek and the gum) and dissolved and absorbed by the **buccal mucosa**. (The **mucosa**, or **mucous membrane**, is the mucus-secreting lining of bodily cavities and canals connected to the external air. For more information on this, see chapter 5.)

Sublingual Tablets. **Sublingual tablets**, such as those used to deliver nitroglycerin, are designed to be dissolved under the tongue (sub = "under"; lingua = "tongue") and absorbed.

Vaginal Tablets. Also known as **vaginal inserts**, **vaginal tablets** are designed to be placed into the vagina by means of an applicator and dissolved and absorbed by the vaginal mucosa.

Tablet Triturates (TT), Hypodermic Tablets, and Dispensing Tablets. These forms, used in the past for compounding, are rarely used in pharmacy today.

Controlled-Release Tablets. A **controlled-release tablet** is one designed to regulate the rate at which a drug is released from the tablet and into the body. For more information on controlled-release dosage forms, see Capsules, p. 73–76.

LIQUID DOSAGE FORMS

Liquid dosage forms consist of one or more active ingredients in a liquid medium, or **vehicle**. These dosage forms can be divided into two major categories: **solutions**, in which active ingredients are dissolved in the liquid vehicle, and **dispersions**, in which undissolved ingredients are dispersed throughout a liquid vehicle.

Solutions

The vehicle that makes up the greater part of a solution is known as a **solvent**. An ingredient dissolved in a solution is known as a **solute**. Solutions may be classified by vehicle as **aqueous** (water-based), **alcoholic** (alcohol-based), or **hydroalcoholic** (water- and alcohol-based). They may be classified by contents as aromatic waters, elixirs, syrups, extracts, fluidextracts, irrigating solutions, liniments, ointments, spirits, and tinctures. They may also be classified by site or method of administration as **topical** (local), **systemic** (throughout the body), **epicutaneous** (on the skin), **percutaneous** (through the skin), **peroral** (for or through the mouth), **otic** (for or through the ear), **ophthalmic** (for the eye), **parenteral** (for injection or intravenous infusion), **rectal** (for or through the rectum), **urethral** (for the urethra), or **vaginal** (for or through the vagina). Chart 4.3 describes some common types of solutions.

Chart 4.3	TYPES OF SOLUTIONS

Aromatic Waters. **Aromatic waters** are solutions of water containing oils or other substances that both have a pungent, and usually pleasing, smell and are **volatile**, or easily released into the air. Rose water is an example.

Collodions. **Collodions** are liquid dosage forms for topical application containing pyroxylin (tiny particles of cellulose derived from cotton) dissolved in a mixture of alcohol and ether, to which medicinal ingredients may be added. On application, the highly volatile alcohol and ether solvent vaporizes, leaving on the skin a film coating containing the medication. Flexible collodion, containing castor oil and camphor, may be applied to bandages or stitches to waterproof them. The product with the brand name Compound W is a collodion containing salicylic acid used to remove corns or warts.

Diluted Acids. **Diluted acids** are aqueous dilutions of concentrated acids. An example is 1% acetic acid solution used as a surgical dressing, irrigating solution, and spermicide.

Elixir. A clear, sweetened, flavored hydroalcoholic solution, containing water and ethanol, is known as an **elixir**. Such a solution can be medicated or nonmedicated. An example of a drug in this dosage form is phenobarbital elixir, containing phenobarbital, orange oil, propylene glycol, alcohol, sorbitol solution, color, and purified water. Children's Tylenol Elixir, a vehicle for acetaminophen, is another example. Elixirs are similar to syrups but, because they are hydroalcoholic, are preferable as vehicles for medications compounded of both water-soluble and alcohol-soluble ingredients. Additional solvents, such as glycerin and propylene alcohol, may be used in elixirs. The choice of sweeteners in an elixir depends on the alcoholic content. If the active ingredients in an elixir are largely water soluble, then a natural sweetener such as sucrose or sorbitol may be used, but if the elixir has high alcohol content, then an artificial sweetener such as saccharin is preferable. In the past, pharmacists often used nonmedicated elixirs as palatable vehicles for unpleasant-tasting drugs.

Enemas. An **enema** is a solution administered rectally for cleansing or drug administration. Enemas generally come in disposable plastic squeeze bottles. A **retention enema** is administered to deliver medication locally or systemically. An **evacuation enema** is administered to clean the bowels.

Extractives. **Extraction** is the process by which desired materials, such as the active ingredients of drugs, are removed from plants or other materials through the application of solvents that place the desired materials in solution. The products of extraction, known as **extractives**, generally contain several ingredients, since several constituents of the plant will be soluble in a given solvent. The process of creating extractives from plants is a central part of so-called Galenical pharmacy (see chapter 1) and was once a major activity of the pharmacist/apothecary. Solvents used for extraction include water, alcohol, hydroalcoholic solutions, and glycerin. Two methods of extraction are commonly employed: maceration and percolation. In the **maceration** method, the crude drug from the plant is **comminuted**, or pulverized, and then soaked in the solvent. In the **percolation** method, the solvent is made to pass slowly, or **percolate**, through a column of the comminuted crude material from which the extraction is being made. Types of extractives include **tinctures** (see "Tinctures," on the next page), fluidextracts, and extracts. **Fluidextracts** are liquid dosage forms prepared by the percolation method from plant sources. They contain the solvent alcohol and 1 g of the drug for each mL of liquid. In current practice, fluidextracts are often flavored and/or sweetened and are not dispensed to patients but rather are used in the formulation of syrups and other dosage forms. **Extracts** are potent dosage forms, from animal or plant sources, from which most or all the solvent has been evaporated to produce a powder, an ointment-like form, or a solid. They are produced from fluidextracts and used in the formulation or compounding of medications.

Irrigating Solutions/Douches. An **irrigating solution**, or **douche**, is any solution for cleansing or bathing an area of the body. Some are used topically, some otically, some ophthalmically, and some for irrigation of bodily tissues exposed by wounds or surgical incisions. The term *douche* is most commonly used for **vaginal douches**, liquid solutions, often reconstituted from powders, administered into the vaginal cavity.

Liniments. **Liniments** are alcoholic or oleaginous (hydrocarbon-containing) solutions or emulsions (see "Emulsions" in Chart 4.4) containing medications and meant for rubbing on the skin.

Parenteral Solutions. **Parenteral solutions** are sterile solutions with or without medication for administration by means of a hollow needle or other device used to place the solution beneath the skin and into the system. There are two major delivery systems for parenteral solutions: intravenous (IV) infusions and injections, which may or may not be intravenous (see "Injections" and "Intravenous Infusions," under "Other Delivery Systems," pp. 86–89). Parenteral solutions must be **stable**. In other words, they must remain effective, without undergoing chemical changes that cause them to degrade, until the time of administration. In addition, parenterals must be **sterile**, or free from all contaminants, including those contaminants known as **pyrogens**, the fever-inducing products of the metabolic action of microorganisms.

Spirits. **Spirits** are alcoholic or hydroalcoholic solutions containing volatile, aromatic ingredients. Examples include camphor spirit and peppermint spirit. Some spirits are used as medicines and some as flavorings.

Chart 4.3
(cont.)

Syrups. A **syrup** is an aqueous solution thickened with a large amount (commonly 60 to 80 percent) of sugar, generally sucrose, or a sugar substitute such as sorbitol or propylene glycol. A simple syrup known as Syrup NF can be made by combining 85 g of sucrose with 100 mL of purified water. Syrups may contain additional flavorings, colors, or aromatic agents. Syrups come in two varieties, **medicated syrups** containing active ingredients, such as Lithium citrate syrup or ipecac syrup; and **nonmedicated syrups,** such as cherry syrup or cocoa syrup, used as vehicles. Because they do not contain alcohol, syrups are often used as vehicles for **pediatric medications** (ones given to children). Syrups are also sometimes used for elderly patients who cannot easily swallow the commonly available solid forms of certain drugs.

Tinctures. Alcoholic or hydroalcoholic solutions of pure chemicals or of extractions from plants are known as **tinctures.** Examples include iodine tincture and belladonna tincture.

Dispersions

Unlike a solution, a **dispersion** is not dissolved in its vehicle. Instead, it is simply distributed throughout. The vehicle for a dispersion is known as the **dispersing phase** or **dispersing medium**. The particulate or liquid dispersed within the vehicle is known as the **dispersed phase**. Dispersions are classified by the size of the dispersed ingredient(s) into suspensions and emulsions, containing relatively large particles, and magmas, gels, and jellies, containing fine particles. If a dispersion contains ultrafine particles, less than a micron in size, it is said to be **colloidal**. One type of colloidal is the **microemulsion**. Dispersions of solids in a liquid are known as **suspensions**. Dispersions of a liquid in a liquid are known as **emulsions**. Some types of dispersions are noted in Chart 4.4.

Chart 4.4

TYPES OF DISPERSIONS

Suspensions. A **suspension** is a type of dispersion in which small particles of a solid, the **suspensoid**, are dispersed in a liquid vehicle. Some suspensions come already prepared. Others come in the form of dry powders that are **reconstituted** (or made again into a fluid), usually with purified water. Suspensions may be classified by route of administration into **oral suspensions** (taken by mouth), **topical suspensions** (such as some lotions that are applied locally, generally to the skin), and **injectable suspensions**. A well-prepared suspension settles slowly, can be redispersed easily throughout the dispersing phase by a gentle shake, and pours easily. A suspension may be a preferred method for dispensing a solid to a young or elderly patient who would find it difficult to swallow a solid dosage form. Examples of suspensions include antacids like the magnesia and alumina oral suspension with the brand name Maalox and the antifungal nystatin oral suspension.

Emulsions. An **emulsion** is a type of dispersion in which one liquid is dispersed in another, **immiscible** liquid (one with which it does not readily mix). Common types of emulsions are of **oil-in-water (O/W)** or **water-in-oil (W/O)**. In addition, emulsions contain a third phase, the **emulsifying agent**, to render the emulsion stable, or not prone to separation or aggregation of the suspended liquid. Emulsions vary in their

viscosity, or rate of flow, from free-flowing liquids such as **lotions** to semisolid preparations such as **ointments** and **creams**.

Lotions. A **lotion** is a liquid for topical application containing insoluble dispersed solids or immiscible liquids. Examples include calamine lotion used for relief of itching and benzoyl peroxide lotion, used to control acne.

Gels and Jellies. Like suspensions, **gels** contain solid particles in liquid, but the particles are ultrafine, of colloidal dimensions, and sufficient in number and so linked as to form a semisolid. The linked particles enclose the liquid, and the liquid is suffused throughout the particles, so much so that the gel is considered a single-phase system. Examples of gels include lidocane gel and the antacid aluminum hydroxide gel. A **jelly** is a gel that contains a high proportion of water, usually formed from a combination of water, a drug substance, and a thickening agent. Antiseptic, antifungal, contraceptive, and lubricant jellies are examples. Jellies are often used as **lubricants**, or substances for reducing friction, for examination of body orifices. Because of their high water content, jellies are subject to bacterial infection and usually contain preservatives.

Magmas and Milks. A **magma**, or **milk**, is similar to a gel in that it contains colloidal particles in liquid, but the particles remain distinct, in a two-phase system. An example is Milk of Magnesia, containing magnesium hydroxide, used to neutralize gastric acid.

Microemulsions. A **microemulsion**, like other emulsions, contains one liquid dispersed in another, but unlike other emulsions, is clear because of the extremely fine size of the droplets of the dispersed phase. An example of a microemulsion is Haley's M-O.

Ointments/Unguents. Ointments, or **unguents**, are semisolid dosage forms meant for topical application. Ointments may be medicated or nonmedicated and may contain various kinds of bases: **oleaginous**, or greasy, bases made from hydrocarbons such as mineral oil or petroleum jelly; water-in-oil emulsions such as anydrous lanolin, lanolin, or cold cream; oil-in-water emulsions such as hydrophilic ointment; and water-soluble or greaseless bases such as polyethylene glycol ointment. Ointments are packaged in jars or tubes.

Pastes. Pastes are like ointments but contain more solid materials and consequently are stiffer and apply more thickly. Examples are zinc oxide paste, an astringent, and acetonide dental paste, an anti-inflammatory preparation.

OTHER DELIVERY SYSTEMS

Bulb Syringe

A **bulb syringe**, consisting of a bulb and a tapering funnel with a hollow end, is used to administer liquids topically, as for irrigation (see Figure 4.15). The bulb is first depressed to expel the air that it contains, and the tip is then inserted into the liquid to be administered. The bulb is released while the end is in the liquid, and liquid rises to fill the vacuum thus created. The end of the bulb is then removed from the liquid, and the liquid is administered by depressing the bulb again.

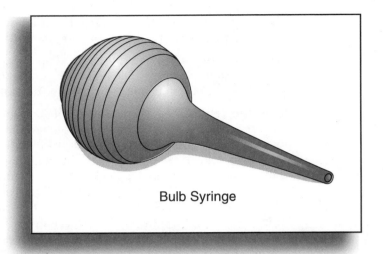

Figure 4.15 A bulb syringe may be used to administer liquids topically.

Bulb Syringe

Dropper

Like a bulb syringe, a **dropper** uses a bulb to create a vacuum for drawing up a liquid. A dropper contains a small, squeezable bulb at one end and a hollow glass or plastic tube with a tapering point. The dropper may be incorporated into the cap of a vial or other container. The **drop**, as a unit of pharmaceutical measurement for droppers or for intravenous infusions, is abbreviated **gt**. Because of the differing **viscosities** (the thicknesses and thus flow characteristics) of differing fluids, the size of a drop is considerably variable from medication to medication. Droppers are often used for **otic** or **ophthalmic** administration of medications.

Glycerogelatins

Glycerogelatins are topical preparations made with gelatin, glycerin, water, and medicinal substances. The hard substance is melted and brushed onto the skin, where it hardens again and is generally covered with a bandage. An example is zinc gelatin, used as a pressure bandage to treat varicose ulcers.

Inhalations

Gases, vapors, drugs, solutions, or suspensions intended to be inhaled via the nasal or oral respiratory routes are known as **inhalations**. Gases such as oxygen and ether are administered by inhalation. Medicated inhalations are often administered via devices such as hand-held, breath-activated, propeller-driven **inhalers** or atomizing machines known as **nebulizers**, which deliver mists containing extremely small, or **micronized**, powders. Common vehicles for inhalation solutions include Sterile Water for Inhalation (USP) and sodium chloride inhalation. Examples of medications delivered by inhalation include isoetharine or isoproterenol inhalation solutions for relief of spasms caused by bronchial asthma, and amyl nitrite as a **vasodilator** (a substance that **dilates**, or expands, vessels, particularly blood vessels). **Vaporizers** and **humidifiers** are machines commonly used to deliver moisture to the air for relief of cold symptoms. Volatile medications can be used with some vaporizers.

Injections

Injections, also known as bolus or intravenous push delivery systems, make use of **syringes**, calibrated devices typically consisting of a **plunger end**, a **plunger**, a flange, a **cannula** (also known as a **barrel** or **shaft**), and a **tip** (see Figure 4.16). Attached to the tip is a hollow needle consisting of a **shaft**, a **bevel**, a **bore** or **lumen**, and a **point** (see Figure 4.17). The thickness of the needle and size of its lumen is referred to as its **gauge**, ranging from 30 gauge (the smallest) to 13 gauge (the largest). Because injections introduce medication into the body, they must be **sterile**, or free from contaminants. Two types of syringes commonly used for injections are **glass syringes**, which are fairly expensive and must be sterilized between uses, and **plastic syringes**, which are easy to handle, disposable, and come from the manufacturer in sterile packaging.

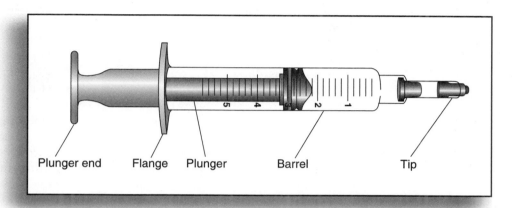

Figure 4.16 A syringe is made up of a plunger and a cannula, or barrel, and is calibrated for the measuring of dosages.

Plunger end   Flange   Plunger   Barrel   Tip

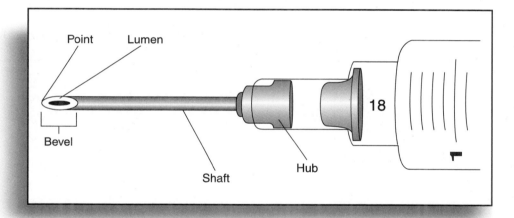

Figure 4.17 The size of the needle used with an injection or intravenous infusion is referred to as its gauge.

Point   Lumen   Bevel   Shaft   Hub   18

Common types of syringes include the **insulin syringe**, used by healthcare professionals and in self-administration by patients of insulin for control of diabetes; the **tuberculin syringe**, with a cannula that contains 0.01 to 1.0 mL of liquid; and the larger **hypodermic syringe**, with a cannula that contains from 3 to 60 mL of liquid. **Unit dose disposable syringes** are prefilled syringes that contain a single premeasured dose of medication and are thrown away after use. Other kinds of syringes not used with needles include the **oral syringe**, used for oral solutions, and the **bulb syringe**, used for topical solutions, as for irrigation. Injections may be administered to almost any organ or part of the body. The most common route is **intravenous (IV) injection**, made into a vein. Also common are **intradermal (ID)** or **intracutaneous injections** made into the skin; **subcutaneous (SC, subq., SQ, hypodermic, or hypo) injections** made under the skin; and **intramuscular (IM) injections** made into a muscle (see Table 4.1 and chapter 5 for more information).

Table 4.1

ROUTES FOR PARENTERAL INJECTION AND INFUSION

Type	Site of Delivery of Parenteral Solution
intra-arterial (IA)	into artery
intra-articular	into joints
intracardiac	into heart
intradermal (intracutaneous) (ID)	into skin
intramuscular (IM)	into muscle
intraspinal	into spinal column
intrathecal (IT)	into spinal fluid
intravenous (IV)	into vein
subcutaneous (SC)	under skin

In addition to syringes, devices available for injection include **patient-controlled analgesia devices**, which are programmable machines that deliver small doses of pain killers on demand; **jet injectors**, which use pressure rather than a needle to deliver the medication; and **ambulatory injection devices** that the patient can wear about. Some injection devices make use of pumps that regulate the amount, rate, and/or timing of injections. Injectables come prefilled or are filled at the time of injection from, most commonly, single or multidose **vials**, small glass or plastic bottles. Sometimes the medication comes in **ampules**, small glass containers that are opened by breaking off the neck of the container (see Figure 4.18). Because of the danger of contaminating the medication with

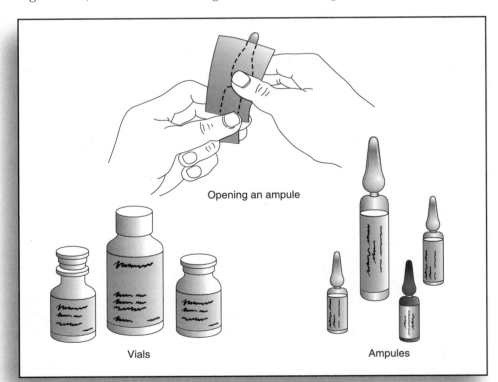

Figure 4.18 Vials and ampules. A piece of paper or, preferably, an alcohol swab is used when opening an ampule to prevent accidental puncturing of the skin.

Opening an ampule

Vials

Ampules

glass particles, medication that comes in ampules must be filtered before it is injected (for more information on injections, see chapter 5).

Intrauterine Delivery Systems

An **intrauterine delivery system** is a drug-releasing device placed into the uterus. One such device is used to release progesterone to prevent pregnancy.

Intravenous Infusions

Intravenous infusion is a method for delivering a large amount of liquid over a prolonged period of time and at a slow, steady rate into the blood system. Infusions are used to deliver blood, water, other fluids, nutrients such as lipids and sugars, electrolytes, and drugs. When drugs are added to an intravenous infusion, they are said to be **piggybacked**. Typical uses of infusions are to deliver pain-killing medications, or **analgesics**; to replenish body fluids; and to deliver nutrients to patients who cannot or will not feed themselves.

Mucilages

A **mucilage** is a viscous, adhesive, semisolid or semiliquid containing a sticky vegetable extractive, with or without additional active ingredients.

Ocular Inserts

Ocular inserts are small, transparent membranes containing medications that are placed between the eye and the lower **conjunctiva** (the mucous membrane on the inside of the eyelid). An example is the product with the brand name Ocusert, used to deliver pilocarpine for the treatment of glaucoma.

Oral Syringes

An **oral syringe** is a calibrated device consisting of a plunger and a cannula, or barrel, used without a needle for administration of precisely measured amounts of medication by mouth (see Figure 4.19).

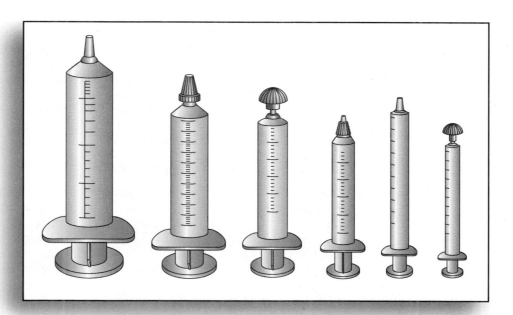

Figure 4.19 Oral syringes come in a number of sizes.

Prefilled Straws

Some hospices and long-term care facilities make use of **straws** (long, hollow tubes) prefilled with medications.

Radiopharmaceuticals

Chemicals containing radioactive isotopes, used diagnostically or therapeutically, are known as **radiopharmaceuticals**. (**Isotopes** are forms of an element that contain the same number of protons but differing numbers of neutrons.) Unstable, or **radioactive**, isotopes give off energy in the form of radiation, measured in rads. One rad is equal to 100 ergs of energy absorbed by 1 g of body tissue. **Nuclear medicine** uses radioactive isotopes such as technetium^{99m} and iodine^{131} for imaging regional function and biochemistry in the body, as in a **PET (Positron Emission Tomography)** or **SPECT (Single Photon Emission Computed Tomography)** scan, and for therapeutic irradiation and destruction of tissue, as in the treatment of hyperthyroidism or, more recently, ovarian and prostate cancer. **Nuclear pharmacy**, which involves the procuring, storage, compounding, dispensing, and provision of information about radiopharmaceuticals, is one possible area of specialization for both pharmacists and pharmacy technicians.

Sponges

One contraceptive commonly used in the past consisted of a polyurethane **sponge** containing a spermicide, nonoxynol 9.

Sprays and Aerosols

A **spray** is a dosage form that consists of a container with a valve assembly that, when activated, generally by depression, emits a fine dispersion of liquid, solid, and/or gaseous material. An **aerosol** is a spray in a pressurized container that contains a **propellant**, an inert liquid or gas under pressure meant to carry the active ingredient to its location of application. Depending on the formulation of the product and on the design of the valve, an aerosol may emit a fine mist, a coarse liquid spray, or a foam. One type of aerosol is the **foam spray aerosol**, which produces a water-in-oil emulsion when the liquid dispersed phase within the spray container vaporizes into the air. Most sprays and aerosols are for topical application to the skin or to mucous membranes, but some are **inhalation aerosols**, meant to be breathed in through the nose or mouth. Sprays and aerosols are commonly used to deliver over-the-counter local anesthetics, antiseptics, deodorants, and, in the case of breath sprays, flavorings. They are also used to deliver prescription drugs. Sprays and aerosols are often used for decongestants and for antiasthmatic and antiallergic drugs.

Transdermal Delivery Systems (TDSs)

A **transdermal delivery system**, or **patch**, is a dosage form meant for delivery **percutaneously** (through the skin) and consists of a backing, a drug reservoir, a control membrane, an adhesive layer, and a protective strip (see Figure 4.20). The strip is removed, and the adhesive layer is attached to the skin. The drug moves by osmosis through the control membrane, delivering medication systemically, rather than locally. In some patches, the rate of drug delivery is controlled by the membrane. In some it is controlled by the skin itself. Examples of drugs administered using transdermal delivery systems include nitroglycerin for relief of angina, clonidine for control of hypertension, estrogen for treatment of menopausal symptoms, testosterone for treatment of testosterone deficiency, and nicotine for relief of cravings for tobacco.

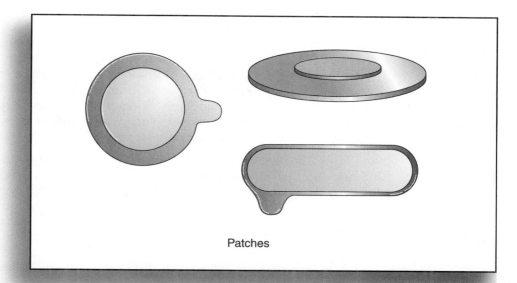

Figure 4.20 A transdermal delivery system, or patch, delivers medication at a controlled rate through the skin.

Patches

chapter summary

Drugs are natural, synthetic, synthesized, or semisynthetic substances, generally compounded and generally taken into or applied to the body to alter biochemical functions and thus to achieve therapeutic, pharmacodynamic, or prophylactic results. Some drugs are used, as well, as diagnostic or destructive agents. Drugs combine active with inert ingredients and can be classified as over-the-counter or legend. Drugs are administered in many dosage forms and using many delivery systems. The dosage form/delivery system is chosen based upon what active ingredient is to be delivered, how much is to be delivered, by what means or route, to what sites, at what rate, over what period of time, and for what purpose.

Solid dosage forms include hard- and soft-shell capsules, effervescent salts, implants or pellets, lozenges, pills, plasters, powders and granules, suppositories, and tablets. Tablets may be single compression, multiple compression, molded, coated, chewable, controlled release, effervescent, and/or formulated for buccal, sublingual, or vaginal use. Tablets used in compounding include tablet triturates, hypodermic tablets, and dispensing tablets. Liquid dosage forms include such solutions as aromatic waters, collodions, diluted acids, elixirs, enemas, extractives such as tinctures and fluidextracts, irrigating solutions or douches, liniments, parenteral solutions, spirits, or syrups, as well as such dispersions as suspensions and emulsions, including gels, jellies, magmas or milks, and microemulsions. Topical solutions include creams, lotions, ointments, and pastes. Other delivery systems/dosage forms include bulb syringes, droppers, glycerogelatins, inhalations, injections, intrauterine delivery systems, intravenous infusions, mucilages, ocular inserts, oral syringes, prefilled straws, radiopharmaceuticals, sponges, sprays and aerosols, and transdermal delivery systems, or patches.

chapter review

Knowledge Inventory

Choose the best answer from those provided.

1. A biochemically reactive component in a drug is known as
   a. an inert ingredient
   b. an active ingredient
   c. a diluent
   d. a vehicle

2. A National Drug Code number does not identify the
   a. product manufacturer
   b. drug
   c. packaging size and type
   d. schedule of the drug

3. A radiopharmaceutical used for imaging is an example of a
   a. therapeutic agent
   b. pharmacodynamic agent
   c. diagnostic agent
   d. prophylactic agent

4. When people use the term *delivery system,* they generally intend, in addition to the dosage form, to refer to the
   a. physical characteristics of the dosage form that determine the method of administration and the site of action of the drug
   b. restrictions placed upon the ordering, storage, and dispensing of the drug due to its classification under the Comprehensive Drug Abuse Prevention and Control Act
   c. chemical composition of the drug, including its active ingredients, inert ingredients, and any colorings, flavorings, preservatives, disintegrants, solubilizers, and emulsifying agents
   d. use of the drug as a therapeutic, pharmacodynamic, diagnostic, prophylactic, or destructive agent

5. A dosage form used in the rectum, vagina, and urethra is the
   a. inhalation aerosol
   b. suppository
   c. elixir
   d. fluidextract

6. Enteric coatings
   a. dissolve in the stomach
   b. dissolve in the intestines
   c. are comprised of sugar for palatability
   d. are made of polymers and form a protective film

7. A solution containing water and ethanol would be described as
   a. hydroalcoholic
   b. aqueous
   c. extractive
   d. immiscible

8. Some examples of dispersions are
   a. suspensions and emulsions
   b. tinctures, fluidextracts, and extracts
   c. aromatic waters and diluted acids
   d. elixirs and syrups

9. Dosage forms that are often or always sweetened include
   a. parenteral solutions, spirits, and tinctures
   b. medicated syrups, elixirs, and fluidextracts
   c. collodions, microemulsions, and unguents
   d. liniments, diluted acids, and extracts

10. Most emulsions are considered dual-phase systems, but one kind of emulsion that is considered single phase is the
    a. milk
    b. gel
    c. jelly
    d. magma

Pharmacy in Practice

1. A mortar and pestle may be made of smooth glass or of rougher porcelain. Experiment with each, triturating some common dried spices such as cloves or fennel seeds. Which device produces the finer trituration? How can you account for your results?

2. Recombinant DNA will, in the future, play a great role in gene therapies, in which recombinant DNA is used to supply the body with genes to supplement or replace the action of the existing genes with which the body is endowed. Do some research on gene therapy for the treatment of cystic fibrosis, the most common of all fatal genetic diseases. Such therapy uses a cold virus containing recombinant DNA that carries a gene called the cystic fibrosis transmembrane regulator. Prepare a brief report explaining how such therapy works. In your report, give particular attention to the pharmaceutical implications of gene therapy. If a missing gene is supplied by means of a virus containing recombinant DNA, what dosage form might be used to deliver this virus ?

3. Practice using the punch technique described in this chapter to fill capsules with granulated sugar and with fine, powdered confectioner's sugar. See chapter 11 for an explanation of aseptic technique for this activity.

4. A tree diagram is a chart that shows a classification system. A single characteristic is used to differentiate the items classified under each node on the chart. For example, a tree chart might classify animals in this way:

ANIMALS	
Vertebrates (with backbones)	**Invertebrates (without backbones)**
mammals	flatworms
reptiles	roundworms
fish	insects
birds	arachnids
amphibians	mollusks

Create tree charts to classify
   a. liquid dosage forms
   b. solutions (by vehicle)
   c. solutions (by contents)
   d. solutions (by site or method of administration)
   e. dispersions (by size of the dispersed ingredients)
   f. dispersions (by type of substance in the dispersed phase)

5. Go to a community or retail pharmacy and make a list of over-the-counter products in as many different dosage forms as you can identify. For each product on your list, give the manufacturer, the brand name, the active ingredient(s), and the dosage form/delivery system.

6. Do some research and write step-by-step instructions for
   a. giving an injection
   b. setting up an intravenous infusion

7. Different dosage forms have different pros and cons. For example, tablets and capsules are premeasured (pro) but may be difficult for some patients to swallow (con). Consider ease of administration, dangers of contamination, shelf-life, ease of obtaining patient compliance, suitability for patients of various ages or conditions, uniformity of dosage size, control of dosage rate,

and site of application, etc. Make a chart listing as many pros and cons as you can think of for each of the following dosage forms:
a. tablets
b. capsules
c. injections and infusions
d. sweetened dosage forms, such as sugar-coated tablets, syrups, and elixirs
e. bulk and divided powders

8. Pharmaceutical manufacturers are continually experimenting with dosage forms and delivery systems. Use an Internet search engine to visit some Web sites belonging to pharmaceutical manufacturers. Explore these sites to find examples of products with controlled-release characteristics. For each product that you find, give the manufacturer, brand name, active ingredient(s), and a description of the method for achieving controlled release.

9. Create a chart illustrating the parts of an intravenous infusion set.

10. Explore news sources for information about product-tampering cases in the past. Identify examples of ways in which the physical construction of a dosage form can inhibit or allow product tampering.

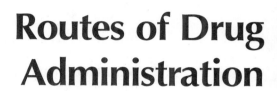

Routes of Drug Administration   **5**

Since ancient times, medications have been administered orally (by swallowing) and topically (by applying them directly to an exterior surface of the body). In the modern era, a wide variety of additional ways to get medications into the body have been developed. This chapter describes those ways.

TERMS TO KNOW

Bolus An injection

Buccal Having to do with the inner lining of the cheek; drugs administered buccally are placed between this lining and the gum, and are absorbed by the buccal mucosa

Compliance The willingness of a patient to take a drug in the amounts and on the schedule prescribed

Conjunctival Having to do with the lining of the inside of the eyelid; drugs administered conjunctivally are placed between this lining and the eye, and are absorbed by the conjunctival mucosa

Epicutaneous Having to do with the surface of the skin; drugs administered epicutaneously are placed upon the surface of the skin and absorbed through the skin into the body

First-pass effect The partial metabolism, or breaking down, of a drug by the liver

Infusion The slow administration of a fluid, with or without added nutrients or drug substances, into the body by means of a catheter or needle placed into a vein

Intrarespiratory Having to do with inhalation into the lungs; drugs administered by the intrarespiratory route are breathed into the lungs

Local Affecting a particular site rather than the entire body or an entire body system

HOW THE ROUTE OF ADMINISTRATION IS CHOSEN

As the previous chapter on dosage forms explained, drugs come in a wide variety of forms. These forms have been designed by pharmaceutical scientists for **administration**, or application, to the body in a wide variety of ways. A choice among the various **routes of administration**, or ways of getting a drug onto or into the body, is made based on many factors, as described in Chart 5.1.

POSSIBLE ROUTES OF ADMINISTRATION

A wide variety of routes of administration are currently employed in medicine. These routes are described in Chart 5.2.

PARENTERAL ADMINISTRATION

Although oral forms of administration are the most common, parenteral forms deserve special attention because of their complexity, their widespread use, and their potential for therapeutic benefit and for danger. The term *parenteral* comes from the Greek words *para*, meaning "outside," and *enteron*, meaning "the intestine." The derivation of the word refers to the fact that this route of administration bypasses the **alimentary canal**, consisting of the mouth, the esophagus, the stomach, the small and large intestines, and the rectum. A parenteral preparation is administered directly into the body, generally, but not always, directly into the bloodstream. Because of this it is relatively irretrievable compared to an oral dosage form. If an adverse reaction occurs to a parenteral, one cannot, as in the case of an oral preparation, induce vomiting to remove it from the system.

CHARACTERISTICS OF PARENTERAL PREPARATIONS

Parenteral preparations must be **sterile**. That is, they must be free of microorganisms and so are prepared using **aseptic techniques** that ensure sterility. They are either **solutions** (in which ingredients are dissolved) or, much less commonly, **suspensions** (in which ingredients are suspended). The body is primarily an **aqueous**, or water-containing, vehicle, and so most parenteral preparations introduced into the body are made up of ingredients placed in sterile water. In the case of intravenous infusions the vehicle is usually dextrose in water, normal saline solution, or dextrose in saline solution. Some parenteral solutions, however, may be **oleaginous**, or oily. For example, an emulsion containing fat may be administered in some cases to supply calories to patients who cannot or will not feed themselves and who need more calories than can be supplied by parenteral administration of water and the sugar known as **dextrose**. Most parenterals are introduced directly into the bloodstream and must be free of air bubbles or particulate matter, known as **emboli** (singular, **embolus**) that might cause an **embolism**, or blockage in a vessel.

Parenteral preparations must also have chemical properties that will prevent damage to vessels or blood cells and that will not alter the chemical properties of the blood serum. Generally speaking, parenterals must be **iso-osmotic** (having the same number of particles in solution per unit volume) and **isotonic** (having the same osmotic pressure) with blood. The **osmolality**, or amount of particulate per unit volume of a liquid preparation, is measured in **milliosmoles** (**mOsm**). The osmolality of blood serum is approximately 285 mOsm/L. Osmolality and tonicity, while similar, are not exactly the same because blood cells are

Ophthalmic Having to do with the eye; a drug administered by the ophthalmic route may be applied directly to the eye or placed against the conjunctiva for absorption by the conjunctival mucosa

Oral Having to do with the mouth; a drug administered orally may be dissolved in the mouth, or swallowed for local effects in the mouth or gastrointestinal tract, or for systemic effects following absorption along the gastrointestinal tract

Otic Having to do with the ear; drugs administered otically are placed into the ear canal

Parenteral Literally, "outside the intestine"; said of drugs administered in solution by injection or infusion using a hollow needle or catheter

Peroral Having to do with the mouth; said of a drug that is swallowed for local application to parts of the gastrointestinal tract or for absorption along that tract into the system

Route of administration A way of getting a drug onto or into the body

Sublingual Having to do with the space beneath the tongue; said of drugs that are administered by placement under the tongue for absorption by the sublingual mucosa

Systemic Affecting the entire body; said of drugs absorbed into the blood and carried throughout the body system

Transdermal Having to do with absorption through the skin; used to describe medicated patches placed on the skin for regular and continued delivery of a drug through the skin

Chart 5.1

FACTORS INFLUENCING THE ROUTE OF ADMINISTRATION CHOSEN

1. **Compliance.** The willingness of a patient to take a drug in the amounts and on the schedule prescribed is called **compliance**. Some drug dosage forms (flavored and sugared syrups or chewable tablets, for example) are specifically designed to improve compliance by patients. In some situations, as when dealing with psychiatric patients who might be a danger to themselves or to others, healthcare professionals must resort to forcing compliance by using a fast-acting route of administration such as injection.

2. **Ease of Administration.** Many people have particular qualities or characteristics that determine to some extent the route of administration chosen. In some situations, patients are unable, because of lack of consciousness, to perform an action such as swallowing a tablet, capsule,

or liquid. A very young or elderly patient might have difficulty swallowing, and in such a case the healthcare provider might have to avoid solid, orally administered dosage forms in favor of oral liquid dosage forms or other, nonoral routes of administration. An oral route of administration might also be inadvisable for a patient experiencing nausea and vomiting, which present the possibility of the drug's being expelled prematurely from the body.

3. **Site of Action.** One obvious factor affecting the route of administration chosen is the desired site of action of the drug. A major distinction can be drawn between drugs intended for local or systemic use. The term *local use* refers to site-specific applications of drugs, for example, when one applies an analgesic ointment to a minor burn or takes an antacid for local relief (in the stomach) of excessive gastric acid. The term *systemic use* refers to the application of a drug by means of absorption into the blood and subsequent transportation throughout the body. Of course, even when a drug is meant for systemic administration, it still is usually targeted to specific sites of action. For example, an **antineoplastic** drug, one that kills newly growing cells, may be administered systemically (by giving the patient an injection or by having him or her swallow a liquid to be absorbed into the system from the gastrointestinal tract), but its intended sites of action are quite specific— it is intended to act on growing tumors. Of course, these sites of action might be scattered throughout the body and might not even be all known, and for this reason the systemic route is chosen.

4. **Rate of Action.** Different routes of administration work more or less quickly. That is, they have different **onset rates**. In general, the fastest method of administration for action within the body is intravenously. The drug is injected or infused directly into the bloodstream and carried immediately throughout the body. Other methods, such as oral administration, are naturally slower.

5. **Duration of Action.** A route of administration may be chosen based on a desire to have the drug act over a long period of time. For example, a transdermal patch can be used to deliver small amounts of a drug, steadily, over a period of many hours. A similar sustained duration effect can be achieved by means of intravenous infusion.

6. **Quantity of Drug.** Sometimes, a route of administration is chosen because of the amount of a drug that must be delivered. A tablet containing a lot of filler, or diluent, might be a preferred method for administering a drug containing a very small amount (0.5 mg, for example) of an active ingredient. Intravenous infusion is an excellent method for delivering large quantities of material, such as blood or glucose, into the system.

7. **Susceptibility to Metabolism by the Liver.** Drugs differ in their resistance to metabolism by the liver. Some drugs, nitroglycerin for example, are given in very small doses and can then be diluted by gastrointestinal fluids and broken down by the liver in what is known as the **first-pass effect**. Such drugs have to be given by a means that bypasses metabolism by the liver.

Chart 5.1
(cont.)

8. **Toxicity. Toxicology** is the study of adverse effects of drugs or other substances on the body. Drugs are potent substances, and often their dangers, or toxicity, must be weighed against their therapeutic benefits. Sometimes the toxicity of a drug directly affects the route of administration chosen. For example, a caustic drug that might cause damage if delivered intravenously might be delivered orally instead.

Chart 5.2

ROUTES OF ADMINISTRATION AND APPLICABLE DOSAGE FORMS

Oral and Peroral

Definition. The term *oral* is used to refer to two very different methods of administration—topical application to the mouth (as for local treatment of a cold sore) and, more commonly, swallowing into the gastrointestinal tract. The latter route of administration, for local application to parts of the gastrointestinal tract or for absorption along that tract into the system, is more properly and precisely referred to as **peroral**.

Dosage Forms. Dosage forms for oral or peroral administration include capsules, elixirs, gels, lozenges (also known as troches or pastilles), magmas, powders, solutions, suspensions, syrups, and tablets.

Advantages and Disadvantages. The peroral route of administration is by far the most common because of the ease and safety of administration. In the case of capsules or tablets, the active ingredient is generally contained in powders or granules that also contain other substances, such as diluents, disintegrants, and colorings. These dissolve or disaggregate in the gastrointestinal tract, and the active ingredient thus becomes available for absorption into the system. Disadvantages of the peroral route include delayed onset, because the drug must often be broken down and then absorbed; "first-pass" metabolism by the liver; and destruction or dilution of the drug by gastrointestinal fluids and/or food or drink present in the stomach or intestines. The peroral route is not indicated in patients who are experiencing nausea or vomiting, or who are comatose, sedated, or otherwise unable to swallow. Most drugs are bitter or otherwise unpleasant in taste, and so another disadvantage of some peroral dosage forms is that the taste must be masked by flavorings to promote compliance.

Sublingual and Buccal

Definition. In **sublingual** administration, the drug is placed under the tongue, where it is absorbed by the **sublingual mucosa**. In **buccal** administration, the drug is placed between the gums and the inner lining of the cheek, in the so-called buccal pouch, where it is absorbed by the **buccal mucosa. Mucosa**, or **mucous membranes**, are the blood- and lymph-vessel rich linings of interior surfaces of the body that are open, via passageways, to the external air.

Dosage Forms. Dosage forms for sublingual and buccal administration include tablets and lozenges.

Advantages and Disadvantages. Sublingual and buccal routes of administration are very rapid in onset (though somewhat slower than intravenous routes) and are thus appropriate for immediate relief, as in use of nitroglycerin for treatment of chest pain due to angina pectoris. However, this route of administration is not appropriate for delivery of medication over an extended period.

Epicutaneous (Topical) or Transdermal

Definitions. **Epicutaneous** administration is the application of a drug directly to the surface of the skin. This route of administration is commonly referred to as topical, although the term *topical* more precisely refers to the application of a drug to any bodily surface. **Transdermal** administration is delivery of a drug via absorption through the skin, especially via a drug-containing patch or disk.

Dosage Forms. Dosage forms for epicutaneous or transdermal administration include aerosols, creams, lotions, ointments, pastes, plasters, powders, and transdermal patches or disks.

Advantages and Disadvantages. The epicutaneous administration route is superb for local effects. Drugs given epicutaneously for local effects include anesthetics, anti-inflammatory drugs, antifungals, antiseptics, astringents, moisturizers, **pediculicides** (for killing lice), protectants (e.g., sunscreen), and **scabicides** (for killing mites). A few drugs, such as nicotine, nitroglycerin, clonidine, and are administered epicutaneously for **percutaneous** (beneath the skin) effects. The skin presents a barrier to ready absorption. However, absorption does occur, slowly, via hair follicles, pores, **sebaceous glands** (glands that secrete a semiliquid, greasy substance known as **sebum**), and sweat glands. Once beneath the skin, the drug can be absorbed by tiny blood vessels known as **capillaries** to be transported systemically. For percutaneous delivery, the epicutaneous route is slow in onset but relatively long lasting.

Ocular, Conjunctival, Nasal, and Otic

Definitions. **Ocular** administration is the application of a drug to the eye. **Conjunctival** administration is the application of a drug to the conjunctival mucosa, the lining of the inside of the eyelid. **Nasal** administration is the application of a drug into the passages of the nose. **Otic** administration is the application of a drug to the ear canal. A drug meant for ocular or conjunctival administration may be called an **ophthalmic** drug.

Dosage Forms. Dosage forms for ocular administration include drug-impregnated contact lenses, solutions, and suspensions. Dosage forms for conjunctival administration include ointments and the Ocusert delivery system, which is an elliptical form for delivery of pilocarpine. Dosage forms for nasal administration include inhalants, ointments, solutions, and sprays. Dosage forms for otic administration include solutions and suspensions.

Advantages and Disadvantages. The ocular, conjunctival, nasal, and otic routes of administration are almost always for local effects, to treat conditions of the eye, the nose or sinuses, or the ear. Sprays for inhalation through the nose, however, may be used for systemic effects.

Rectal

Definition. **Rectal** administration is the application of a drug to or within the rectum.

Dosage Forms. Dosage forms for rectal administration include ointments, solutions, and suppositories.

Advantages and Disadvantages. A major disadvantage of the rectal route of administration is its inconvenience. Another disadvantage is that absorption

Chart 5.2
(cont.)

by the rectal mucosa is erratic and unpredictable. However, such a route is, of course, preferable for local effects (for example, for cleansing the rectum, administration of laxatives or cathartics, treatment of hemorrhoids, or delivery of barium prior to radiographic examination of the gastrointestinal tract). This may be a preferred method of delivery for systemic drugs in situations in which the drug might be destroyed or diluted by gastrointestinal fluids, in which an oral dosage form is precluded by lack of consciousness or nausea and vomiting, or in which the drug might be too readily metabolized by the liver. **Suppositories**, solid forms that melt or dissolve in the rectum, may be used to promote discharge of the bowels or to deliver a drug. The large number of blood and lymph vessels lining the walls of the rectum make drug absorption at this administration site quite good, though irregular. Ointments are used for local effects. Rectal solutions, or **enemas**, are used for cleansing and as laxatives or cathartics.

Vaginal and Urethral

Definitions. The **vaginal** route of administration is application of a drug within the canal of the vagina. The **urethral** route of administration is application of a drug to or within the urethra.

Dosage Forms. Dosage forms for vaginal administration include emulsion foams, inserts, ointments, solutions, sponges, suppositories, and tablets. Dosage forms for urethral administration include solutions and suppositories.

Advantages and Disadvantages. Generally speaking, these routes of administration are for local effects such as cleansing (e.g., douches), contraception, or treatment of infection.

Intrarespiratory

Definitions. The **intrarespiratory** route of administration is application of a drug through inhalation into the lungs. Typically, this inhalation occurs through the mouth.

Dosage Forms. The usual dosage form for intrarespiratory administration is gas or aerosol. However, volatile liquids can also be used in this manner.

Advantages and Disadvantages. The lungs are designed for absorption of gas (oxygen) into the bloodstream. Therefore, they are an excellent site for absorption of gases or drugs. Entry into the bloodstream is extremely rapid, second only to direct injection or infusion. The intrarespiratory route is used to deliver bronchodilaters to asthma sufferers, to provide oxygen to those suffering from oxygen deprivation, and to deliver general anesthetics.

Parenteral

Definitions. Parenteral administration is injection or infusion by means of a needle or catheter placed into the body. The parenteral route, because of its complexity, is discussed in detail in the next section.

Dosage Forms. Injection or infusion of sterile solutions or suspensions.

Advantages and Disadvantages. The parenteral route is the fastest of all methods for delivering systemic drugs, but it has associated dangers, including traumatic injury from the insertion of the needle or catheter into the body and the potential for introducing, by this means, toxic agents, microbes, or **pyrogens** (fever-producing agents produced by microbial metabolism).

more or less permeable by various chemical substances. A parenteral solution of greater than normal **tonicity**, or ability to permeate blood cells due to osmotic pressure and other characteristics, is said to be **hypertonic**. One of less than normal tonicity is said to be **hypotonic**. Pharmacists sometimes have to adjust the tonicity of parenteral preparations to ensure that they are not hypertonic or hypotonic. On occasion, it is necessary to administer hypertonic solutions, but this must be done very slowly and cautiously. The degree of acidity or alkalinity of a solution is known as its **pH value**. If a solution has a pH of less than 7, it is **acidic**. If it has a pH value of more than 7, it is **alkaline**. Blood plasma has a pH of 7.4. In other words, it is slightly alkaline. Parenteral solutions, if they are not to alter the acidity or alkalinity of the blood, must have a close to neutral pH value.

Injections

The **bolus**, or **injection**, is one of the most common routes of administration. The injection is performed using a syringe (see Figure 4.16). These days, many injectables come prepackaged in the form of filled, disposable plastic syringes. At other times, the injectable drug must be taken up into the syringe from a single-dose or multi-dose glass or plastic vial, or from a glass ampule. In some cases, as with lypholized powder, the solid drug in the vial has to be reconstituted by addition of a liquid (generally sterile water for injection) before use. A vial may be clear or light amber in color (to protect the drug from exposure to light). To fill a syringe from a vial, one generally follows the steps outlined in Chart 5.3.

Chart 5.3	USING A SYRINGE TO DRAW LIQUID FROM A VIAL

1. Choose the smallest gauge needle appropriate for the task (needles vary from 30 gauge [the smallest] to 13 gauge [the largest]) to avoid coring the rubber top of the vial and introducing particulate into the liquid within.

2. Attach the needle to the syringe.

3. Draw into the syringe an amount of air equal to the amount of drug to be drawn from the vial.

4. Swab or spray the top of the vial with alcohol; allow the alcohol to dry. Puncture the rubber top of the vial with the needle bevel up. Then bring the syringe and needle straight up, penetrate the stopper, and depress the plunger of the syringe, emptying the air into the vial.

5. Draw up from the vial the amount of liquid required, and withdraw the needle from the vial. In the case of a multi-dose vial, the rubber cap will close, sealing the contents of the vial.

6. Remove and dispose of the needle, and attach a new needle with which to do the injection.

When filling a syringe from an ampule, one must first break the top off the ampule. The glass around the base of the top is scored to make such breaking easy and clean; still, one should protect oneself against being cut by the breaking glass when breaking off the top by placing an alcohol swab between the fingers and the ampule, or by using an ampule-breaking device. Then, when filling the syringe, one should use a needle equipped with a filter for filtering out any tiny glass particles that may have fallen into the ampule. Before injecting the contents of a syringe into an IV, change the needle to avoid introducing glass into the admixture.

Injections may be made into almost any part of the body. The most common sort of injection is one done by the **intravenous (IV)** route, directly into a vein. However, **intradermal (ID)** or **intracutaneous** injections made into the skin, **subcutaneous (SC, subq., SQ, hypodermic, or hypo)** injections made under the skin, and **intramuscular (IM)** injections made into a muscle are also common (see Figure 5.1).

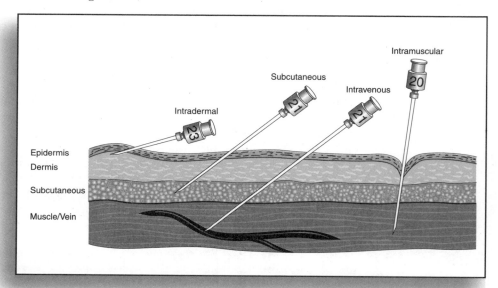

Figure 5.1 Routes of parenteral administration.

Intravenous drug administration, by injection or by infusion is an extremely fast-acting route because the drug goes directly into the bloodstream for transport throughout the system. Because of their rapid delivery, intravenous injection and infusion are often used in emergency situations. Commonly, intravenous injections and infusions, which can vary in amount from a few to thousands of milliliters, are given into the superficial veins of the arm on the side opposite the elbow, though other sites are occasionally used.

Intramuscular injections, appropriate in most cases for no more than 5 mL of drug, are slower in delivery but longer in duration than intravenous ones. Care must be taken with deep intramuscular injections to avoid hitting a vein, artery, or nerve. In adults, intramuscular injections are generally given into the upper, outer portion of the gluteus maximus, the large muscle on either side of the buttocks. Another common site, especially for children, is the deltoid muscles of the shoulders.

Subcutaneous injections, usually of very small amounts (less than 2 mL), are given just beneath the skin, usually on the outside of the upper arm, the top of the thigh, or the lower portion of the abdomen. Insulin, the most common of subcutaneous injections, is given using 25 to 28 gauge needles, and the site is varied from injection to injection. A special **insulin syringe** is used, which has a short needle and measures **units (U)** of insulin (see Figure 5.2).

Intradermal injections, given into the more capillary-rich layer just below the epidermis, are given for local anesthesia and for various diagnostic tests and immunizations. A typical site for such injections is the upper forearm, below the area where intravenous injections are given.

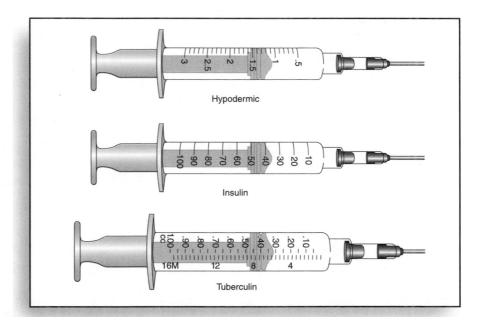

Figure 5.2 Types of syringes include the hypodermic, the insulin syringe, and the tuberculin syringe.

Hypodermic

Insulin

Tuberculin

Infusions

Not much will be said of parenteral infusions here, as these are treated in detail in chapter 9. **Intravenous infusions**, or **IVs**, deliver large amounts of liquid, over prolonged periods, into the bloodstream. This route of administration is used to deliver blood, water, other fluids, nutrients such as lipids and sugars, electrolytes, and drugs. Infusions are administered using sterile, pyrogen-free IV containers and IV sets. The **IV container**, which holds the fluid to be administered, is a vented or unvented glass bottle or a flexible, vented plastic bottle (see Figure 5.3). The **IV set**, or **IV administration set**, is a sterile, pyrogen-free, disposable unit. The set may be sterilized before use by means of radiation or ethylene oxide, or it may come in sterile packaging with a peel-off top cardboard and a sealed plastic wrap. Some IV set packaging has a clear wrap for viewing the contents, while other packaging employs a diagram of the enclosed set printed on the outside of the packaging. Sets do not carry expiration dates but do carry the legend "Federal law restricts this device to sale by or on the order of a physician."

Regardless of manufacturer, sets have certain basic components, which include a **spike** to pierce the rubber stopper or port on the IV container, a **drip chamber** for trapping air and adjusting flow rate, a **control clamp** for adjusting flow rate or shutting down the flow, flexible **tubing** to convey the fluid, and a **needle adapter** for attaching a needle or a catheter (see Figure 5.4). A **catheter**, or tube, may be implanted into the patient and fixed with tape to avoid having to repuncture the patient each time an infusion is given. In addition to these parts, most IV sets contain a **Y-site**, or **injection port**, a rigid piece of plastic with one arm terminating in a resoluble port that is used for adding medication to the IV. Some IV sets also contain **resealable inline filters** that offer protection for the patient against particulates, including bacteria and emboli. Intravenous infusion may employ any of a variety of **pumps** to regulate amount, rate, and timing of flow. Pharmacists and pharmacy technicians are often called upon to prepare intravenous admixtures for infusion. The procedures for doing this are treated in chapter 9.

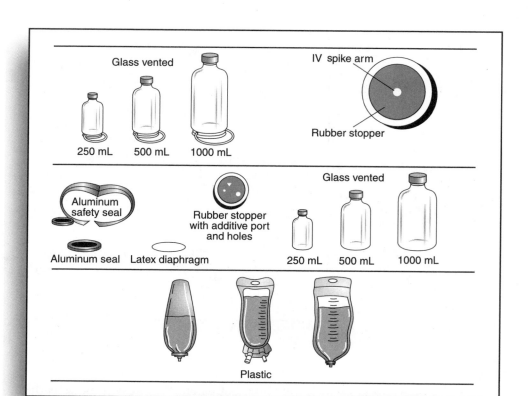

Figure 5.3 IV containers.

Glass vented

250 mL   500 mL   1000 mL

IV spike arm

Rubber stopper

Aluminum safety seal

Aluminum seal   Latex diaphragm

Rubber stopper with additive port and holes

Glass vented

250 mL   500 mL   1000 mL

Plastic

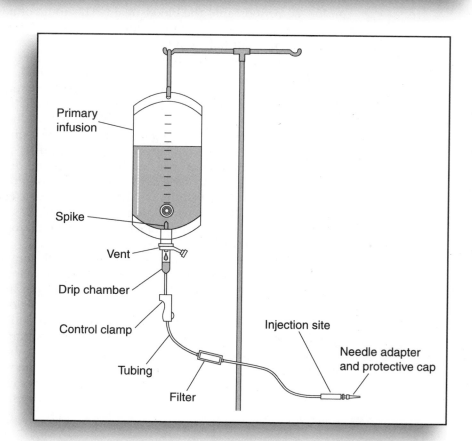

Figure 5.4 Upright IV set.

Primary infusion

Spike

Vent

Drip chamber

Control clamp

Tubing

Filter

Injection site

Needle adapter and protective cap

chapter summary

Many factors influence the decision about which of the many possible routes of administration is chosen in order to deliver a particular drug or combination of drugs. These factors include compliance, ease of administration, site of action (local or systemic), rate of onset of action, duration of action, the quantity to be administered, the susceptibility of the drug to first-pass metabolism by the liver, and the toxicology of the drug. Possible routes of administration are the oral and peroral, the sublingual, the buccal, the epicutaneous (including the transdermal), the ophthalmic (ocular or conjunctival), the nasal, the otic, the rectal, the vaginal, the urethral, the intrarespiratory, and the parenteral. Types of parenterals include injections and intravenous infusions.

Parenterals are sterile, pyrogen and embolus free, and are usually aqueous solutions. Parenterals for intravenous injection or infusion generally have an osmolality, tonicity, and pH value similar to that of blood. Because they are injected directly into the bloodstream, special precautions must be taken in the preparation and administration of intravenous parenterals. Injections are typically given intravenously, intradermally, subcutaneously, or intramuscularly. Infusions for a variety of purposes, including delivery of fluids, nutrients, and drugs, are administered by means of IV sets.

chapter review

Knowledge Inventory

Choose the best answer from those provided.

1. The willingness of a patient to take a drug in the amounts and on the schedule prescribed is called
   a. ease of administration
   b. compliance
   c. route of administration
   d. factor of administration

2. Nausea and vomiting might preclude the use of
   a. a parenteral route of administration
   b. an epicutaneous route of administration
   c. a peroral route of administration
   d. a urethral route of administration

3. The most common route of administration is the
   a. parenteral route of administration
   b. epicutaneous route of administration
   c. peroral route of administration
   d. intravenous route of administration

4. In the first-pass effect, some drugs taken orally are rapidly metabolized, or broken down, by the
   a. spleen
   b. bowels
   c. liver
   d. kidneys

5. A tablet placed between the gums and the inner lining of the cheek is dissolved by the
   a. conjunctival mucosa
   b. sublingual mucosa
   c. vaginal mucosa
   d. buccal mucosa

6. Suppositories are *not* used for
   a. rectal administration
   b. urethral administration
   c. buccal administration
   d. vaginal administration

7. The word *parenteral* means, literally, "outside the
   a. stomach"
   b. intestine"
   c. mouth"
   d. liver"

8. A solution with a pH of 8 would be
   a. acidic
   b. alkaline
   c. hypertonic
   d. hypotonic

9. When opening an ampule, one uses an alcohol wipe to
   a. sterilize the fingers
   b. protect the fingers from being cut
   c. force open the top if it will not break easily
   d. swab the site of injection

10. A transdermal patch makes use of the
    a. percutaneous route of administration
    b. ophthalmic route of administration
    c. otic route of administration
    d. conjunctival route of administration

Pharmacy in Practice

1. Nitroglycerin is an example of a drug that comes in a wide variety of dosage forms appropriate for a wide variety of routes of administration. Do some research on the different routes of administration used for nitroglycerin. Refer to sites on the World Wide Web, to reference works, and to healthcare professionals. Pose the following questions: What are the dosage forms of nitroglycerin? What routes of administration are used? Why do people choose one route of administration over another? For what purposes are the various routes of administration used?

2. The label on a medication contains directions for using the medication, including amounts to be taken, times when these should be taken, and any other information that the prescriber deems necessary. Write a brief report explaining why it is important for a pharmacist to counsel customers or patients with regard to taking medications. How can such counseling improve compliance?

3. Hold a discussion in class on the advantages and disadvantages of the various routes of administration. Which are the most convenient? Which are the safest? Which are the fastest acting? Which provide for controlled release? Which last a long time? Which pose compliance problems?

4. Create a chart with a schematic diagram of the human body, illustrating the various routes of administration described in this lesson.

5. Do some research into the history of parenterals. When were they first used? By whom? What difficulties did they present to the people who first experimented with parenteral administration? How have these difficulties been overcome? Present your findings in a report or class discussion.

Sources of Information

6

Pharmacy is a complex, technical field. No single individual can possibly learn all that he or she needs to know in order to perform pharmacy duties correctly. Even if a person could do so, at least some of what he or she had learned would become obsolete in a short time. For these reasons, it is extremely important for people in the profession to become familiar with the major reference works available. Fortunately, a large body of pharmacy literature exists, offering precise, accurate, timely information to workers in the profession. This chapter will survey some of the most important references available.

Learning Objectives

- List the major pharmacy organizations and their journals
- Identify important general references in medicine and anatomy
- Identify important general references on drugs, dosage forms, patient counseling, pharmacology, and adverse reactions
- Identify important references on filling prescriptions, compounding, calculations, and preparing parenteral admixtures
- Identify important references on pharmaceutical law, regulation, ethics, communication, and economics
- Identify important works on technician training and certification
- Explain the contents of a package insert

TERMS TO KNOW

American Association of Pharmacy Technicians (AAPT) National organization representing pharmacy technicians

American Pharmaceutical Association (APhA) Largest of the national pharmacy organizations

American Society of Health-System Pharmacists (ASHP) Large organization representing pharmacists who practice in hospitals and other institutions

Drug Enforcement Administration (DEA) Federal agency that enforces laws and regulations related to controlled substances

Food and Drug Administration (FDA) Federal agency charged with primary responsibility for creating regulations governing the safety of foods, drugs, and cosmetics

National Association of Boards of Pharmacy (NABP) Association of state boards of pharmacy

PHARMACY ORGANIZATIONS AND THEIR JOURNALS

Since the days of the medieval guilds, when craftspeople and artisans such as silversmiths and carpenters joined together to oversee apprenticeships, training, and business affairs, professional people have created organizations or associations to advance the purposes of their professions. Contemporary pharmacy is no exception. Listed below are some of the most important organizations in the pharmacy profession.

American Association of Colleges of Pharmacy (AACP) The AACP, founded in 1900, represents all 79 pharmacy colleges and schools in the United States and is the national organization representing the interests of pharmaceutical education and educators. The AACP publishes the journals *American Journal of Pharmaceutical Education, Roster of Faculty and Professional Staff, Profile of Pharmacy Faculty, Profile of Pharmacy Students,* and a monthly newsletter, the *AACP News.* The address of the AACP on the World Wide Web is http://www.aacp.org.

American Association of Pharmaceutical Scientists (AAPS) The AAPS, formerly an academy of the APhA, represents pharmaceutical scientists employed in academia, industry, government, and other research institutions. It has sections related to such fields as pharmaceutical quality, biotechnology, medicinal and natural products chemistry, pharmaceutics and drug delivery, pharmacokinetics, pharmacodynamics, and regulatory affairs. Its publications include the journals *Pharmaceutical Research, Pharmaceutical Development and Technology, Journal of Pharmaceutical and Biomedical*

Analysis, Journal of Pharmaceutical Marketing and Management, and the *AAPS Newsletter.* The address of the AAPS on the World Wide Web is http://www.aaps.org.

American Association of Pharmacy Technicians (AAPT) Formerly called the APT, the AAPT, founded in 1979, is a national organization, with chapters in many states, representing pharmacy technicians and promoting certification of technicians. The association has established a Code of Ethics for Pharmacy Technicians. The address of the national headquarters is P.O. Box 1447, Greensboro, NC 27402. Its telephone numbers are (910) 275-1700 (voice) and (910) 275-7222 (fax).

American College of Apothecaries (ACA) The ACA, a professional association representing community-based pharmacists, publishes the quarterly ***Voice of the Pharmacist*** and the ***ACA Newsletter.***

American College of Clinical Pharmacy (ACCP) The ACCP is a professional and scientific society that provides leadership, education, advocacy, and resources for clinical pharmacists. The ACCP publishes the journal ***Pharmacotherapy***. The address of the ACCP on the World Wide Web is http://www.accp.com.

American Council on Pharmaceutical Education (ACPE) Founded in 1932, the ACPE is the national accrediting agency for pharmacy education programs recognized by the Secretary of Education. The ACPE is located in Chicago, Illinois, and can be reached at (312) 664-3575.

American Pharmaceutical Association (APhA) The largest of the national pharmacy organizations, the APhA consists of three academies: the Academy of Pharmacy Practice and Management (APhA-APPM), the Academy of Pharmaceutical Research and Science (APhA-APRS), and the Academy of Students of Pharmacy (APhA-ASP). The APhA publishes the bimonthly ***Journal of the American Pharmaceutical Association,*** the monthly ***Pharmacy Today*** newsletter, and the monthly ***Journal of Pharmaceutical Sciences***. The APhA also operates a political action committee, or PAC. According to the APhA, its mission is "to advocate the interests of pharmacists; influence the profession, government, and others in addressing vital pharmaceutical care issues; promote the highest professional and ethical standards; and foster science and research in support of the practice of pharmacy." The address of the APhA on the World Wide Web is http://www.aphanet.org.

American Society of Consultant Pharmacists (ASCP) The ASCP is a professional organization representing consultant pharmacists, practitioners who provide, on a contractual basis, medication distribution and pharmacy expertise to nursing homes and other long-term care facilities, including subacute care and assisted living facilities, psychiatric hospitals, facilities for the mentally retarded, correctional facilities, adult day care centers, hospices, alcohol and drug rehabilitation centers, ambulatory and surgical care centers, and home care providers. The ASCP publishes a journal, ***The Consultant Pharmacist,*** and ***Update—The Monthly Newsletter of the American Society of Consultant***

Pharmacists. The address of the ASCP on the World Wide Web is http://www.ascp.com.

American Society of Health-System Pharmacists (ASHP) The ASHP is a large organization that represents pharmacists who practice in hospitals, health maintenance organizations (HMOs), long-term care facilities, home care agencies, and other institutions. The ASHP is a national accrediting organization for pharmacy residency and pharmacy technician training programs. The ASHP publishes the *American Journal of Health-System Pharmacy*. The address of the ASHP on the World Wide Web is http://www.ashp.org. The society's Practice Standards are available online at http://www.figleaf.com/production/ashp/practicestandards.

Drug Enforcement Administration (DEA) The DEA enforces federal laws and regulations related to controlled substances. The address of the DEA on the World Wide Web is http://www.usdoj.gov/dea.

Food and Drug Administration (FDA) The FDA is the federal government agency charged with primary responsibility for creating regulations governing the safety of foods, drugs, and cosmetics. The FDA enforces the Food, Drug, and Cosmetic Act of 1938 and its subsequent amendments, oversees new drug development, approves or disapproves applications to market new drugs, monitors reports of adverse reactions, and has the authority to recall drugs deemed dangerous. The address of the FDA on the World Wide Web is http://www.fda.gov.

National Association of Boards of Pharmacy (NABP) The NABP is an association of state boards of pharmacy. State boards of pharmacy are the organizations, in the individual states, with the responsibility of licensing pharmacists, conducting inspections, and ensuring compliance with regulations and ethical standards. The NABP supports the rights of states to determine their own pharmacy regulations and guidelines but has worked toward standardizing licensing, especially through the promotion of a national licensing examination, the North American Pharmacist Licensure Examination, or NABPLEX. The address of the NABP is 700 Busse Highway, Park Ridge, Illinois 60068. The telephone number is (847) 698-6227.

National Association of Chain Drug Stores (NACDS) Founded in 1933, the NACDS is an association representing the large number of community pharmacies that are parts of chain retail operations. This well-funded public relations and political action organization includes as members chief executives of retail chains that include pharmacies. The address of the NACDS on the World Wide Web is http://www.nacds.org.

National Association of Pharmaceutical Manufacturers (NAPM) The NAPM is an industry association representing manufacturers of pharmaceuticals and related products. This association lobbies government agencies and legislators regarding legislation and regulations affecting the pharmaceuticals industry. The address of the NAPM is 320 Old Country Road, Suite 205, Garden City, NY 11530-1752. The telephone number is   (516) 741-3699.

National Community Pharmacists Association (NCPA) Formerly known as the National Association of Retail Druggists, or NARD, the NCPA is an association representing independent community pharmacies. The NCPA publishes *America's Pharmacist, NCPA Newsletter, Inside Pharmacist Care, Alternate Site Pharmacist,* and *Regimen: An Update on Long-Term Care Drug Therapy*. The address of the NCPA on the World Wide Web is http://www.ncpanet.org.

National Home Infusion Association (NHIA) Located in Alexandria, Virginia, this association, created by NARD (now NCPA), provides information and support related to the fast-growing field of home infusion. The address of the NHIA on the World Wide Web is http://www.geohealthweb.com/GHW/public/NIHA/niha.html.

National Pharmaceutical Association (NPA) The NPA is the professional organization representing the community pharmacies of Great Britain. Its address on the World Wide Web is http://www.npa.co.uk.

National Wholesale Druggists' Association (NWDA) The NWDA is an association representing those companies that provide pharmacies with drugs and supplies. The address of the NWDA on the World Wide Web is http://www.nwda.org.

Pharmaceutical Research and Manufacturers of America (PhRMA) PhRMA is an association of companies involved in pharmaceutical research. The address of PhRMA on the World Wide Web is http://www.phrma.org.

Pharmacy Technician Certification Board (PTCB) The PTCB publishes the Pharmacy Technician Certification Examination, or PTCE, for those wishing to become Certified Pharmacy Technicians (CPhTs). The PTCE has been taken, voluntarily, by thousands of technicians around the country and is required for certification in some states. In addition to publishing the PTCE, the PTCB oversees a recertification program for technicians. The address of the PTCB is 2215 Constitution Avenue, NW, Washington, DC, 20037. The telephone number is (202) 429-7576. The address of the PTCB on the World Wide Web is http://www.ptcb.org.

Pharmacy Technician Educators Council (PTEC) PTEC is an association of educators who prepare people for careers as pharmacy technicians. Its official publication is the *Journal of Pharmacy Technology*. The PTEC address on the World Wide Web is http://www.mbnet.mb.ca/ptec.

Proprietary Association of Great Britain (PAGB) The PA is a British association representing manufacturers of over-the-counter medications and related products. The address of the PA on the World Wide Web is http://www.asa.org.uk/bcasp/r_pagb.htm.

United States Pharmacopeial Convention (USP) The USP is a nonprofit organization that sets standards for the identity, strength, quality, purity, packaging, and labeling of drug products. The address of the USP on the World Wide Web is http://www.usp.org. The USP provides an online drug information service at http://www.usp.org/toolbar/search.htm#check.

REFERENCE WORKS

A wide variety of reference works on topics related to pharmacy are available. A complete description of these references is beyond the scope of this book. However, some of the most important reference works are described under appropriate topical headings below.

General References: Medicine and Anatomy

A.D.A.M. Interactive Anatomy. **CD-ROM. Atlanta, GA. A.D.A.M. Software, 1998.** A new, professional version of the acclaimed human anatomy software. Less expensive teaching versions of this software are available. See the company's site on the World Wide Web at http://www.adam.com.

The Charles Press Handbook of Current Medical Abbreviations. **Philadelphia: Charles Press, 1997.** A standard reference work on symbols and abbreviations used in medicine. The address of the Charles Press on the World Wide Web is http://www.charlespresspub.com.

Davis, Neil M. *Medical Abbreviations: 12,000 Conveniences at the Expense of Communications and Safety.* **8th ed. Huntingdon Valley, PA: N.M. Davis Assoc., 1997.** A guide to medical abbreviations.

Dorland's Illustrated Medical Dictionary. **28th ed. Philadelphia: Saunders, 1994.** A standard medical dictionary. W. B. Saunders can be reached at (800) 545-2522.

Gray's Anatomy: The Anatomical Basis of Medicine and Surgery. **38th ed. New York: Churchill Livingstone, 1995.** The classic reference work on human anatomy.

Harrison's Principles of Internal Medicine. **14th ed. New York: McGraw-Hill, 1998.** A standard, authoritative overview of the field of internal medicine. See McGraw-Hill Professional Publications on the World Wide Web at http://www.pbg.mcgraw-hill.com.

The Merck Manual of Diagnosis and Therapy. **16th ed. Whitehouse Station, NJ: Merck, 1992.** This comprehensive survey of diseases, diagnosis, prevention, symptoms, and treatments is now somewhat out of date, but a new edition is due in 1999. The manual is available in book form; in a free, searchable online edition at http://www.merck.com//!!uwVil1oMiuwVj10qmQ/pubs/mmanual; on CD-ROM or diskette from Keyboard Publishing at http://www.kbpub.com or (610) 832-0945; and in a handheld electronic version from Franklin Electronic Publishers at http://www.franklin.com or (800) 266-5626.

The Merck Manual of Medical Information: Home Edition. **Whitehouse Station, NJ: Merck, 1997.** A simplified and updated version of the Merck Manual for use by lay people. See the company's World Wide Web site at http://www.merck.com.

Nelson Textbook of Pediatrics. **15th ed. Philadelphia: W.B. Saunders, 1996.** A standard textbook on pediatric medicine. W.B. Saunders can be reached at (800) 545-2522.

Stedman's Medical Dictionary: Illustrated in Color. **26th ed. Baltimore: Williams & Wilkins, 1995.** A standard medical dictionary. The address of Williams & Wilkins on the World Wide Web is http://www.wwilkins.com.

General References: Drugs, Dosage Forms, Patient Counseling, Pharmacology, and Adverse Reactions

American Drug Index 1998. **St. Louis, MO: Facts and Comparisons, 1997.** This standard reference work contains more than 20,000 entries on drugs and drug products, including alphabetically listed drug names, cross-indexing, phonetic pronunciations, brand names, manufacturers, generic and/or chemical names, composition and strength, pharmaceutical forms available, package size, use, and common abbreviations. It also contains a listing of orphan drugs. The work is available in hardbound and CD-ROM editions. The address of Facts and Comparisons on the World Wide Web is http://www.fandc.com.

American Hospital Formulary Service Drug Information (AHFS). Bethesda, MD: American Society of Health-System Pharmacists, 1998. The complete text of roughly 1,400 monographs covering about 50,000 commercially available and experimental drugs, including information on uses, interactions, pharmacokinetics, dosage, and administration. The address of the American Society of Health-System Pharmacists on the World Wide Web is http://www.ashp.org.

Ansel, Howard C., et al. *Pharmaceutical Dosage Forms and Drug Delivery Systems.* 6th ed. Baltimore: Williams & Wilkins, 1995. A superb survey of contemporary dosage forms and delivery systems. The address of Williams & Wilkins on the World Wide Web is http://www.wwilkins.com.

Drugdex. Englewood, CO: Micromedex. This is a computerized drug information system.

Drug Facts and Comparisons. 52nd ed. St. Louis, MO: Facts and Comparisons, 1997. This comprehensive source of information about 16,000 prescription and 6,000 over-the-counter drugs contains monographs about individual drugs and groups of related drugs; product listings in table format providing information on dosage forms and strength, distributor names, costs, package sizes, product identification codes, flavors, colors, and distribution status; and information on therapeutic uses, interactions, and adverse reactions. The publication includes an index of manufacturers and distributors and controlled substance regulations. This reference work is available in hardbound form, on CD-ROM, or in a loose-leaf form that is updated monthly. The address of Facts and Comparisons on the World Wide Web is http://www.fandc.com.

Drug Information Fulltext (DIF). Norwood, MA: Silverplatter. A searchable computer database combining two publications: the *American Hospital Formulary Service Drug Information* and the *Handbook on Injectable Drugs.* This database is available on a hard disk, on CD-ROM, or via the Internet. Silverplatter's address on the World Wide Web is http://www.silverplatter.com.

Drug Interaction Facts. 6th ed. St Louis, MO: Facts and Comparisons, 1997. This reference, available as a hardbound book, CD-ROM, or loose-leaf book that is updated quarterly, provides comprehensive information on potential interactions that can be reviewed by drug class, generic drug name, or trade name. Provides information on drug/drug and drug/food interactions. The address of Facts and Comparisons on the World Wide Web is http://www.fandc.com.

Food and Drug Administration. *Approved Drug Products with Therapeutic Equivalence Evaluations.* Washington, DC: U.S. Government Printing Office. Revised annually, with monthly updates, this source lists drug products approved for use in the United States. Also known as the *Orange*

Book because of its orange-colored cover. The address of the FDA on the World Wide Web is http://www.fda.gov.

Fudyuma, Janice. *What Do I Take? A Consumer's Guide to Nonprescription Drugs.* New York: HarperCollins, 1997. A simple-to-read guide to over-the-counter drugs.

Goodman & Gilman's The Pharmacological Basis of Therapeutics. **9th ed. New York: McGraw-Hill, 1996.** An authoritative text on pharmacology and therapeutics containing 67 articles by leading experts in the field. This text provides information for pharmacists to help them answer clinical questions about how drugs work under different conditions in the body. See McGraw-Hill Professional Publications on the World Wide Web at http://www.pbg.mcgraw-hill.com.

Graedon, Joe, and Teresa Graedon. *Deadly Drug Interactions: The People's Pharmacy Guide: How to Protect Yourself from Harmful Drug/Drug, Drug/Food, Drug/Vitamin Combinations.* **New York: St. Martin's Press, 1997.** An easy-to-read guide to dangerous drug interactions.

Koda-Kimble, Maryanne, and Lloyd Yee Young. *Applied Therapeutics: The Clinical Use of Drugs.* **6th ed. Vancouver, WA: Applied Therapeutics Inc., 1995.**

Index Nominum. **Geneva: Swiss Pharmaceutical Society, 1995.** A compilation of synonyms, formulas, and therapeutic classes of over 7,000 drugs and 28,000 proprietary preparations from 27 countries. Available in text and CD-ROM formats.

The International Pharmacopoeia. **3rd ed. New York: World Health Organization, 1994.** Recommended production methods and specifications for drugs, in four volumes. The World Health Organization is on the World Wide Web at http://www.who.ch.

MedCoach CD-ROM **(Windows, NT, & Macintosh). Rockville, MD: United States Pharmacopeial Convention, 1997.** A database of information for patients on over 6,000 generic and brand-name drug products, over-the-counter drugs, nutritional and home infusion items, test devices, and infant formulas. Provides information for patients on proper drug use and preparation, drug and food interactions, side effects/adverse effects, therapeutic contraindications, and product storage. Information is tailored to particular patients' needs (pediatric, male or female, geriatric, etc.). Subscription includes quarterly updates. The address of the United States Pharmacopeial Convention on the World Wide Web is http://www.usp.org.

Orange Book. See Food and Drug Administration.

Patient Drug Facts, 1996: Professionals Guide to Patient Drug Facts. **St. Louis, MO: Facts and Comparisons, 1996.** This is a comprehensive guide to patient counseling about drugs, available in loose-leaf format for verbal patient counseling and in PC format (on disk) for creation of patient handouts. The address of Facts and Comparisons on the World Wide Web is http://www.fandc.com.

Physician's Desk Reference (PDR). **52nd ed. Oradell, NJ: Medical Economics, 1998.** Available in hardbound and CD-ROM form, with two supplements published twice a year, this standard reference work contains information from package inserts (see below) for more than 4,000 prescription drugs, as well as information on 250 drug manufacturers. The address of Medical Economics on the World Wide Web is http://www.medec.com.

Smith, C. G. *The Process of New Drug Discovery and Development.* **Boca Raton, FL: CRC Press, 1992.** Description of the process by which new drugs are developed, tested, and approved for clinical trials and marketing.

Stringer, Janet L. *Basic Concepts in Pharmacology: A Student's Survival Guide.* **New York: McGraw-Hill, 1995.** Survey of basic pharmacological concepts for students. See McGraw-Hill Professional Publications on the World Wide Web at http://www.pbg.mcgraw-hill.com.

United States Pharmacopeia, 23rd Rev.—National Formulary. **18th ed. Rockville, MD: United States Pharmacopeial Convention, 1995.** Combined compendium of monographs setting official national standards for drug substances and dosage forms (*United States Pharmacopeia*) and standards for pharmaceutical ingredients (*National Formulary*). Available in book or CD-ROM form and in English- and Spanish-language editions. The address of the United States Pharmacopeial Convention on the World Wide Web is http://www.usp.org.

USP Dictionary of USAN and International Drug Names. **Rockville, MD: United States Pharmacopeial Convention, 1997.** An authoritative guide to drug names, including chemical names, brand names, manufacturers, molecular formulas, therapeutic uses, and chemical structures. The address of the United States Pharmacopeial Convention on the World Wide Web is http://www.usp.org.

USP Drug Information (USP DI). Vol. I. Drug Information for the Health Care Professional. **Rockville, MD: United States Pharmacopeial Convention, 1997.** A comprehensive source of in-depth drug information, available in book or CD-ROM form and in English- and Spanish-language editions. Describes medically accepted uses of more than 11,000 generic and brand-name products. The address of the United States Pharmacopeial Convention on the World Wide Web is http://www.usp.org.

USP Drug Information (USP DI). Vol. II. Advice for the Patient. **Rockville, MD: United States Pharmacopeial Convention, 1997.** Contains monographs corresponding to those in the *USP DI*, Vol. I, but simplified for the purpose of patient education and counseling. Available in English- and Spanish-language editions. The address of the United States Pharmacopeial Convention on the World Wide Web is http://www.usp.org.

USP Drug Information (USP DI). Vol. III. Approved Drug Products and Legal Requirements. **Rockville, MD: United States Pharmacopeial Convention, 1997.** Therapeutic equivalence information and selected federal requirements that affect the prescribing and dispensing of prescription drugs and controlled substances. Includes the FDA *Orange Book;* USP-NF requirements for labeling, storage, packaging, and quality; federal Food, Drug, and Cosmetic Act provisions relating to drugs for human use; portions of the Controlled Substance Act Regulations; and the FDA's Good Manufacturing Practice regulations for finished pharmaceuticals. The address of the United States Pharmacopeial Convention on the World Wide Web is http://www.usp.org.

Filling Prescriptions, Compounding, Calculations, Preparing Parenteral Admixtures, Drug Interactions, and Toxicology

Allan, E., et al. "Dispensing Errors and Counseling in Community Practice." *American Pharmacy* NS35(12) (1995): 25–33. Information on avoiding dispensing errors.

Benitz, William E., and David S. Tatro. *The Pediatric Drug Handbook.* St. Louis, MO: Mosby-Year Book, 1995. Information on drugs, dosage forms, and administration for pediatric patients. The address of Mosby on the World Wide Web is http://www.mosby.com.

Davies, D. M. *Textbook of Adverse Drug Reactions.* 4th ed. New York: Oxford University Press, 1991. A standard textbook on the subject. The address of Oxford University Press on the World Wide Web is http://www.oup-usa.org.

Goldfrank's Toxicologic Emergencies. 6th ed. New York: Appleton & Lange, 1998. Information on treating toxicologic emergencies. The address of Appleton & Lange on the World Wide Web is http://www.appleton-lange.com.

Handbook of Nonprescription Drugs. 2 vols. 11th ed. Washington, DC: American Pharmaceutical Association, 1996-1997. A reference work on over-the-counter medications. The address of the American Pharmaceutical Association on the World Wide Web is http://www.aphnet.org.

Hunt, Max L., Jr. *Training Manual for Intravenous Admixture Personnel.* 5th ed. Chicago: Bonus Books, 1995. A manual for training people to create parenteral preparations.

The King Guide to Parenteral Admixtures. Napa, CA: King Guide Publications, 1998. Available in four loose-leaf volumes, on microfiche, and on CD-ROM, the *King Guide* provides 350 monographs on compatibility and stability information critical to determining the advisability of preparing admixtures of drugs for parenteral administration. The guide is updated quarterly. The address of King Publications on the World Wide Web is http://www.kingguide.com.

Nahata, Milap C., and Thomas F. Hipple. *Pediatric Drug Formulations.* 3rd ed. Cincinnati, OH: Harvey Whitney, 1997. Information on formulation and compounding of drugs for pediatric patients. You can e-mail Harvey Whitney Books at hwb@eos.net.

POISINDEX System. Englewood, CO: Micromedex. A computerized poison information system. The address of Micromedex on the World Wide Web is http://www.mdx.com.

The Pharmacy Certified Technician Calculations Workbook. Lansing: Michigan Pharmacists Association, 1997. A companion workbook to the *Pharmacy Certified Technician Training Manual* (see Reference Works on Training and Certification of Pharmacy Technicians, below). This book is distributed by the American Pharmaceutical Association (APhA). The address of the APhA on the World Wide Web is http://www.aphanet.org.

Remington's Pharmaceutical Sciences: The Science and Practice of Pharmacy. 18th ed. Easton, PA: MacK Publishing, 1990. The compounding "bible" of the pharmacy profession.

Stephens, M. D. B. *Detection of New Adverse Drug Reactions.* 4th ed. New York: Wiley, 1993. Information on recognizing adverse drug reactions. The address of John Wiley & Sons on the World Wide Web is http://www.wiley.com.

Stoklosa, Mitchell J., and Howard C. Ansel. *Pharmaceutical Calculations.* 10th ed. Baltimore, MD: Williams & Wilkins, 1996. A clear, concise, thorough introduction to pharmaceutical mathematics. The address of Williams & Wilkins on the World Wide Web is http://www.wwilkins.com.

"Tips for Avoiding Errors in Your Pharmacy." *Pharmacy Today* 2 (10) (1996): 11. Information on avoiding dispensing errors.

Trissel, Lawrence A. *Handbook on Injectable Drugs, with Supplement.* 9th ed. Bethesda, MD: American Society of Health-System Pharmacists, 1996. Provides information on stability and compatibility of injectable drug products, including formulations, concentrations, and pH values. The address of the American Society of Health-System Pharmacists on the World Wide Web is http://www.ashp.org.

Understanding and Preventing Errors in Medication Orders and Prescription Writing. Bethesda, MD: United States Pharmacopeial Convention, 1998. An education resource, consisting of lecture materials, videotapes, and 35 mm slides describing medication errors that arise from poorly written orders and prescriptions, using examples of actual reports received through the USP Medication Errors Reporting Program. Contains recommendations for preventing errors. The address of the United States Pharmacopeial Convention on the World Wide Web is http://www.usp.org.

Pharmaceutical Law, Regulation, Ethics, Communication, and Economics

Abood, Richard R., and David B. Brushwood. *Pharmacy Practice and the Law.* 2nd ed. Gaithersburg, MD: Aspen, 1997. A survey of contemporary pharmacy law, covering the entire range of legal issues in pharmacy, including major acts, regulations, regulatory agencies, torts, malpractice liability, and legal issues related to hospital pharmacies, long-term care, third-party prescription programs, and managed care, with cases. The address of Aspen Publishers on the World Wide Web is http://www.aspenpub.com.

Code of Federal Regulations (CFR), Title 21, Food and Drugs. Washington, DC: U.S. Government Printing Office, Superintendent of Documents. Annually revised compilation of federal Food and Drug Administration regulations. The address of the Government Printing Office on the World Wide Web is http://www.access.gpo.gov.

Cramer, Joyce A., and Bert Spilker. *Quality of Life and Pharmacoeconomics: An Introduction.* Philadelphia: Lippencott-Raven, 1997. A general survey of the economics of pharmacy. The address of Lippencott-Raven on the World Wide Web is http://www.lrpub.com.

Federal Register. Washington, DC: U. S. Government Printing Office, Superintendent of Documents. Daily publication listing new federal regulations. The address of the Government Printing Office on the World Wide Web is http://www.access.gpo.gov.

Practice Standards of ASHP, 1997–1998. **Bethesda, MD: American Society of Health-System Pharmacists, 1997.** Standards for hospital pharmacy practice. The address of the American Society of Health-System Pharmacists on the World Wide Web is http://www.ashp.org.

Smith, Mickey, et al. *Pharmacy Ethics.* **Binghamton, NY: Haworth Press, 1991.** The address of Haworth Press on the World Wide Web is http://www.haworth.com.

Tootelian, Dennis H., and Ralph M. Gaedeke. *Essentials of Pharmacy Management.* **St. Louis, MO: Mosby-Year Book, 1993.** Information on managing a retail pharmacy operation. The address of Mosby on the World Wide Web is http://www.mosby.com.

Vivian, J. C., and D. B. Brushwood. "Monitoring Prescriptions for Legitimacy," *American Pharmacy* NS31 (9) (1991): 32–33. Information on spotting falsified prescriptions.

Reference Works on Training and Certification of Pharmacy Technicians

Ballington, Don A., and Mary M. Laughlin. *Pharmacology for Technicians.* **St. Paul, MN: EMC/Paradigm, 1999.** Presents the basic principles of pharmacology and the essential characteristics of commonly prescribed drug classes. The address of EMC/Paradigm on the World Wide Web is http://www.emcp.com.

Ballington, Don A., and Mary M. Laughlin. *Pharmacy Math for Technicians.* **St. Paul, MN: EMC/Paradigm, 1999.** Offers a review of basic mathematics as applied to common pharmaceutical calculations. The address of EMC/Paradigm on the World Wide Web is http://www.emcp.com.

Idsvoog, Peter B. *Manual for Hospital Pharmacy Technicians: A Programmed Course in Basic Skills.* **Bethesda, MD: American Society of Health-System Pharmacists, 1977.** The address of the American Society of Health-System Pharmacists on the World Wide Web is http://www.ashp.org.

Keresztes. *Manual for the Pharmacy Technician.* **Philadelphia: W.B. Saunders, 1998.** A handbook for pharmacy technicians. W.B. Saunders can be reached at (800) 545-2522.

Manual for Pharmacy Technicians. **2d ed. Bethesda, MD: American Society of Health-System Pharmacists, 1998.** The address of the American Society of Helath-System Pharmacists on the World Wide Web is http://www.ashp.org.

Moss, Susan. *Pharmacy Technician Certification Quick Study Guide.* **Washington, DC: American Pharmaceutical Association, 1995.** A study guide for the Pharmacy Technician Certification Examination. The address of the American Pharmaceutical Association on the World Wide Web is http://www.aphanet.org.

Pharmacy Certified Technician Training Manual. **Lansing: Michigan Pharmacists Association, 1997.** A manual for technicians wishing to study for the Pharmacy Technician Certification Examination. This book is distributed by the American Pharmaceutical Association (APhA) The address of the APhA on the World Wide Web is http://www.aphanet.org.

Pharmacy Technician Workbook: A Self-Instructional Approach. Bethesda, MD: **American Society of Health-System Pharmacists, 1994.** The address of the American Society of Hospital Pharmacists on the World Wide Web is http://www.ashp.org.

Reifman, Noah. *Certification Review for Pharmacy Technicians.* 3rd ed. **Brooklyn: Certification Review, 1997.**

Reilly, Robert. *The Pharmacy Tech: Basic Pharmacology & Calculations.* **Englewood, CO: Skidmore-Roth, 1994.** Introductory information on drug effects and pharmaceutical mathematics for technicians in training. Skidmore-Roth's World Wide Web address is http://www.skidmore-roth.com.

Rudman, Jack. *Pharmacy Technician (Career Examination Series, Vol. C-3822).* **Sussosett, NY: National Learning Corporation, 1997.** Guide to taking a pharmacy technician civil service examination.

Stoogenke, Marvin M. *The Pharmacy Technician.* **2nd ed. Englewood Cliffs, NJ: Prentice Hall, 1997.** The address of Prentice Hall on the World Wide Web is http://www.prenhall.com.

Other References

Gerson, Cyrelle K. *More Than Dispensing: A Handbook on Providing Pharmaceutical Services to Long Term Care Facilities.* **Washington, DC: American Pharmaceutical Association, 1980.** The address of the American Pharmaceutical Association on the World Wide Web is http://www.aphanet.org.

Journal of Pharmacy Technology is the official publication of the Pharmacy Technician Educators Council. This journal is published by Harvey Whitney Books, which can be contacted by e-mail at hwb@eos.net, by telephone at (513) 793-3555, or by fax at (513) 793-3600.

Meldrum, Helen. *Interpersonal Communication in Pharmaceutical Care.* **Binghamton, NY: Haworth Press, 1994.** The address of the Haworth Press on the World Wide Web is http://www.haworth.com.

Pharmaceutical Information Network, or **PharmInfoNet,** publishes online information, including the *Medical Sciences Bulletin,* on pharmacology and therapeutics; *PNN Pharmacotherapy Line: A One-Dose Shot of Information,* a daily newsletter distributed by fax, mail, and e-mail; and *MedWatch News,* including alerts and medical advisory notices from the Food and Drug Administration. The address of the PharmInfoNet on the World Wide Web is http://pharminfo.com.

RxTrek, a Web site providing information and links for pharmacy technicians, is located at http://ourworld.compuserve.com/homepages/RxTrek/homepage.htm.

The World Wide Web Virtual Library maintains a large list of pharmacy links at http://157.142.72.77/pharmacy/pharmint.html.

Individual **drug manufacturers, colleges of pharmacy,** and **state pharmacy boards** also have Web sites of interest to pharmacy technicians. To identify these sites, use a search engine such as Yahoo!, Infoseek, Lycos, or Excite.

PACKAGE INSERTS

Another source of information for the pharmacy technician is the **package inserts** included by manufacturers with prescription drug products. Legally, these package inserts are extensions of the labeling on the drug product, and laws and regulations involving misbranding or mislabeling apply to them. These inserts are required by FDA regulation to contain the following information listed in Table 6.1 in the order shown.

Table 6.1

INFORMATION IN PACKAGE INSERTS FOR PRESCRIPTION DRUGS

- Description
- Clinical pharmacology
- Indications and usage
- Contraindications
- Warnings
- Precautions
- Adverse reactions
- Drug abuse and dependence
- Overdosage
- Dosage and administration
- How supplied
- Date of the most recent revision of the labeling

The Physician's Desk Reference, published by Medical Economics of Oradell, New Jersey, is primarily a compilation of package inserts. It provides, in an easily accessed form, a great deal of information about prescription drugs.

chapter summary

To perform pharmacy duties correctly, it is important to become a lifelong learner, capable of assimilating new information in this fast-changing field and of turning to reliable sources when the need for information arises. Excellent sources of information for the pharmacist and pharmacy technician include professional organizations such as the American Pharmaceutical Association and the American Association of Pharmacy Technicians; the journals published by such organizations, such as *Pharmacy Today* and the *Journal of Pharmacy Technology;* federal and state agencies; reference works such as *Drug Facts and Comparisons,* the *USP DI,* and Remington's *Pharmaceutical Sciences;* and package inserts.

In recent years, journals and text-based references have been supplemented by new technologies, including CD-ROMs and databases available via the Internet. These sources of information help to ensure that pharmacists and pharmacy technicians will have the information they need, when they need it, to perform their jobs with the high level of accuracy required.

chapter review

Knowledge Inventory

Choose the best answer from those provided.

1. The largest of the national pharmacy organizations is the
   a. American Pharmaceutical Association
   b. American Society of Health-System Pharmacists
   c. Food and Drug Administration
   d. National Pharmaceutical Association

2. The organization that administers the Pharmacy Technician Certification Examination is the
   a. Pharmacy Technician Educators Council
   b. Pharmacy Technician Certification Board
   c. United States Pharmacopeial Convention
   d. American Association of Colleges of Pharmacy

3. The agency that enforces laws related to controlled substances is the
   a. Food and Drug Administration
   b. United States Pharmacopeial Convention
   c. Drug Enforcement Administration
   d. National Association of Boards of Pharmacy

4. A source of information on preparing infusions is
   a. *Facts and Comparisons*
   b. *Approved Drug Products with Therapeutic Equivalence Evaluations*
   c. *The King Guide to Parenteral Admixtures*
   d. *USP Drug Information for the Health Care Professional*

5. A comprehensive source of information about prescription and over-the-counter drugs is
   a. *The Pediatric Drug Handbook*
   b. *Facts and Comparisons*
   c. *The King Guide to Parenteral Admixtures*
   d. *USP Drug Information for the Health Care Professional*

6. An excellent source for drug information for patients is
   a. *USP DI, Vol. I*
   b. *USP DI, Vol. II*
   c. *USP DI, Vol. III*
   d. *United States Pharmacopeia*

7. An excellent source of information on compounding a medication is
   a. *Remington's Pharmaceutical Sciences*
   b. *Facts and Comparisons*
   c. *Pharmaceutical Dosage Forms and Drug Delivery Systems*
   d. *Approved Drug Products with Therapeutic Equivalence Evaluations*

8. Package inserts are required by
   a. DEA regulation
   b. FDA regulation
   c. USDA regulation
   d. APhA regulation

9. A package insert contains information on
   a. indications and usage
   b. contraindications, warnings, precautions, and adverse reactions
   c. drug abuse and dependence, overdosage, and dosage and administration
   d. all of the above

10. The *Physician's Desk Reference* is a collection of
    a. clinical monographs
    b. pharmacological monographs
    c. adverse reaction reports
    d. package inserts

Pharmacy in Practice

1. Locate a package insert for a widely used prescription medication, or look up this information in a current edition of the *Physician's Desk Reference*. Write a brief report on the medication describing its uses, how it is administered, what dosage forms it is available in, its contraindications, and its potential for abuse or dependence.

2. Using *Remington's Pharmaceutical Sciences,* look up, and then describe in writing, how to compound a standard rectal suppository.

3. Using *The King Guide to Parenteral Admixtures,* look up, and then describe in writing, how to prepare a standard intravenous admixture for total parenteral nutrition.

4. Look up the drug chlorambucil in the *United States Pharmacopeia, 23rd Rev.* Answer the following questions:
   a. What is the chemical formula of the drug?
   b. What precautions should be taken when handling this drug?
   c. How should the drug be packaged and stored?
   d. How can the drug be identified?

5. Using reference works described in this chapter, find a recent journal article on the subject of recertification of pharmacy technicians. What is the title of the article, and who is (are) its author(s)? Read the article, then write a few paragraphs explaining the point of view of the article, and giving reasons for your agreement or disagreement with it.

Basic Pharmaceutical Measurements and Calculations

7

The daily activities of pharmacists and pharmacy technicians, including the compounding of drugs and the preparation of parenteral infusions, require making precise measurements of amounts, or **quantities**, and doing calculations that involve manipulations of those quantities. A mistake in calculation can have severe consequences. Therefore, it is essential for practicing pharmacists and technicians to grasp the basic measurement systems and mathematical techniques used in the field. This chapter introduces you to the basic systems and methods used in pharmacy.

Learning Objectives

- Describe four systems of measurement commonly used in pharmacy
- Explain the meanings of the prefixes most commonly used in metric measurement
- Convert metric measurements to express different metric units (e.g., grams to milligrams)
- Convert Roman numerals to Arabic numerals
- Distinguish among proper, improper, and compound fractions
- Perform basic operations with fractions, including finding the least common denominator; converting fractions to decimals; and adding, subtracting, multiplying, and dividing fractions
- Perform basic operations with proportions, including identifying equivalent ratios and finding an unknown quantity in a proportion
- Convert percentages to and from fractions and ratios and convert percentages to decimals
- Perform elementary dosage calculations, calculations of IV rate and administration, and calculations necessary for solution preparation

TERMS TO KNOW

Area A measurement of extension in space in two dimensions
Decimal notation Mathematical system in which units are described in multiples of ten
Fraction A number expressed as the quotient of two whole numbers, as in 1/2 or 33/79
Gram 1000 milligrams, or one thousandth of a kilogram
Kilogram 1000 grams
Least common denominator (LCD) The smallest number that is evenly divisible by all the denominators in a group of numbers expressed as fractions

SYSTEMS OF PHARMACEUTICAL MEASUREMENT

Systems of measurement are widely accepted standards used to determine such quantities as area, distance (or length), temperature, time, volume, and weight. Of these, temperature, distance, volume, and weight are the most important for the pharmacy profession. Quantities of temperature and weight are unproblematic and intuitively obvious. **Distance**, of course, is a measurement of extension in space in one dimension. **Area** is a measurement of extension in space in two dimensions. **Volume**, the least obvious of these quantities, is a measurement of extension in space in three dimensions.

The Metric System

Figure 7.1 shows an example of measurements of distance, area, and volume using the **metric system**, the system most commonly used today for pharmaceutical measurement and calculation. Developed in France in the 1700s, the metric system became, in 1893, the legal standard of measure in the United States, the system to which other measurements are compared for legal purposes. Still, the United States remains practically alone in the industrialized world in its widespread popular use of so-called common measure, described below.

The metric system has several distinct advantages over other measurement systems. First, the metric system is based on **decimal notation**, in which units are described as multiples of ten (.001, .01, .1, 1, 10, 100, 1000, and so on), and this decimal notation makes calculation simple. Second, the system contains clear correlations among the units of measurement of length, volume, and weight, again simplifying calculation. For example, the standard metric unit for volume, the **liter**, is almost exactly equivalent to 1000 cubic **centimeters** (a metric unit of length). Third, with slight variations in notation, the metric system is used worldwide, especially in scientific measurement, and so is, like music, a "universal language."

Like languages, measurement systems tend to develop evolutionarily by folk processes. Thus a foot was, originally, a length approximately equal to that of the foot on which one walks. Later, these systems become standardized by governments and professional organizations. The modern metric system makes use of the standardized units of the **Système International (SI)**, adopted by agreement among governments worldwide in 1960. Three basic units in this system are the **meter**, the **liter**, and the **gram**:

$$\text{Meter} = \text{unit of length}$$
$$\text{Liter} = \text{unit of volume}$$
$$\text{Gram} = \text{unit of weight}$$

To specify a particular measure, one can add **prefixes**—syllables placed at the beginnings of words—to these basic units. Because SI is a decimal system, the prefixes denote powers of ten, as shown in Table 7.1.

Figure 7.1
Measurements of distance, area, and volume using the metric system.

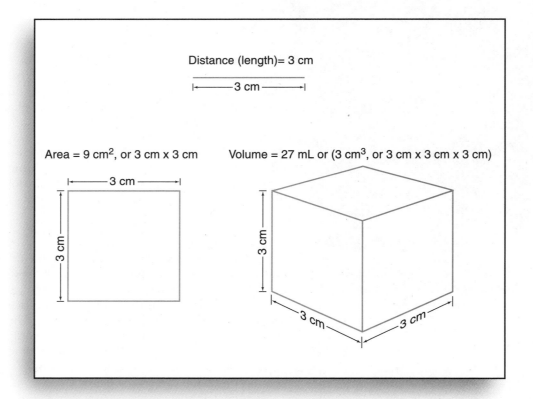

The metric units most commonly used in pharmacy practice, along with their abbreviations, are given in Table 7.2. Note that the same abbreviations are used for both singular and plural (1 g, 3 g).

Table 7.1

SYSTÈME INTERNATIONAL (SI) PREFIXES	
Prefix	**Meaning**
pico–	one trillionth (basic unit x 10^{-12}, or unit x .000,000,000,001)
nano–	one billionth (basic unit x 10^{-9}, or unit x .000,000,001)
micro–	one millionth (basic unit x 10^{-6}, or unit x .000,001)
milli–	one thousandth (basic unit x 10^{-3}, or unit x .001)
centi–	one hundredth (basic unit x 10^{-2}, or unit x .01)
deci–	one tenth (basic unit x 10^{-1}, or unit x .1)
Base Unit (for example, grams or milliliters)	
deka–	ten times (basic unit x 10^{1}, or unit x 10)
hecto–	one hundred times (basic unit x 10^{2}, or unit x 100)
kilo–	one thousand times (basic unit x 10^{3}, or unit x 1,000)
myria–	ten thousand times (basic unit x 10^{4}, or unit x 10,000)
mega–	one million times (basic unit x 10^{6}, or unit x 1,000,000)
giga–	one billion times (basic unit x 10^{9}, or unit x 1,000,000,000)
tera–	one trillion times (basic unit x 10^{12}, or unit x 1,000,000,000,000)

Table 7.2

COMMON METRICAL UNITS	
Weight: Basic Unit, the Gram	
1 milligram (mg)	= 1000 micrograms (μg, mcg, or γ),* one thousandth of a gram
1 gram (g)	= 1000 milligrams (mg)
1 kilogram (kg)	= 1000 grams (g)
Area: Basic Unit, the Meter	
1 millimeter (mm)	= one thousandth of a meter, 1000 micrometers, or microns (μm)
1 centimeter (cm)	= one hundredth of a meter, 10 millimeters
1 meter (m)	= 100 centimeters (cm)
Volume: Basic Unit, the Liter	
1 milliliter (mL)	= one thousandth of a liter, 1000 microliters (μL)
1 liter	= 1000 milliliters (mL)

*These abbreviations make use of the Greek letters μ, or mu, and γ, or gamma.

In prescriptions using the metric system, numbers are expressed as decimals rather than fractions. Weights are generally given in grams, and volumes in milliliters. For numbers less than 1, a 0 is placed before the decimal to prevent misreading, as in

R   Phenobarbital 0.46 g

Note that an error of a single decimal place is an error by a factor of 10! It is therefore extremely important that decimals be written properly.

To convert from one metric unit to another, simply move the decimal place to the left (to convert to larger units) and to the right (to convert to smaller units). The most common metric calculations in pharmacy involve conversions to and from milliliters and liters, and to and from grams, milligrams, and kilograms. Table 7.3 shows how to do these conversions.

Table 7.3

CONVERSION TABLE FOR KILOGRAMS/GRAMS/MILLIGRAMS AND LITERS/MILLILITERS

kilograms (kg) to grams (g)	multiply by 1000 (move decimal three places to the right) 6.25 kg = 6250 g
grams (g) to milligrams (mg)	multiply by 1000 (move decimal three places to the right) 3.56 g = 3560 mg
milligrams (mg) to grams (g)	multiply by 0.001 (move decimal three places to the left) 120 mg = 0.120 g
liters (L) to milliliters (mL)	multiply by 1000 (move decimal three places to the right) 2.5 L = 2500 mL
milliliters (mL) to liters (L)	multiply by 0.001 (move decimal three places to the left) 238 mL = 0.238 L

Common Measure

In addition to the metric system, pharmacy makes use of older systems of measure that together make up **common measure**. The term *common measure* refers to the fact that these measurement systems were once commonly employed. They are not widely used in pharmacy today, but since they do crop up from time to time, it is a good idea to become familiar with the most standard measurement units in these systems.

Three types of common measure sometimes encountered are **apothecary measure**, **avoirdupois measure**, and **household measure**. Table 7.4 gives conversion equivalents for common units in these systems.

Note that the only equivalent common unit in the apothecary and avoirdupois systems is the unit of dry measure known as the **grain**. This is the most commonly encountered nonmetric unit in pharmacy practice. Pharmacists

Table 7.4

UNITS IN COMMON MEASURE WITH METRIC EQUIVALENTS

APOTHECARY FLUID MEASURE (VOLUME)

Measurement Unit	Equivalent in System	Metric Equivalent
1 minim (♏)		0.0616 mL
1 fluiddrachm or fluidram (℥)	60 minims (♏)	3.6966 mL
1 fluidounce (℥)	8 fluidrachms (℥)	0.0296 L or 30 mL
1 pt (pt or O)	16 fluidounces (℥)	0.4732 L
1 quart (qt)	2 pints (pt), 32 fluidounces (℥)	0.9464 L
1 gallon (gal or C)	4 quarts (qt), 8 pints (pt)	3.7856 L

APOTHECARY DRY MEASURE (WEIGHT)

Measurement Unit	Equivalent in System	Metric Equivalent
1 grain (gr)		0.0648 g or 65 mg
1 scruple (℈)	20 grains (gr)	1.296 g
1 drachm or dram (℥)	3 scruples (℈), 60 grains (gr)	3.888 g

1 ounce (℥)	8 drachms (ℨ), 480 grains (gr)	31.1035 g
1 pound (#)	12 ounces (℥), 5760 grains (gr)	373.24 g
2.2 pounds	26.4 ounces (℥), 12,672 grains (gr)	1 kg

AVOIRDUPOIS DRY MEASURE (WEIGHT)

Measurement Unit	Equivalent in System	Metric Equivalent
1 grain (gr)		0.0648 g or 65 mg
1 ounce (oz.)	437.5 grains (gr)	28.3495 g
1 pound (lb.)	16 ounces (oz), 7000 grains (gr)	453.59 g or 0.45 kg

HOUSEHOLD MEASURE

Measurement Unit	Equivalent in System	Metric Equivalent
1 teaspoon		approximately 5 mL
1 tablespoon (Tbs)	3 teaspoons (tsp)	approximately 15 mL
1 fluid ounce	2 tablespoons (Tbs)	approximately 30 mL
1 cup	8 fluid ounces	approximately 240 mL
1 pint	2 cups	0.4732 L
1 quart	2 pints	0.9464 L
1 gallon	4 quarts	3.7854 L

sometimes make use of apothecaries' weights that come in 5-grain, 4-grain, 3-grain, 2-grain, 1-grain, and 1/2-grain units.

A prescription written using apothecary measure commonly uses **Roman numerals** that follow rather than precede the unit of measurement. Thus aspirin gr vi means six grains of aspirin. Roman numerals are also sometimes used to express other quantities, as in tablets no. C (100 tablets) or Tbs iii (three tablespoons). Table 7.5 summarizes the Roman numeral system and gives equivalents in Arabic numerals.

Table **7.5**

UNDERSTANDING ROMAN NUMERALS

BASIC UNITS

Roman	Arabic	Roman	Arabic	Roman	Arabic
ss	.5 or ½	x (X)	10	d (D)	500
i (I)	1	l (L)	50	m (M)	1000
v (V)	5	c (C)	100		

Rules for Interpretation of Roman Numerals

When the letters are successively equal or smaller in value, then their quantity equals the sum of their values. Thus iii = 3 and xi = 11.

In other cases, a series of letters is equal to the sum of their values after the value of each smaller letter has been subtracted from the value of each larger letter that follows it.

Thus iv = 4 and xxiv = 24.

SOME BASIC MATHEMATICS USED IN PHARMACY

Many tasks in pharmacy—determining dosages, compounding medications, and preparing solutions, for example—involve simple calculations of the units of measure given in the preceding section. If you are fairly confident about your basic mathematical skills, you may wish to skip this section. However, it never hurts to review fundamental principles before undertaking mathematical work. Pharmacy work often requires performing fundamental operations involving fractions, decimals, ratios, proportions, and percentages.

Fractions

A **fraction** consists of two numbers, a **numerator** (the number on the top) and a **denominator** (the number on the bottom).

$$\frac{1}{2} \quad \begin{array}{l} \text{numerator} \\ \text{denominator} \end{array}$$

A fraction is simply a convenient way of representing an operation, the division of the numerator by the denominator. Thus the fraction ⅔ equals 6 divided by 3, or 2. The fraction ⅞ is 7 divided by 8, or 0.875. The number that you get when you divide the numerator by the denominator is the **value** of the fraction. Fractions with the same value are said to be **equivalent fractions**:

$$\text{equivalent fractions: } \frac{1}{2} = \frac{2}{4} = \frac{4}{8} = 0.5$$

$$\frac{3}{16} = \frac{12}{64} = 0.1875$$

Notice that in the decimal expansion of a fraction, a zero (0) is placed before the decimal point if the number is less than 1. Using the zero helps to prevent errors in reading decimals.

A fraction may be **proper** (less than 1) or **improper** (more than 1):

$$\text{proper fractions: } \quad \frac{3}{8}, \frac{1}{4}$$

$$\text{improper fractions: } \frac{3}{2}, \frac{138}{17}$$

A **compound fraction** is one that contains both a whole number and a fraction:

$$\text{compound fractions: } 3\frac{3}{8}, 2\frac{3}{4}$$

In pharmaceutical work, it is especially important not to misread a compound fraction as a simple one:

$$3\frac{3}{8}, \text{ not } \frac{33}{8}$$

To add or subtract fractions, first convert any compound fractions to improper fractions containing no whole numbers. To do this, multiply the whole number part of the compound fraction by the denominator and add the result to the numerator.

Example: Converting Compound Fractions

$$3\frac{3}{8} = \frac{(3 \times 8) + 3}{8} = \frac{27}{8} \qquad\qquad 4\frac{1}{3} = \frac{(4 \times 3) + 1}{3} = \frac{13}{8}$$

The next step in adding or subtracting fractions is to look to see if the denominators are equal. If all the fractions have the same denominator, you can proceed. If not, you need to convert each fraction to an equivalent fraction that has the same denominator as each of the other fractions. To do that, you will first have to find the least common denominator of the fractions. The **least common denominator**, or **LCD**, of a group of fractions is the smallest number that is evenly divisible by all the denominators. To find the least common denominator, follow the procedure shown in Table 7.6.

Table 7.6

FINDING THE LEAST COMMON DENOMINATOR

1. Find the prime factors (numbers divisible only by one and themselves) of each denominator.
2. Make a list of all the different prime factors that you find. Include in the list each different factor as many times as the factor occurs for any one of the denominators of the given fractions.
3. Multiply all the prime factors on your list. The result of this multiplication is the least common denominator.

Example:

Find the least common denominator of $\frac{9}{28}$ and $\frac{1}{6}$.

The prime factors of 28 are 2, 2, and 7 (because 2 x 2 x 7 = 28).

The prime factors of 6 are 2 and 3 (because 2 x 3 = 6).

The number 2 occurs twice in one of the denominators, so it must occur twice in the list. The list will also include the unique factors 3 and 7:

2, 2, 3, 7

Multiplying these, we get the least common denominator:

2 x 2 x 3 x 7 = 84

To convert the fractions to equivalents with a common denominator, first divide the least common denominator by the denominator of each fraction. Then multiply both the numerator and denominator by the result.

Example: Converting Fractions to Equivalents with Common Denominators

Convert $\frac{9}{28}$ and $\frac{1}{6}$ to equivalent fractions with common denominators.

The least common denominator of $\frac{9}{28}$ and $\frac{1}{6}$ is 84.

Dividing 84 by 28, we get 3. So, we multiply both the numerator and the denominator by this number:

$$\frac{9}{28} = \frac{9 \times 3}{28 \times 3} = \frac{27}{84}$$

Dividing 84 by 6, we get 14. Again, we multiply both the numerator and the denominator by this number:

$$\frac{1}{6} = \frac{1 \times 14}{6 \times 14} = \frac{14}{84}$$

So, the equivalent fractions are $\frac{27}{84}$ and $\frac{14}{84}$.

Once fractions are converted to contain equivalent denominators, adding or subtracting them is easy. Simply add or subtract the numerators.

Table **7.6**

(cont.)

Examples: Adding and Subtracting Fractions

$$\frac{9}{28} + \frac{1}{6} = \frac{27}{84} + \frac{14}{84} = \frac{41}{84}$$

$$\frac{9}{28} - \frac{1}{6} = \frac{27}{84} - \frac{14}{84} = \frac{13}{84}$$

To multiply fractions, (a) multiply the numerators and write the product as the numerator of the result, and (b) multiply the denominators and write the product as the denominator of the result.

Example: Multiplying Fractions

$$\frac{3}{4} \times \frac{12}{17} = \frac{3 \times 12}{4 \times 17} = \frac{36}{68} = \frac{9}{17}$$

To divide by a fraction, simply invert the fraction and multiply. The inverted fraction is known as the **reciprocal**.

Example: Dividing Fractions

$$\frac{3}{4} \div \frac{1}{3} = \frac{3}{4} \times \frac{3}{1} = \frac{3 \times 3}{4 \times 1} = \frac{9}{4} = 2\frac{1}{4}$$

Decimals

A **decimal** is any number that can be written in decimal notation, using the integers 0, 1, 2, 3, 4, 5, 6, 7, 8, and 9 and a point (.) to divide the one's place from the tenth's place.

> Decimals: 0.131313   2.09   43.0

As you have already seen, a fraction can be expressed as a decimal by simply dividing the numerator by the denominator:

> 1/2 = 1 divided by 2 = .5
>
> 1/3 = 1 divided by 3 = 0.33333. . .
>
> 438/64 = 438 divided by 64 = 6.84375

So, one way to add, subtract, multiply, or divide fractions is first to convert each fraction to a decimal equivalent and then perform the operation.

Example: Multiplying Fractions by Converting to Decimals

Find $\frac{24}{3} \times \frac{22}{4}$

$$\frac{24}{3} = 24 \div 3 = 8$$

$$\frac{22}{4} = 22 \div 4 = 5.5$$

$$\frac{24}{3} \times \frac{22}{4} = 8 \times 5.5 = 44$$

The metric system makes use of numbers that are expressed as decimals. Any decimal can be expressed as a **decimal fraction**, which contains a power of 10 as its denominator (see Table 7.7).

Table **7.7**

DECIMALS AND EQUIVALENT DECIMAL FRACTIONS

$$0.00001 = 1/100,000$$
$$0.0001 = 1/10,000$$
$$0.001 = 1/1,000$$
$$0.01 = 1/100$$
$$0.1 = 1/10$$
$$1 = 1/1$$

To express a decimal number as a fraction, simply remove the decimal point and use the resulting number as the numerator and use as the denominator a 1 followed by the number of places in the decimal:

$$2.33 = \frac{233}{100}$$

$$0.1234 = \frac{1234}{10,000}$$

$$0.00367 = \frac{367}{100,000}$$

A decimal fraction can then be reduced to a common fraction:

$$0.84 = \frac{84}{100} = \frac{21}{25} \qquad 0.1234 = \frac{1234}{10,000} = \frac{617}{5,000}$$

Ratios and Proportions

A **ratio** is a comparison of two like quantities and can be expressed in a fraction or in ratio notation. For example, if a beaker contains two parts water and three parts alcohol, then the ratio of water to alcohol in the beaker can be expressed as the fraction 2/3 or as the ratio 2:3. The ratio is read not as a value (2 divided by 3) but by the expression "a ratio of 2 to 3."

One common use of ratios is to express in the numerator the number of parts of one thing contained in a certain quantity of another, expressed in the denominator. Suppose that 60 mL of sterile solution contains 3 mL of tetrahydrozoline hydrochloride. This could be expressed as the ratio 3/60, or 1/20. In other words, the ratio of the active ingredient to the sterile solution is 1 to 20, or 1 part in 20.

Two ratios that have the same value, such as 1/2 and 2/4, are said to be **equivalent ratios**. When ratios are equivalent, the product of the numerator of the first ratio and denominator of the second ratio is equal to the product of the denominator of the first ratio and numerator of the second ratio:

$$\frac{2}{3} = \frac{6}{9} \quad \text{and} \quad 2 \times 9 = 3 \times 6 = 18$$

The same thing is true of the reciprocals:

$$\frac{3}{2} = \frac{9}{6} \quad \text{and} \quad 3 \times 6 = 2 \times 9 = 18$$

Two equivalent ratios are said to be in the same **proportion.** Equivalent, or proportional, ratios can be expressed in three different ways:

$$\text{a/b} = \text{c/d} \qquad (\text{example: } 1/2 = 2/4)$$

$$a{:}b = c{:}d \qquad \text{(example: } 1{:}2 = 2{:}4\text{)}$$
$$a{:}b :: c{:}d \qquad \text{(example: } 1{:}2 :: 2{:}4\text{)}$$

The outer members of a proportion are known as the **extremes**. The inner members are known as the **means**. An extremely useful fact about proportions is that when you multiply the extremes by one another and the means by one another, you get the same result. In other words, the product of the extremes equals the product of the means. If the proportion is expressed as a relationship between fractions, one can say that the numerator of the first fraction times the denominator of the second is equal to the denominator of the first fraction times the numerator of the second. In other words,

$$\text{If } \frac{a}{b} = \frac{c}{d} \text{, then } a \times d = b \times c$$

The equation just given proves extremely valuable because it can be used to calculate an unknown quantity when the other three variables in a proportion are known. In math, it is common to express unknown quantities using letters from the lower end of the alphabet, especially x, y, and z.

Example: Finding the Unknown Quantity in a Proportion

Given the equivalent ratios $\frac{2}{7}$ and $\frac{x}{35}$, find the value of x.

By the rule given above, $7x = 70$.

Dividing both sides by 7, we get the value for x, which is 10.

When using proportions, it is important to remember that the numerators of both fractions must be in the same units, and the denominators of both fractions must also be in the same units. Otherwise, one would be in the position of comparing apples and oranges (or, more precisely, grams and grains, ounces and pounds).

Percentages

The word *percent* comes from the Latin words *per centum,* meaning "for, to, or in one hundred." A **percentage** is a given part or amount in a hundred. Percentages can be expressed in many ways:

As a percentage (example: 3% or 3 percent)

As a fraction with 100 as the denominator (example: $\frac{3}{100}$)

As a decimal (example: 0.03)

As a ratio (example 3:100)

Return for a moment to the proportion example given earlier. If 60 mL of a sterile solution contains 3 mL of tetrahydrozoline hydrochloride, what is the percentage of Tetrahydrozoline Hydrocloride in the solution? By the rule for equivalent ratios given above, we know that

$$\frac{3 \text{ mL}}{60 \text{ mL}} = \frac{x \text{ mL}}{100 \text{ mL}} \qquad 60x = 300 \qquad x = 5$$

Solving for x, we find that the percentage of tetrahydrozoline hydrochloride in the solution is 5/100, or 5 percent.

SOME COMMON PROBLEMS IN PHARMACEUTICAL CALCULATION

Conversion Between Units and Measurement Systems

Many situations in pharmacy practice call for conversion of quantities within one measurement system or between measurement systems. Consider the examples in Chart 7.1.

Chart 7.1

CONVERSION OF QUANTITIES WITHIN OR BETWEEN MEASUREMENT SYSTEMS

Conversion Problem 1—Metric Volume. Three liters of solution are on hand. This solution is to be used to fill hypodermics containing 60 mL each. How many hypodermics can be filled with the three liters of solution?

Solution: From Table 7.3, you know that 1 L = 1000 mL. The available supply is therefore 3 x 1000, or 3000 mL. Dividing 3000 by 60, you arrive at the answer, 50 hypodermics.

Conversion Problem 2—Household Measure to Metric. You are to dispense 300 mL of a liquid preparation. If the dose is 2 tsp., how many doses will there be in the whole preparation?

Solution: From Table 7.4, you know that 1 tsp. = approximately 5 mL. Therefore, 1 dose = 10 mL. Dividing 300 mL by 10 mL, you get the number of doses, 30.

Conversion Problem 3—Metric to Apothecary Measure. A prescription calls for acetaminophen 400 mg. How many grains of acetaminophen should be used in the prescription?

Solution: From Table 7.4, you know that 1 gr = 0.0648 g, or 65 mg (the value commonly used in pharmaceutical calculation). Using this information, you can set up a proportion:

$$\frac{1 \text{ gr}}{65 \text{ mg}} = \frac{x}{400 \text{ mg}}$$

In other words, 1 grain is to 65 milligrams as the unknown number of grains is to 400 milligrams. Cross-multiplying, you get 65x = 400 mg. Dividing each side by 65, you get 6.17, or approximately 6 grains.

Conversion Problem 4—Apothecary Measure to Metric. A physician desires that a patient be given 0.8 mg of nitroglycerin. On hand are tablets containing nitroglycerin 1/150 gr. How many tablets will the patient be given?

Solution: From Table 7.5, you know that 1 gr = 0.0648 g, or 65 mg. To determine the number of grains in .8 mg, you can use this proportion:

Chart 7.1

(cont.)

$$\frac{1 \text{ gr}}{65 \text{ mg}} = \frac{x \text{ gr}}{0.8 \text{ mg}}$$

Cross multiplying, you get 65x gr = .8. Dividing each side by 65, you get x gr = .0123. To determine the number of tablets that the patient should receive, you can use this proportion:

$$\frac{1 \text{ tablet}}{1/150 \text{ gr}} = \frac{x \text{ tablets}}{0.0123 \text{ gr}}$$

Cross multiplying, you get 0.0123 = 1/150x. To determine x, you must divide both sides by 1/150. Dividing by the fraction 1/150 is the same as multiplying by 150/1, or 150. Therefore, x = 150 x 0.0123, or 1.845 tablets, which is approximately 2 tablets.

Calculation of Dosages

One of the most common problems in pharmacy practice is the calculation of dosages. The supply on hand contains a ratio of some active ingredient to some carrier vehicle:

$$\frac{\text{Active Ingredient (on hand)}}{\text{Vehicle (on hand)}}$$

The prescription gives the amount of the active ingredient to be administered. The unknown quantity to be calculated is the amount of the carrier vehicle to be administered in order to achieve the desired dosage of the active ingredient.

$$\frac{\text{Active Ingredient (to be administered)}}{\text{Vehicle (to be administered)}}$$

The problem is to determine the amount of the carrier vehicle to be delivered in order for the two ratios to be equal:

$$\frac{\text{Active Ingredient (on hand)}}{\text{Vehicle (on hand)}} = \frac{\text{Active Ingredient (to be administered)}}{\text{Vehicle (to be delivered)}}$$

Consider the examples in Chart 7.2.

Chart 7.2

CALCULATION OF DOSAGES

Dosage Problem 1. You have a stock solution that contains 10 mg of active ingredient per 5 mL of carrier vehicle. The physician orders a dose of 4 mg. How many mL of the stock solution will have to be administered?

Solution: Using the information provided, set up a proportion:

$$\frac{10 \text{ mg}}{5 \text{ mL}} = \frac{4 \text{ mg}}{x \text{ mL}}$$

Cross multiplying, you arrive at the equation 10x = 20. Dividing both sides by 10, you arrive at the solution, x = 2 mL.

Dosage Problem 2. An order calls for Demerol 75 mg IM q.4h. p.r.n. pain. (If you find it necessary, review the pharmaceutical abbreviations given in chapter 3.) The supply available is Demerol 100 mg/mL syringes. How many mL will the nurse give?

Solution: Using the information provided, set up a proportion:

$$\frac{100 \text{ mg}}{1 \text{ mL}} = \frac{75 \text{ mg}}{x \text{ mL}}$$

Cross multiplying, you arrive at the equation $75 = 100x$. Solving for x, you get 0.75 mL.

Dosage Problem 3. An average adult has a body surface area of 1.72 m² and requires an adult dosage of 12 mg of a given medication. The same medication is to be given to a child in a pediatric dosage. If the child has a body surface area of 0.60 m², and if the proper dosage for pediatric and adult patients is a linear function of the body surface area, what is the proper pediatric dosage?

Solution: Using the information provided, set up a proportion:

$$\frac{12 \text{ mg}}{1.72 \text{ m}^2} = \frac{x \text{ mg}}{0.60 \text{ m}^2}$$

Cross multiplying, you get $1.72x = 12 \times 0.60$, or $1.72x = 7.2$. Solving for x, you find that the child's dosage is 4.19 mg.

Calculation of IV Rate and Administration

Another common problem in pharmacy practice is the calculation of the rate of flow for intravenous infusions. Intravenous flow rates are usually described as mL/hr or as drops (gtt) per minute. Pharmacy usually uses the mL/hr method. Nursing generally uses drops per minute. The most common intravenous sets dispense at a rate of 10 gtt/mL, 15 gtt/mL, and 60 gtt/mL. Consider the examples in Chart 7.3.

| Chart 7.3 | CALCULATION OF IV RATE |

IV Flow Rate Problem. A physician orders 4000 mL of 5% dextrose and normal saline (D$_5$NS) IV over a 36-hour period. If the IV set will deliver 15 drops per milliliter, how many drops must be administered per minute?
Solution: First, determine the number of mL that the patient is to receive each hour.

$$\frac{4000 \text{ mL}}{36 \text{ hr}} = 111.11 \text{ mL/hr}$$

Dividing 4000 by 36, you find that the patient is to receive 111.11 mL/hr.

Second, use this formula to determine the number of milliliters that the patient will receive each minute:

Chart 7.3
(cont.)

$$\frac{(mL/hr) \times (gtt/mL)}{60 \ min} = gtt/min$$

Substituting our figures in the formula gives us:

$$\frac{111.11 \ mL/hr \times 15 \ gtt/mL}{60 \ min} = 27.75 \ gtt/min \ (rounded \ down \ from \ 27.77)$$

IV Administration Problem. A liter IV is running at 125 mL/hr. How often will a new bag have to be administered?

Solution: The number of hours that the IV will last can be determined by dividing the size of the IV bag (1 L, or 1000 mL) by the volume per hour (125 mL/hr):

$$\frac{1000 \ mL}{125 \ mL/hr} = 8 \ hr$$

Preparation of Solutions

When solutions are prepared, you must remember that although we refer to the active ingredient in terms of weight, that active ingredient also occupies a certain amount of space. This space is referred to as the **powder volume**. Powder volume can be defined as the difference between the amount of diluent added and the final volume. See the examples in Chart 7.4.

Chart 7.4

SOLUTION PREPARATION

Solution Preparation Problem 1. A solution must be prepared containing a dry powder antibiotic that occupies 0.5 mL. The total volume of the prepared solution is to be 10 mL. Determine the volume of space taken up by the amount of diluent needed. What will be the percentage of antibiotic in the prepared solution?

Solution: The total volume of the prepared solution is to be 10 mL. The diluent volume to be added (dv) can be calculated by subtracting the dry powder volume in the solution (pv) from the total final volume of the solution (fv):

dv = fv – pv

x = 10 mL – 0.5 mL

x = 9.5 mL

(A variation of the same formula can be used to determine powder volume if diluent volume is already known: pv = fv – dv.)

To determine the percentage of antibiotic in the prepared solution, you can set up a proportion:

$$\frac{x}{100} = \frac{0.5 \ mL}{9.5 \ mL}$$

Cross multiplying, you get 9.5x = 50. Solving for x, one finds that this is a 5.26% solution of the antibiotic.

Solution Preparation Problem 2. You must prepare 250 mL of solution containing 7.5% dextrose. On hand you have solutions containing 5% dextrose (solution 1) and 50% dextrose (solution 2). How many mL of each stock solution must you use?

Solution: Begin by determining the parts of each solution on hand to be used in the prepared solution. Write down two pairs of numbers, each consisting of the percentage of the solution on hand and the percentage of the solution to be prepared:

> 5% (solution 1, on hand), 7.5% (prepared solution)
>
> 50% (solution 2, on hand), 7.5% (prepared solution)

Then, determine the parts of each solution to be used by subtracting the larger number in each pair from the smaller number:

> 7.5 – 5 = 2.5 parts of solution 1
>
> 50 – 7.5 = 42.5 parts of solution 2
>
> Total number of parts = 2.5 parts + 42.5 parts = 45 parts

Then, determine the volume of each solution to be used by doing a proportional analysis for each solution:

For solution 1:

$$\frac{45 \text{ parts}}{250 \text{ mL}} = \frac{42.5 \text{ D}_5\text{W}}{\text{x mL}}$$

For solution 2:

$$\frac{45 \text{ parts}}{250 \text{ mL}} = \frac{42.5 \text{ D}_{50}\text{W}}{\text{x mL}}$$

Solving each equation, you get x = 236.11 mL for solution 1 and x = 13.89 mL for solution 2.

Do a quick check to make sure that the two volumes equal the desired volume of the prepared solution:

> 236.11 mL + 13.89 mL = 250.00 mL

A more precise method for checking the calculation is to determine the volume of dextrose in each constituent solution and to see if those volumes, when added up, equal the volume of dextrose in the prepared solution:

> 236.1 mL x 0.05 = 11.805
>
> 13.89 mL x 0.50 = 6.945
>
> 250 mL x 0.075 = 18.750

chapter summary

The daily activities of pharmacists and pharmacy technicians often require measurement and calculation. Pharmacy typically employs the metric system of measurement, which makes use of decimal units, including the basic units of the gram (for weight), the meter (for length and area), and the liter (for volume). Pharmacy also makes use of so-called common measure, including the apothecary, avoirdupois, and household measurement systems.

The most widely used units of measure in pharmacy are the metric units of milligrams, grams, kilograms, milliliters, and liters, and the apothecary/avoirdupois unit known as the grain. Pharmacy technicians should be able to convert between these units and should be conversant with the standard prefixes for abbreviating metric quantities.

To move between units in the metric system, one simply moves the decimal to the right to go from larger to smaller units and to the left to go from smaller to larger units. Technicians should also be conversant with the basic rules for adding, subtracting, multiplying, and dividing fractions; with the basic principles for manipulating decimals; and with procedures for calculating ratios and proportions. Of particular use to the technician is the ability to find an unknown quantity in a proportion when three elements of the proportion are known.

These basic mathematical principles and procedures are used in a wide variety of pharmaceutical calculations, including those for calculating dosages; size, period, and rates of flow for intravenous solutions; and amounts of ingredients in dry and liquid admixtures.

chapter review

Knowledge Inventory

1. The modern metric system makes use of the standardized units of the
   a. avoirdupois system
   b. Système International (SI)
   c. Système Quebecois
   d. apothecaries' system

2. The metric prefix meaning one millionth is
   a. nano-
   b. micro-
   c. milli-
   d. deci-

3. A gram is equal to
   a. 1000 micrograms
   b. 1000 milligrams
   c. 1000 centigrams
   d. 1000 nanograms

4. The liter is a standard measurement of
   a. distance
   b. area
   c. volume
   d. weight

5. 1/2 is a fraction, and 2/1 is its
   a. equivalent fraction
   b. value
   c. reciprocal
   d. least common denominator

6. The decimal fraction has as its denominator a power of
   a. 2
   b. 5
   c. 10
   d. 25

7. 58 percent means 58 out of one
   a. hundred
   b. thousand
   c. million
   d. billion

8. To find out if two fractions are equivalent, one can
   a. cross multiply them and check to see if the products of the multiplications are equal
   b. multiply their denominators and check to see if the products are equal
   c. multiply their numerators and check to see if the products are equal
   d. invert them, then cross multiply them and check to see if the products of the multiplications are equal

9. Intravenous flow rates are usually described as mL/hr or as
   a. mL/min
   b. gtt/min
   c. gtt/hr
   d. mL/sec

10. The proper pediatric dosage of a medication depends upon the child's
    a. body mass
    b. weight
    c. body surface area
    d. none of the above

Pharmacy in Practice

1. Convert the following:
   a. 34.6 g to milligrams
   b. 735 mg to grams
   c. 3400 mL to liters
   d. 1.2 L to milliliters
   e. 7.48 kg to grams
   f. 4.27 mL to liters

2. Convert the following:
   a. 24 oz. to pints
   b. 40 gr to scruples
   c. 6 oz. (avoirdupois) to pounds (avoirdupois)
   d. 6.25 tablespoons to teaspoons
   e. 8 quarts to gallons
   f. viii to Arabic numerals
   g. C to Arabic numerals

3. Solve the following conversion problems.
   a. You have 2 L of solution in stock. The solution is to be used to fill vials containing 40 mL each. How many vials can you fill with the 2 L of solution?
   b. The patient has received a bottle containing 400 mL of a liquid medication. The patient is to take 3 teaspoons of the medication per day. How many days will the bottle last?
   c. A prescription calls for codeine sulfate 40 mg. How many grains of codeine sulfate should be used in the prescription?
   d. A patient takes two 1/150 gr nitroglycerin tablets per day. How many mg of nitroglycerin does the patient receive each day?

4. Solve the following dosage problems.
   a. In stock, you have a solution that contains 8 mg of active ingredient per 10 mL of solution. A customer has a prescription calling for 4 doses of 6 mg each of the active ingredient. How many mL of the solution should the customer be given?
   b. A medication order calls for phenobarbital 60 mg. The supply available is phenobarbital 100 mg/mL of solution. How many milliliters of the solution will the patient be given?
   c. If the adult dose of a medication is 30 mg and the average adult body surface area is 1.72 m^2, what would be the appropriate pediatric dosage for a child with a body surface area of 0.50 m^2?

5. Solve the following IV rate and administration problems.
   a. A physician orders 3000 mL of 10% dextrose and normal saline ($D_{10}NS$) IV over a 48-hour period. If the IV set will deliver 15 drops per milliliter, how many drops must be administered per minute?
   b. A 1/2 liter IV is running at a rate of 100 mL/hr. How long will the bag last?

6. Solve the following solution preparation problems.
   a. You have been asked to prepare a solution containing a powder with a volume of 0.7 mL. The total volume of the solution that you are to prepare should be 30 mL. How much diluent will you use in the solution, and what will be the percentage, by volume, of the powder in the solution?
   b. You must prepare 300 mL of solution containing 4.25% dextrose. In stock you have solutions containing 5% dextrose (solution 1) and 50% dextrose (solution 2). How many mL of each stock solution must you use in the solution that you prepare?

Dispensing, Billing, and Inventory Management

8

The primary role of the pharmacy, of course, is to dispense medications safely, accurately, and in accordance with the law. In this chapter you will learn some of what is involved in the dispensing of medications. The chapter also treats the mechanics of billing, purchasing, receiving, and inventory management.

COMMUNITY PHARMACY OPERATIONS

Community pharmacies sell both **over-the-counter (OTC)** and **legend drugs**. The former are drugs that can be legally sold without a prescription. The latter are drugs that, under the Durham-Humphrey Amendment of 1951, are required to bear on their labeling the legend, "Caution: Federal law prohibits dispensing without a prescription." Community pharmacies are generally organized into a **front area**, where OTC drugs, toiletries, cosmetics, greeting cards, and other merchandise are sold and an R_x **area**, where prescription merchandise and related items are sold. For obvious reasons, the R_x area is off limits to customers and may be entered only by authorized employees.

Technician Duties Related to Dispensing Over-the-Counter Drugs

Increasingly, customers are turning to products that they can purchase at will for self administration. The increase in use of over-the-counter drugs is related to a number of factors, including the increased cost of visits to physicians and the rising cost of prescription medications. In addition, many drugs that once could be purchased only with a prescription are now available over the counter. Although over-the-counter medications may be purchased without a prescription, the active ingredients in these medications are sometimes the same as those found in higher-strength prescription versions. The FDA generally approves an over-the-counter preparation only when the approval process leaves no doubt that the dosage strength is beneficial but unlikely to cause harm when taken as directed. These days, pharmacists devote a greater percentage of their time to recommending over-the-counter products to their customers and to counseling customers about their proper use. Over-the-counter drugs are also becoming an increasingly important part of the technician's responsibilities. Technicians often carry out such functions as stocking over-the-counter drugs, taking inventory of these drugs, removing drugs from stock when they have expired, and helping customers to locate drugs on the shelves. However, technicians should avoid counseling customers with regard to use of over-the-counter drugs unless directed to do so by the pharmacist. Questions about the applications, effects, and administration of such drugs may be referred to the pharmacist.

Technician Duties Related to Dispensing Prescription Drugs

With regard to legend, or prescription, drugs, the technician may carry out a number of different duties, including greeting customers and receiving from them written prescriptions, answering the telephone and referring call-in prescriptions to the pharmacist, calling up the patient's profile on the computer or retrieving it from files, retrieving products from storage in the Rx area, assisting the pharmacist with compounding (in some states), packaging of products, preparing labels for prescriptions, entering billing information into the computer, and third-party billing. These duties are described in the following sections.

RECEIVING AND REVIEWING PRESCRIPTIONS

Prescriptions come into a pharmacy in a variety of ways. Most often, of course, customers carry in written prescriptions or physicians phone them in. A technician may, by law, receive a written prescription from a customer. However, he or she cannot take a prescription by telephone and reduce it to writing. Taking telephone prescriptions, by law, can only be done by a licensed pharmacist, although taking prescription refill information by telephone is, in many instances, considered acceptable.

When taking a written prescription from a customer, first review it to make sure that it looks legitimate. A physician legally must write a prescription out entirely by hand. However, almost always, the prescription will be on a **preprinted prescription form** bearing the name, address, and telephone number of the prescribing physician (see Figure 8.1). If you have any doubts about the authenticity of a prescription, mention these to the pharmacist. A phone call from the pharmacist to the prescribing physician might be in order. Of course, prescriptions can come into a pharmacy by other means as well. A physician might fax a prescription. In some drugstore chains, a prescription may be entered into a central database and be accessed at a store other than the one where the prescription was originally received. It is important for pharmacy technicians to be aware of state laws regarding prescription faxing and the transferring of prescriptions via a database.

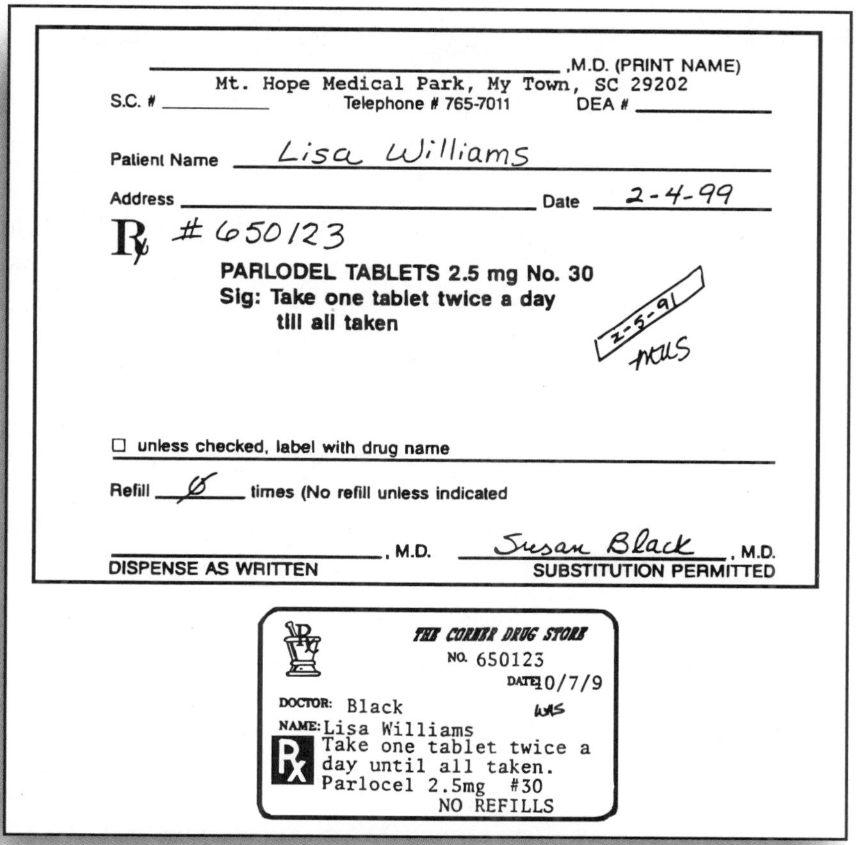
________________________ ,M.D. (PRINT NAME)
Mt. Hope Medical Park, My Town, SC 29202
S.C. # __________ Telephone # 765-7011 DEA # __________

Patient Name Lisa Williams

Address ______________________ Date 2-4-99

℞ # 650123

PARLODEL TABLETS 2.5 mg No. 30
Sig: Take one tablet twice a day
till all taken

2-5-91

☐ unless checked, label with drug name

Refill Ø times (No refill unless indicated

__________, M.D. Susan Black, M.D.
DISPENSE AS WRITTEN SUBSTITUTION PERMITTED

THE CORNER DRUG STORE
NO. 650123
DATE 10/7/9
DOCTOR: Black
NAME: Lisa Williams
Rx Take one tablet twice a day until all taken.
Parlocel 2.5mg #30
NO REFILLS

Figure 8.1 A completed prescription on a preprinted prescription form. A label based on this prescription.

The Parts of a Prescription

Chart 8.1 lists the components generally found on a prescription.

Chart 8.1

PARTS OF A PRESCRIPTION

1. **Prescriber information:** The name, address, telephone number, and other information identifying the prescriber
2. **Date:** The date on which the prescription was written
3. **Patient information:** The name, address, and other pertinent information about the patient receiving the prescription. If the patient is an infant, a toddler, an elderly person, or someone else with special needs, the prescription may include such information as the age, weight, and **body surface area (BSA)** of the patient, information needed by the pharmacist in order to calculate appropriate dosages. To assist the pharmacist, the pharmacy technician may query the customer about this information and add it to the prescription.
4. **℞:** The symbol **℞**, for the Latin word *recipe*, meaning "take"
5. **Inscription:** The medication or medications prescribed, including generic or brand names, strengths, and amounts. States and most institutions have regulations and policies allowing pharmacists to

Chart 8.1

(cont.)

substitute cheaper **generic equivalents** of brand name medications when appropriate. Appendix A of this textbook lists commonly prescribed medications and intravenous admixtures by category.

6. **Subscription:** Instructions to the pharmacist on dispensing the medication, including such information as compounding or packaging instructions, labeling instructions, instructions on allowable refills, and, when a generic equivalent may not be substituted, instructions to that effect (e.g., "No substitutions," "No substitutions allowed," or "Dispense as Written)

7. **Signa:** Directions for the patient to follow

8. **Additional instructions:** Any additional instructions that the prescriber deems necessary

9. **Signature:** The signature of the prescriber

Abbreviations used on prescriptions are covered in chapter 3. You may wish to review that chapter or refer to it as you look at the sample prescriptions in the rest of this chapter.

The following are some general guidelines with regard to reviewing prescriptions:

1. The patient's name should be given in full, including at least the full first and last names. Initials alone are not acceptable. If necessary, rewrite the patient's name, in full, above the name on the prescription.

2. The patient's address is needed for patient records. In most states, the address is required for all prescriptions. Federal law requires addresses on prescriptions for **controlled substances** (substances with a high potential for abuse that are governed by the Controlled Substances Act—see chapter 4); they must be, for such prescriptions, a resident address, not a post office box number.

3. Preprinted prescriptions often contain a space for the patient's birth date. If this space is not filled in, you should ask for the information. The patient's birth date is helpful for third-party billing (discussed below) and for distinguishing among patients with the same name. Knowing the patient's age also helps the pharmacist evaluate the appropriateness of the drug, quantity, and dosage form prescribed.

4. The date is the date when the physician wrote the prescription. For pharmacy records, the date when the prescription is received should be written on the prescription as well. State regulations may dictate the length of time a controlled-substance prescription is valid, for example, six months from the date of issue. The date received is especially important for prescriptions for controlled substances, especially **Schedule II controlled substances**, which are drugs with accepted medical uses that have high potential for abuse. State regulations may control the time period for filling a controlled-substance prescription. In some states, a Schedule II must be filled within seven days of issue. Prescriptions for Schedule II controlled substances may be handwritten or typed. Signatures on such prescriptions must be handwritten, not stamped. In an emergency situation, a person with the legal authority to issue prescriptions for controlled substances may provide oral, rather than written authorization for the prescription.

However, the amount prescribed must not exceed the amount necessary for treatment during the emergency period, and the prescriber must provide a written prescription within 72 hours of the oral authorization.

5. If the prescription is for a controlled substance, the quantity must be limited in some states to 120 units or a 30-day supply or, depending on the state, 34 days or 120 units, whichever is less. A prescription for a Schedule II drug is not refillable. A prescription for a Schedule III or IV drug may be refilled up to five times, but these refills must occur within a 6-month period, after which time a new prescription is required. A prescription for a Schedule V controlled substance may be refilled only if authorized by a prescribing physician.

6. Drugs may be listed on prescriptions using brand names or generic names. A **brand**, **proprietary**, or **trademark name** is a name given to a product by a manufacturer, which is the property of that manufacturer. A **generic name** is a nonproprietary, or nontrademark, name that identifies a drug substance. A given drug (that is, one with a particular generic name) may be marketed under various brand names. For example, NitroBid and Nitrostat are two brand names under which nitroglycerin is marketed. A **generic drug** is one that is marketed under the generic name rather than under a brand name. Generic drugs are often cheaper than brand name drugs and are often substituted, under regulations now existing in every state, for brand name drugs. Such substitutions can be made, of course, only if the generic drug and the brand name drug are **therapeutically equivalent**, that is, if they have the same consequences for the treatment of the patient. If the prescription for a brand name drug is filled with a generic equivalent, then the name, strength, and manufacturer of the generic substitution must be written on the prescription.

7. The **signa**, or directions for use, from the prescription must be placed on the label produced for the medication. The label should read exactly as indicated on the prescription. Any signa comments written on the prescription must be included on the label.

8. If the refill blank on the prescription is left blank, then there can be no refill for the prescription. The words "No Refill" will appear on the prescription label, and an indication of *No Refill* will be entered into the patient's record. If the refill blank on the prescription indicates "**as needed**" (**PRN**), then this is not construed as indicating an unlimited duration. Most pharmacies require at least yearly updates on PRN prescriptions.

9. Prescriptions should generally be refilled, if refills are called for, one or two days before the customer's supply will run out, although this is not a hard-and-fast rule. In some circumstances—as, for example, when a customer is leaving on vacation—an early refill might be in order.

10. Regulations in a given state may require two signature lines at the bottom of the prescription, one reading "Dispense as Written," and the other reading "Substitution Permitted." If the "Dispense as Written" line is signed, then substitution of a generic equivalent is not permitted.

11. The space for **DEA number** on the prescription form is for the number issued to the physician authorizing him or her to prescribe controlled substances (see Figure 8.2). Pharmacy personnel can check for falsified DEA numbers by following this procedure:

a. Add the first, third, and fifth digits of the DEA number.

b. Add the second, fourth, and sixth digits of the number and multiply the sum by two.

c. Add the two results from steps a and b. The last digit of this sum should be the same as the last digit of the DEA number.

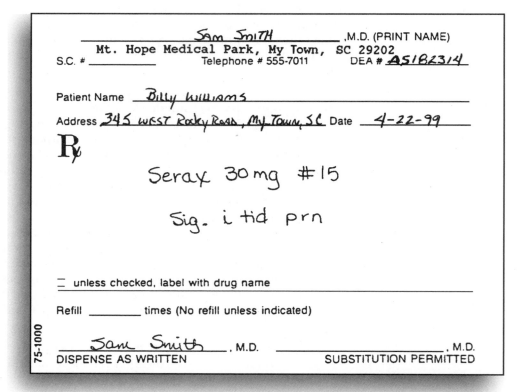

Figure 8.2 Prescription for a controlled substance. Note the DEA number in the upper right-hand corner of the prescription form.

12. The patient should be asked whether he or she has any known allergies to drugs or foods. If the answer is negative, the notation **NKA**, for **No Known Allergies**, should be made on the back of the prescription form and on the patient profile (see next section). If the answer is positive, the allergy should be listed on the back of the prescription form and on the patient profile.

PREPARING, CHECKING, AND UPDATING THE PATIENT PROFILE

A **patient profile** is a paper form (hardcopy) or a computerized record that contains a record of the patient's prescriptions and other relevant information. If the patient is a previous customer, he or she may already have a profile on file that the technician will retrieve. If not, then a new profile will have to be created. Figure 8.3 is an example of a hardcopy patient profile. Figure 8.4 shows a computerized profile.

PATIENT PROFILE

Patient Name

_____ _____ _____
        Last   First   Middle Initial

•••

_____
        Street or PO Box

_____ _____ _____
      City   State   Zip

•••

Phone   **Date of Birth**   **Social Security No.**
( ) __ __   _____   ☐ Male ☐ Female   ___ __ _____
         Month   Day   Year

☐ Yes, I would like medication dispensed in a child-resistant container.
☐ No, I do not want medication dispensed in a child-resistant container.

Medication Insurance   Card Holder Name _____
☐ Yes   ☐ No   ☐ Card Holder   ☐ Child   ☐ Disabled Dependent
                          ☐ Spouse   ☐ Dependent Parent   ☐ Full Time Student

MEDICAL HISTORY

HEALTH

		ALLERGIES AND DRUG REACTIONS
☐ Angina	☐ Epilepsy	☐ No known drug allergies or reactions
☐ Anemia	☐ Glaucoma	
☐ Arthritis	☐ Heart Condition	☐ Aspirin
☐ Asthma	☐ Kidney Disease	☐ Cephalosporins
☐ Blood Clotting Disorders	☐ Liver Disease	☐ Codeine
☐ High Blood Pressure	☐ Lung Disease	☐ Erythromycin
☐ Breast Feeding	☐ Parkinson's Disease	☐ Penicillin
☐ Cancer	☐ Pregnancy	☐ Sulfa Drugs
☐ Diabetes	☐ Ulcers	☐ Tetracyclines

Other Conditions _____   ☐ Xanthines
_____   **Other Allergies/Reactions** _____
_____   _____

Prescription Medication Being Taken   **OTC Medication Currently Being Taken**
_____   _____
_____   _____
_____   _____

Would You Like Generic Medication Where Possible? ☐ Yes ☐ No
_____

Comments
_____

Health information changes periodically. Please notify the pharmacy of any new medications, allergies, drug reactions, or health conditions.

_____ **Signature** _____ **Date** ☐ I do not wish to provide this information.

167-B

Figure 8.3 A hardcopy patient profile.

```
04-21-1999                    PATIENT MEDICATION PROFILE          DR: JONES

NAME: SMITH, GEORGE                    ROOM: 276              SEX: M      HT:  73 IN
DIAGNOSIS: PNEUMONIA                                          AGE:  46    WT: 195 LB
ALLERGIES: NKA
COMMENTS:

          ********************************* ACTIVE MEDICATIONS *********************
          ********** MEDICATIONS PRECEDED BY '*' WILL BE STOPPED TODAY UNLESS REORDER

          MEDICATION        STRENGTH    FORMULARY        RT   DOSAGE   FREQUENCY      START  R
          ================  =========   ==============   ==   ======   ============   =====  =
          APRESOLINE        75MG        HYDRALAZINE      PO   TAB      TID            04/21
          ASA EC                        ACETYL SALICYL   PO   TAB      QD             04/21
          LANOXIN           .125MG      DIGOXIN          PO   TAB      QD             04/21
          MAALOX            30ML                         PO   LIQ      Q4H            04/21
          TYLENOL           650MG       ACETAMINOPHEN    PO   CAPLET   Q4H PRN        04/21
          ZANTAC            150MG       RANITIDINE       PO   TAB      BID            04/21
          --------------------------------------------------------------------------------


          ****************** INACTIVE MEDICATIONS (STOPPED WITHIN LAST THREE DAYS) ****

          --------------------------------------------------------------------------------
```

Figure 8.4 A computerized patient profile.

The Parts of the Patient Profile

The patient profile will generally contain the information listed in Chart 8.2.

Chart 8.2

PARTS OF THE PATIENT PROFILE

1. **Identifying information:** This part of the profile includes the patient's full name, including the middle initial; address; telephone number; social security number; birth date; and gender.

2. **Insurance/billing information:** This part of the profile records information necessary for billing. If the patient has prescription insurance, this should be indicated, along with information such as the name of the insurer, the group number, the patient's ID or card number, the effective date and expiration date of the insurance, the cardholder's name, the persons covered by the insurance, and other relevant information.

3. **Medical history:** Information on existing conditions (such as epilepsy or glaucoma) and on known allergies and adverse drug reactions the patient has experienced. An **allergy** is a hypersensitivity to a specific substance that is manifested in a physiological disorder. Common allergic reactions include sweating, rashes, swelling, and difficulty in breathing. In extreme cases, allergic reactions can lead to shock, coma, or death. An **adverse drug reaction** is any negative consequence to any individual from taking a particular drug. The pharmacist reviews the medical history information on the profile to make sure that the prescription is safe to fill for a given patient.

4. **Medication/prescription history:** Describes any prescription and OTC medications currently being taken and provides a list of previous prescriptions filled for this patient, including information on refills. The pharmacist reviews this information to make sure that the prescription will not cause **adverse drug interactions**, negative consequences due to the combined effects of drugs and/or drugs and foods.

5. **Prescription preferences:** The profile may also indicate patient preferences with regard to his or her prescriptions, such as child-resistant or non–child-resistant containers (see below) or generic substitutions.

6. **Refusal of information:** The profile may provide, for the protection of the pharmacy, a section for the patient to fill out if he or she refuses to provide any or all of the above information.

Policies and Procedures for Patient Profiles

Different pharmacies follow different policies and procedures, generally explained in a **policies and procedures manual**. This manual reflects not only the requirements of the relevant state laws and regulations but also the guidelines for safe and effective operation established by the pharmacy itself. Part of the technician's job, as described in the policies and procedures manual, might be to enter data from a new prescription into the patient profile. Completing a patient profile might require asking questions related to each of the items indicated above.

Updating the Patient Profile

When the prescription is filled, the patient profile must be updated to reflect that prescription. A technician who has received sufficient training may be given the task of recording the new prescription in the profile to provide such information as the prescription number; the name of the drug prescribed; the dosage form; the quantity; the number of refills authorized, if any; and the charge for the prescription.

COMPUTER SYSTEMS

Contemporary pharmacies, both community and institutional, often use computer systems to carry out a wide variety of functions, such as checking and updating patient profile information, checking for possible allergies and drug interactions, printing labels, calculating charges, and completing automated third-party billing. From their beginnings as simple order input devices, pharmacy computer systems have evolved into complex systems offering a wide range of functions. Today, some systems are capable of such functions as tracking expenses, doing pharmacokinetic calculations, tracking inventory, generating controlled substances reports, retrieving literature, and controlling automatic or robotic dispensing and compounding devices. Systems vary from pharmacy to pharmacy. A computer system within an institution is often networked with other departments, such as nursing, laboratory, and administration, thus providing the opportunity for transmitting and sharing of information, including patient data, medication orders, pharmacy literature, and adverse reaction reports.

Because of the widespread use of computers in pharmacy, the aspiring technician should familiarize himself or herself with computer systems and how they work. This section provides some elementary information about computer systems, but a thorough introduction to computers is beyond the scope of this book. The reader should consult a general text such as Shepherd, Robert D., *Introduction to Computers and Technology*. St. Paul: Paradigm, 1998.

The Parts of a Computer System

A **computer** is an electronic device for inputting, storing, processing, and/or outputting information. A **digital computer** represents information internally using **binary numbers**, which are constructed of strings of ones and zeros. Many types of digital computers exist today. In order of size and power, some types of computers available today include supercomputers, mainframe computers, minicomputers, workstations, personal computers, network computers, laptop computers, and handheld or palmtop computers. Some of the more important parts of a typical computer system include the following:

1. one or more **input devices**, such as a **keyboard**, a **mouse**, or a **touch screen**, for getting information into the computer

2. a **central processing unit (CPU)** for processing (manipulating) data that is input prior to output or storage

3. one or more **storage devices**, such as a **floppy disk drive**, **hard drive**, **tape drive**, or **removable disk drive** (such as a **Zip**, **Jaz**, **Syquest**, **Bernoulli**, or **optical drive**), for storing information that has been input into the computer

4. **random-access memory (RAM)**, which is the temporary, nonpermanent memory of the computer in which information is held while it is being input and processed

5. **read-only memory (ROM)**, which is permanent memory containing essential operating instructions for the computer

6. a **monitor**, or **display**, providing a visual representation of data that has been input and/or processed

7. a **printer**, for creating hardcopy, or paper output, such as patient profiles, medication labels, and receipts

8. a **modem**, a device for connecting a computer to a remote network via telephone lines

9. an **operating system**, a software program that performs essential functions such as maintaining a list of file names, issuing processing instructions, and controlling output

10. **applications**, software programs that perform particular functions, such as word processing. An application that allows one to enter, retrieve, and query records is known as a **database management system**, or **DBMS**. Database management systems are the kind of application most commonly used in pharmacy. Often the DBMS used in a particular community or institutional pharmacy was specifically written and/or altered to meet the needs of the pharmacy. Such a program, which meets a wide variety of needs within an organization from customer record keeping to inventory control and billing, is known as a **vertically integrated application**. Often, the pharmacy DBMS is **menu-driven**, allowing the operator to choose functions from a menu of options on the screen by typing a single number, letter, or function key on the keyboard.

How Pharmacy Computer Systems Work

In many pharmacies the operator works at a **dumb terminal**, a computer device that contains a keyboard and a monitor but does not contain its own storage and processing capabilities. A terminal is connected to a remote computer—often a minicomputer or a mainframe—where data is stored and processed.

Pharmacy computer systems differ dramatically from one another. In large retail chains, it is not uncommon for computers to be connected to a single large mainframe system at the company headquarters or home office. In such systems, customer records are stored remotely and backed up at the home office computer site and are accessed via **telecommunications**, connecting to the remote computer via telephone lines or wireless connections. Wireless communications involve the transmission of data or voice signals through the air and involve transmitters, receivers, and often, satellites.

As you have seen above, pharmacy computer systems often allow the operator to call up patient profiles onscreen and to enter new prescription information. A hardcopy patient profile might then be generated for backup filing. In addition, the system may automatically print labels containing information keyed into the profile for a given prescription. Many systems in use today contain automatic warning capabilities to indicate, based on the patient profile and new prescription information entered, possible adverse drug interactions or potential problems with allergic reactions to a given prescription (see Figure 8.5). Such systems typically prevent the filling of an order until a pharmacist provides appropriate intervention. In no situation should a pharmacy technician override such a warning on his or her own initiative. In all cases, the pharmacist should review the warning and make the decision as to whether the prescription should be filled. Drugs are generally identified on computer screens using the product name, manufacturer, strength, and unique **National Drug Code (NDC) number**.

Figure 8.5 Many pharmacy computer systems contain features that will warn, automatically, of possible allergic reactions or adverse food or drug interactions based on information in the patient profile and on a database of known contraindications for given medications.

DRUG INTERACTIONS

PHARMACY
PATIENT: George Smith
PHYSICIAN: Jones
ALLERGIES: NKA

SIGNIFICANCE RATING 1 Drug interactions have been identified (1 interaction)

    1. ASA interacts with coumadin

REFERENCE: 'Drug Interaction Facts' by Facts and Comparsions

Computers (see Figure 8.6) are fallible machines. They often break down and are susceptible to such problems as power failures and surges. Therefore, it is important that copies, or **backups**, of all data be made at regular intervals. Often, pharmacy computer systems make use of tape backup devices. A **tape backup device** stores backup data on reels or cassettes of magnetic tape.

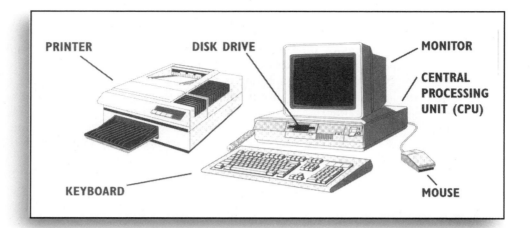

Figure 8.6 A desktop computer system, consisting of a CPU, a keyboard, and a mouse for input and a printer for output.

PRINTER DISK DRIVE MONITOR

CENTRAL PROCESSING UNIT (CPU)

KEYBOARD

MOUSE

PRODUCT SELECTION AND PREPARATION

After the information for a new prescription or refill has been entered into the patient profile, the customer is given a time at which the prescription will be ready for pickup, and the prescription is ready to be filled. A given prescription may require either dispensing of drugs that come prepackaged in given dosage forms (e.g., tablets, prefilled capsules, transdermal patches, etc.) or compounding prior to dispensing.

Extemporaneous Compounding

In some cases, filling the prescription requires **extemporaneous compounding**, the actual preparation of the medication by pharmacy personnel. Compounding might involve, for example, mixing a powdered active ingredient with a diluent powder and filling a given number of capsules with the combined materials, which is known as an **admixture**. The pharmacy technician may be required to retrieve from storage in the pharmacy area the necessary constituents of a compound (liquids, powders, capsules, containers, etc.), to prepare necessary equipment for the compounding process, to count or weigh materials, to compound the prescription, and to return products and clean up the compounding area and equipment after the procedure. In any case, compounding duties undertaken by the technician must be directly supervised and checked by the pharmacist. Extemporaneous compounding is treated in chapter 9.

Dispensing of Prepackaged Drugs

Filling a prescription often involves simply retrieving from stock a drug with the right name, manufacturer, and strength. Sometimes, drugs come in prepackaged, unit dose form (a **unit dose** is a single dose of a drug). This is true, for example, of transdermal patches, of tablets, and of prefilled capsules. Filling the prescription thus amounts to little more than locating the correct drug, in the correct strength, in storage; counting out the number of doses called for by the prescription; and, if necessary, placing these in a container with a label. Sometimes filling a prescription involves retrieving a **multiple-dose container** of a premixed drug and then measuring out the prescribed quantity and placing it into a container with a label. This would be true, for example, of some powders and liquids. Again, the pharmacist must verify that the proper drug, in the proper dosage form, in the proper amount, in the proper container, and with the proper label has been chosen and prepared.

Choosing Containers

Pediatric medications should always be dispensed in **child-resistant containers**, which are designed to be difficult for children to open. The Poison Prevention Packaging Act of 1970 requires, with some exceptions, that prescription drugs be packaged in child-resistant containers but states that a non–child-resistant container may be used if the physician prescribing the drug or the patient receiving it makes a request for such a container. The regulations of a given state may require the patient to make a special request for dispensing a prescription in a non–child-resistant container. Some pharmacies allow patients to complete a blanket request form for non–child-resistant containers. Others require patients to sign such a request for each prescription. Often pharmacies make use of a stamp on the back of the prescription for this purpose.

PREPARING LABELS

From a technical, legal point of view, a label consists of all information provided with a drug by a manufacturer or pharmacist, including the label on the container and the **package insert** (see Figure 8.7), which contains information on the product's pharmacological properties and uses, as well as contraindications and side effects. Before or after the preparation of the order, according to the policy of the individual pharmacy, a **container label** must be generated. This label may either be affixed directly to the container by the person generating the label, or it may be kept separate for review by the pharmacist before being affixed.

As was indicated above, many pharmacies generate labels by computer. In other cases, labels are typed. Less commonly, preprinted labels are used, requiring that information for a specific prescription be added, checked, or circled. Preprinted labels are generally discouraged because of the potential for labeling error. It is too easy to check the wrong box on a preprinted label.

The information required on a label depends upon the laws and regulations of a given state. As was indicated above, manufacturers' labels for prescription medications must carry the legend, "Caution: Federal law prohibits dispensing without a prescription." Typical information required on a container label prepared by a pharmacy includes the following:

Chart 8.3	LABEL INFORMATION

1. Date when the prescription was filled

2. Serial number of the prescription

3. Name and address of the pharmacy

STERILE METHYLPREDNISOLONE ACETATE SUSPENSION, USP

FOR INTRAMUSCULAR, INTRASYNOVIAL, SOFT TISSUE AND INTRALESIONAL USE
Not For Intravenous Use

DESCRIPTION: Sterile methylprednisolone acetate suspension contains methylprednisolone acetate which is the 6-methyl derivative of prednisolone. Methylprednisolone acetate is a white or practically white, odorless, crystalline powder which melts at about 215° with some decomposition. It is soluble in dioxane, sparingly soluble in acetone, in alcohol, in chloroform, and in methanol, and slightly soluble in ether. It is practically insoluble in water. The chemical name for methylprednisolone acetate is pregna-1,4-diene-3,20-dione,21-(acetyloxy)-11, 17-dihydroxy-6-methyl-,(6α, 11β)-and the molecular weight is 416.51. The structural formula is represented as follows:

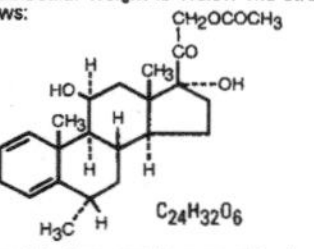

$C_{24}H_{32}O_6$

Sterile methylprednisolone acetate suspension is an anti-inflammatory glucocorticoid, for intramuscular, intrasynovial, soft tissue or intralesional injection. It is available in two strengths: 40 mg/mL and 80 mg/mL.

Each mL of these preparations contains:

Methylprednisolone Acetate	40 mg	80 mg
Polyethylene Glycol 3350	29 mg	28 mg
Sodium Chloride	8.7 mg	8.5 mg
Myristyl-gamma-picolinium Chloride		0.19 mg
Water for Injection	q.s.	

Sodium Hydroxide and/or Hydrochloric Acid may have been used to adjust pH. The pH of the finished product remains within the USP specified range; ie, 3.5 to 7.0.

CLINICAL PHARMACOLOGY: Naturally occurring glucocorticoids (hydrocortisone), which also have salt-retaining properties, are used in replacement therapy in adrenocortical deficiency states. Their synthetic analogs are used primarily for their potent anti-inflammatory effects in disorders of many organ systems.

Glucocorticoids cause profound and varied metabolic effects. In addition, they modify the body's immune response to diverse stimuli.

INDICATIONS AND USAGE: A. FOR INTRAMUSCULAR ADMINISTRATION: When oral therapy is not feasible and the strength, dosage form, and route of administration of the drug reasonably lend the preparation to the treatment of the condition, the intramuscular use of sterile methylprednisolone acetate suspension is indicated as follows:

1. Endocrine Disorders: Primary or secondary adrenocortical insufficiency (hydrocortisone or cortisone is the drug of choice; synthetic analogs may be used in conjunction with mineralocorticoids where applicable; in infancy, mineralocorticoid supplementation is of particular importance).

Acute adrenocortical insufficiency (hydrocortisone or cortisone is the drug of choice; mineralocorticoid supplementation may be necessary, particularly when synthetic analogs are used).

Preoperatively and in the event of serious trauma or illness, in patients with known adrenal insufficiency or when adrenocortical reserve is doubtful.

Congenital adrenal hyperplasia   Nonsuppurative thyroiditis
Hypercalcemia associated with cancer

2. Rheumatic Disorders: As adjunctive therapy for short-term administration (to tide the patient over an acute episode or exacerbation) in:

Post-traumatic osteoarthritis	Epicondylitis
Synovitis of osteoarthritis	Acute nonspecific
Rheumatoid arthritis, including juve-	tenosynovitis
nile rheumatoid arthritis (selected	Acute gouty arthritis
cases may require low-dose	Psoriatic arthritis
maintenance therapy)	Ankylosing spondylitis
Acute and subacute bursitis	

3. Collagen Diseases: During an exacerbation or as maintenance therapy in selected cases of:

Systemic lupus erythematosus	Acute rheumatic carditis
Systemic dermatomyositis (polymyositis)	

4. Dermatologic Diseases:

Pemphigus	Bullous dermatitis herpetiformis
Severe erythema multiforme	Severe seborrheic dermatitis
(Stevens-Johnson syndrome)	Severe psoriasis
Exfoliative dermatitis	Mycosis fungoides

5. Allergic States: Control of severe or incapacitating allergic conditions intractable to adequate trials of conventional treatment in:

Bronchial asthma	Drug hypersensitivity reactions
Contact dermatitis	Urticarial transfusion reactions
Atopic dermatitis	Acute noninfectious laryngeal edema
Serum sickness	(epinephrine is the drug of first choice)
Seasonal or perennial allergic rhinitis	

6. Ophthalmic Diseases: Severe acute and chronic allergic and inflammatory processes involving the eye, such as:

Herpes zoster ophthalmicus	Sympathetic ophthalmia
Iritis, iridocyclitis	Anterior segment inflammation
Chorioretinitis	Allergic conjunctivitis
Diffuse posterior uveitis	Allergic corneal marginal ulcers
and choroiditis	Keratitis
Optic neuritis	

7. Gastrointestinal Diseases: To tide the patient over a critical period of the disease in:

Ulcerative colitis (systemic therapy)	Regional enteritis (systemic therapy)

8. Respiratory Diseases:

Symptomatic sarcoidosis	Loeffler's syndrome not
Berylliosis	manageable by other means
Fulminating or disseminated	Aspiration pneumonitis
pulmonary tuberculosis when	
used concurrently with appropriate	
antituberculous chemotherapy	

9. Hematologic Disorders:

Acquired (autoimmune) hemolytic anemia	Erythroblastopenia (RBC anemia)
Secondary thrombocytopenia in adults	Congenital (erythroid) hypoplastic anemia

10. Neoplastic Diseases: For palliative management of:

Leukemias and lymphomas in adults	Acute leukemia of childhood

11. Edematous States: To induce diuresis or remission of proteinuria in the nephrotic syndrome, without uremia, of the idiopathic type or that due to lupus erythematosus.

12. Nervous System: Acute exacerbations of multiple sclerosis.

13. Miscellaneous: Tuberculous meningitis with subarachnoid block or impending block when used concurrently with appropriate antituberculous chemotherapy.

Trichinosis with neurologic or myocardial involvement.

B. FOR INTRASYNOVIAL OR SOFT TISSUE ADMINISTRATION: (See WARNINGS) Methylprednisolone acetate is indicated as adjunctive therapy for short-term administration (to tide the patient over an acute episode or exacerbation) in:

Synovitis of osteoarthritis	Epicondylitis
Rheumatoid arthritis	Acute nonspecific tenosynovitis
Acute and subacute bursitis	Post-traumatic osteoarthritis
Acute gouty arthritis	

C. FOR INTRALESIONAL ADMINISTRATION: Methylprednisolone acetate is indicated for intralesional use in the following conditions:

Keloids	Discoid lupus erythematosus
Localized hypertrophic,	Necrobiosis lipoidica diabeticorum
infiltrated, inflammatory lesions of:	Alopecia areata
lichen planus, psoriatic plaques,	
granuloma annulare, and lichen	
simplex chronicus (neurodermatitis)	

Methylprednisolone acetate also may be useful in cystic tumors of an aponeurosis or tendon (ganglia).

CONTRAINDICATIONS: Methylprednisolone acetate is contraindicated in systemic fungal infections and patients with known hypersensitivity to the product and its constituents.

WARNINGS: Multidose use of sterile methylprednisolone acetate suspension from a single vial requires special care to avoid contamination.

Although initially sterile, any multidose use of vials may lead to contamination unless strict aseptic technique is observed. The preservative in sterile methylprednisolone acetate suspension will prevent growth of most pathogenic organisms, but certain ones (e.g., *Serratia marcescens*) may remain viable. Particular care, such as use of disposable sterile syringes and needles is necessary. Multidose use of methylprednisolone acetate from vials is not recommended for intrasynovial injection.

While crystals of adrenal steroids in the dermis suppress inflammatory reactions, their presence may cause disintegration of the cellular elements and physiochemical changes in the ground substance of the connective tissue. The resultant infrequently occurring dermal and/or subdermal changes may form depressions in the skin at the injection site. The degree to which this reaction occurs will vary with the amount of adrenal steroid injected. Regeneration is usually complete within a few months or after all crystals of the adrenal steroid have been absorbed.

In order to minimize the incidence of dermal and subdermal atrophy, care must be exercised not to exceed recommended doses in injections. Multiple small injections into the area of the lesion should be made whenever possible. The technique of intrasynovial and intramuscular injection should include precautions against injection or leakage into the dermis. Injection into the deltoid muscle should be avoided because of a high incidence of subcutaneous atrophy.

It is critical that, during administration of methylprednisolone acetate, appropriate technique be used and care taken to assure proper placement of drug.

Sterile methylprednisolone acetate suspension is Not Recommended For Intrathecal Administration.

In patients on corticosteroid therapy subjected to any unusual stress, increased dosage of rapidly acting corticosteroids before, during, and after the stressful situation is indicated.

Corticosteroids may mask some signs of infection, and new infections may appear during their use. There may be decreased resistance and inability to localize infection when corticosteroids are used. Do not use intra-articularly, intrabursally or for intratendinous administration for *local* effect in the presence of acute infection.

Corticosteroids are drugs which suppress the immune system are more susceptible to infections than healthy individuals. Chickenpox and measles, for example, can have a more serious or even fatal course in non-immune children or adults on corticosteroids. In such children or adults who have not had these diseases, particular care should be taken to avoid exposure. How the dose, route and duration of corticosteroid administration affects the risk of developing a disseminated infection is not known. The contribution of the underlying disease and/or prior corticosteroids treatment to the risk is also not known. If exposed to chickenpox, prophylaxis with varicella zoster immune globulin (VZIG) may be indicated. If exposed to measles, prophylaxis with pooled intramuscular immunoglobulin (IG) may be indicated. (See respective package inserts for complete VZIG and IG prescribing information). If chickenpox develops, treatment with antiviral agents may be considered.

Prolonged use of corticosteroids may produce posterior subcapsular cataracts, glaucoma with possible damage to the optic nerves, and may enhance the establishment of secondary ocular infections due to fungi or viruses.

Usage in Pregnancy: Since adequate human reproduction studies have not been done with corticosteroids, the use of these drugs in pregnancy, nursing mothers, or women of childbearing potential requires that the possible benefits of the drug be weighed against the potential hazards to the mother and embryo or fetus. Infants born of mothers who have received substantial doses of corticosteroids during pregnancy should be carefully observed for signs of hypoadrenalism.

Average and large doses of cortisone or hydrocortisone can cause elevation of blood pressure, salt and water retention, and increased excretion of potassium. These effects are less likely to occur with the synthetic derivatives except when used in large doses. Dietary salt restriction and potassium supplementation may be necessary. All corticosteroids increase calcium excretion.

While on corticosteroid therapy patients should not be vaccinated against smallpox. Other immunization procedures should not be undertaken in patients who are on corticosteroids, especially in high doses, because of possible hazards of neurological complications and lack of antibody response.

The use of methylprednisolone acetate in active tuberculosis should be restricted to those cases of fulminating or disseminated tuberculosis in which the corticosteroid is used for the management of the disease in conjunction with appropriate antituberculous regimen.

If corticosteroids are indicated in patients with latent tuberculosis or tuberculin reactivity, close observation is necessary as reactivation of the disease may occur. During prolonged corticosteroid therapy, these patients should receive chemoprophylaxis.

Because rare instances of anaphylactoid reactions have occurred in patients receiving parenteral corticosteroid therapy, appropriate precautionary measures should be taken prior to administration, especially when the patient has a history of allergy to any drug.

Allergic skin reactions have been reported apparently related to the excipients in the formulation (See DESCRIPTION). Rarely has skin testing demonstrated a reaction to methylprednisolone acetate, per se.

PRECAUTIONS: General: Drug-induced secondary adrenocortical insufficiency may be minimized by gradual reduction of dosage. This type of relative insufficiency may persist for months after discontinuation of therapy; therefore, in any situation of stress occurring during that period, hormone therapy should be reinstituted. Since mineralocorticoid secretion may be impaired, salt and/or a mineralocorticoid should be administered concurrently.

When multidose vials are used, special care to prevent contamination of the contents is essential. There is some evidence that benzalkonium chloride is not an adequate antiseptic for sterilizing sterile methylprednisolone acetate suspension multidose vials. A povidone-iodine solution or similar product is recommended to cleanse the vial top prior to aspiration of contents. (See WARNINGS).

There is an enhanced effect of corticosteroids in patients with hypothyroidism and in those with cirrhosis.

Corticosteroids should be used cautiously in patients with ocular herpes simplex for fear of corneal perforation.

The lowest possible dose of corticosteroid should be used to control the condition under treatment, and when reduction in dosage is possible, the reduction must be gradual.

Figure 8.7 A package insert (front).

Psychic derangements may appear when corticosteroids are used, ranging from euphoria, insomnia, mood swings, personality changes, and severe depression to frank psychotic manifestations. Also, existing emotional instability or psychotic tendencies may be aggravated by corticosteroids.

Aspirin should be used cautiously in conjunction with corticosteroids in hypoprothrombinemia.

Steroids should be used with caution in nonspecific ulcerative colitis, if there is a probability of impending perforation, abscess or other pyogenic infection. Caution must also be used in diverticulitis, fresh intestinal anastomoses, active or latent peptic ulcer, renal insufficiency, hypertension, osteoporosis, and myasthenia gravis, when steroids are used as direct or adjunctive therapy.

Growth and development of infants and children on prolonged corticosteroid therapy should be carefully followed.

The following additional precautions apply for parenteral corticosteroids.

Intrasynovial injection of a corticosteroid may produce systemic as well as local effects.

Appropriate examination of any joint fluid present is necessary to exclude a septic process.

A marked increase in pain accompanied by local swelling, further restriction of joint motion, fever, and malaise are suggestive of septic arthritis. If this complication occurs and the diagnosis of sepsis is confirmed, appropriate antimicrobial therapy should be instituted.

Local injection of a steroid into a previously infected joint is to be avoided.

Corticosteroids should not be injected into unstable joints.

The slower rate of absorption by intramuscular administration should be recognized.

Although controlled clinical trials have shown corticosteroids to be effective in speeding the resolution of acute exacerbations of multiple sclerosis, they do not show that corticosteroids affect the ultimate outcome or natural history of the disease. The studies do show that relatively high doses of corticosteroids are necessary to demonstrate a significant effect. (See DOSAGE AND ADMINISTRATION).

Since complications of treatment with glucocorticoids are dependent on the size of the dose and the duration of treatment, a risk/benefit decision must be made in each individual case as to dose and duration of treatment and as to whether daily or intermittent therapy should be used.

Convulsions have been reported with concurrent use of methylprednisolone and cyclosporin. Since concurrent use of these agents results in a mutual inhibition of metabolism, it is possible that adverse events associated with the individual use of either drug may be more apt to occur.

Information for Patients: Persons who are on immunosuppressant doses of corticosteroids should be warned to avoided exposure to chickenpox or measles. Patients should also be advised that if they are exposed, medical advice should be sought without delay.

ADVERSE REACTIONS:

Fluid and electrolyte disturbances
Sodium retention
Fluid retention
Congestive heart failure in susceptible patients
Potassium loss
Hypokalemic alkalosis
Hypertension

Musculoskeletal
Muscle weakness
Steroid myopathy
Loss of muscle mass
Osteoporosis
Vertebral compression fractures
Aseptic necrosis of femoral and humeral heads
Pathologic fracture of long bones
Gastrointestinal
Peptic ulcer with possible subsequent perforation and hemorrhage
Pancreatitis
Abdominal distention
Ulcerative esophagitis

Dermatologic
Impaired wound healing
Thin fragile skin
Petechiae and ecchymoses
Facial erythema
Increased sweating
May suppress reactions to skin tests.

Neurological
Convulsions
Increased intracranial pressure with papilledema (pseudotumor cerebri) usually after treatment
Vertigo
Headache

Endocrine
Menstrual irregularities
Development of Cushingoid state
Suppression of growth in children
Secondary adrenocortical and pituitary unresponsiveness, particularly in times of stress, as in trauma, surgery or illness
Decreased carbohydrate tolerance
Manifestations of latent diabetes mellitus
Increased requirements for insulin or oral hypoglycemic agents in diabetes

Ophthalmic
Posterior subcapsular cataracts
Increased intraocular pressure
Glaucoma
Exophthalmos

Metabolic
Negative nitrogen balance due to protein catabolism

The following *additional* adverse reactions are related to parenteral corticosteroid therapy:
Anaphylactic reaction
Allergic or hypersensitivity reactions
Urticaria
Hyperpigmentation or hypopigmentation
Subcutaneous and cutaneous atrophy
Sterile abscess
Injection site infections following non-sterile administration (See WARNINGS)
Postinjection flare, following intrasynovial use
Charcot-like arthropathy

Adverse Reactions Reported with the Following Routes of Administration:

Intrathecal/Epidural
Arachnoiditis
Meningitis
Paraparesis/paraplegia
Sensory disturbances
Bowel/bladder dysfunction
Headache
Seizures

Ophthalmic
Temporary/permanent visual impairment including blindness
Increased intraocular pressure
Ocular and periocular inflammation including allergic reactions
Infection
Residue or slough at injection site

Intranasal
Temporary/permanent visual impairment including blindness
Allergic reactions
Rhinitis

Miscellaneous injection sites (scalp, tonsillar fauces, sphenopalatine ganglion)-blindness.

DOSAGE AND ADMINISTRATION: Because of possible physical incompatibilities, sterile methylprednisolone acetate suspension should not be diluted or mixed with other solutions.

A. Administration for Local Effect: Therapy with sterile methylprednisolone acetate suspension does not obviate the need for the conventional measures usually employed. Although this method of treatment will ameliorate symptoms, it is in no sense a cure and the hormone has no effect on the cause of the inflammation.

1. Rheumatoid and Osteoarthritis: The dose for intra-articular administration depends upon the size of the joint and varies with the severity of the condition in the individual patient. In chronic cases, injections may be repeated at intervals ranging from one to five or more weeks depending upon the degree of relief obtained from the initial injection. The doses in the following table are given as a general guide:

Size of Joint	Examples	Range of Dosage
Large	Knees Ankles Shoulders	20 to 80 mg
Medium	Elbows Wrists	10 to 40 mg
Small	Metacarpophalangeal Interphalangeal Sternoclavicular Acromioclavicular	4 to 10 mg

Procedure: It is recommended that the anatomy of the joint involved be reviewed before attempting intra-articular injection. In order to obtain the full anti-inflammatory effect it is important that the injection be made into the synovial space. Employing the same sterile technique as for a lumbar puncture, a sterile 20 to 24 gauge needle (on a dry syringe) is quickly inserted into the synovial cavity. Procaine infiltration is elective. The aspiration of only a few drops of joint fluid proves the joint space has been entered by the needle. *The injection site for each joint is determined by that location where the synovial cavity is most superficial and most free of large vessels and nerves.* With the needle in place, the aspirating syringe is removed and replaced by a second syringe containing the desired amount of sterile methylprednisolone acetate suspension. The plunger is then pulled outward slightly to aspirate synovial fluid and to make sure the needle is still in the synovial space. After injection, the joint is moved gently a few times to aid mixing of the synovial fluid and the suspension. The site is covered with a small sterile dressing.

Suitable sites for intra-articular injection are the knee, ankle, wrist, elbow, shoulder, phalangeal, and hip joints. Since difficulty is not infrequently encountered in entering the hip joint, precautions should be taken to avoid any large blood vessels in the area. Joints not suitable for injection are those that are anatomically inaccessible such as the spinal joints and those like the sacroiliac joints that are devoid of synovial space. Treatment failures are most frequently the result of failure to enter the joint space. Little or no benefit follows injection into surrounding tissue. If failures occur when injections into the synovial spaces are certain, as determined by aspiration of fluid, repeated injections are usually futile. Local therapy does not alter the underlying disease process, and whenever possible comprehensive therapy including physiotherapy and orthopedic correction should be employed.

Following intra-articular steroid therapy, care should be taken to avoid overuse of joints in which symptomatic benefit has been obtained. Negligence in this matter may permit an increase in joint deterioration that will more than offset the beneficial effects of the steroid.

Unstable joints should not be injected. Repeated intra-articular injection may in some cases result in instability of the joint. X-ray follow-up is suggested in selected cases to detect deterioration.

If a local anesthetic is used prior to injection of sterile methylprednisolone acetate suspension, the anesthetic package insert should be read carefully and all the precautions observed.

2. Bursitis: The area around the injection site is prepared in a sterile way and a wheal at the site made with 1 percent procaine hydrochloride solution. A 20 to 24 gauge needle attached to a dry syringe is inserted into the bursa and the fluid aspirated. The needle is left in place and the aspirating syringe changed for a small syringe containing the desired dose. After injection, the needle is withdrawn and a small dressing applied.

3. Miscellaneous: Ganglion, Tendinitis, Epicondylitis: In the treatment of conditions such as tendinitis or tenosynovitis, care should be taken, following application of a suitable antiseptic to the overlying skin, to inject the suspension into the tendon sheath rather than into the substance of the tendon. The tendon may be readily palpated when placed on a stretch. When treating conditions such as epicondylitis, the area of greatest tenderness should be outlined carefully and the suspension infiltrated into the area. For ganglia of the tendon sheaths, the suspension is injected directly into the cyst. In many cases, a single injection causes a marked decrease in the size of the cystic tumor and may effect disappearance. The usual sterile precautions should be observed, of course, with each injection.

The dose in the treatment of the various conditions of the tendinous or bursal structures listed above varies with the condition being treated and ranges from 4 to 30 mg. In recurrent or chronic conditions, repeated injections may be necessary.

4. Injections for Local Effect in Dermatologic Conditions: Following cleansing with an appropriate antiseptic such as 70% alcohol, 20 to 60 mg of the suspension is injected into the lesion. It may be necessary to distribute doses ranging from 20 to 40 mg by repeated local injections in the case of large lesions. Care should be taken to avoid injection of sufficient material to cause blanching since this may be followed by a small slough. One to four injections are usually employed, the intervals between injections varying with the type of lesion being treated and the duration of improvement produced by the initial injection.

When multidose vials are used, special care to prevent contamination of the contents is essential. (See WARNINGS).

B. Administration for Systemic Effect: The intramuscular dosage will vary with the condition being treated. When employed as a temporary substitute for oral therapy, a single injection during each 24-hour period of a dose of the suspension equal to the total daily oral dose of methylprednisolone is usually sufficient. When a prolonged effect is desired, the weekly dose may be calculated by multiplying the daily oral dose by 7 and given as a single intramuscular injection.

Dosage must be individualized according to the severity of the disease and response of the patient. For infants and children, the recommended dosage will have to be reduced, but dosage should be governed by the severity of the condition rather than by strict adherence to the ratio indicated by age or body weight.

Hormone therapy is an adjunct to, and not a replacement for, conventional therapy. Dosage must be decreased or discontinued gradually when the drug has been administered for more than a few days. The severity, prognosis and expected duration of the disease and the reaction of the patient to medication are all factors in determining dosage. If a period of spontaneous remission occurs in a chronic condition, treatment should be discontinued. Routine laboratory studies, such as urinalysis, two-hour postprandial blood sugar, determination of blood pressure and body weight, and a chest X-ray should be made at regular intervals during prolonged therapy. Upper GI X-rays are desirable in patients with an ulcer history or significant dyspepsia.

In patients with the adrenogenital syndrome, a single intramuscular injection of 40 mg every two weeks may be adequate. For maintenance of patients with rheumatoid arthritis, the weekly intramuscular dose will vary from 40 to 120 mg. The usual dosage for patients with dermatologic lesions benefited by systemic corticoid therapy is 40 to 120 mg of methylprednisolone acetate administered intramuscularly at weekly intervals for one to four weeks. In acute severe dermatitis due to poison ivy, relief may result within 8 to 12 hours following intramuscular administration of a single dose of 80 to 120 mg. In chronic contact dermatitis, repeated injections at 5 to 10 day intervals may be necessary. In seborrheic dermatitis, a weekly dose of 80 mg may be adequate to control the condition.

Following intramuscular administration of 80 to 120 mg to asthmatic patients, relief may result within 6 to 48 hours and persist for several days to two weeks. Similarly, in patients with allergic rhinitis (hay fever), an intramuscular dose of 80 to 120 mg may be followed by relief of coryzal symptoms within six hours persisting for several days to three weeks.

If signs of stress are associated with the condition being treated, the dosage of the suspension should be increased. If a rapid hormonal effect of maximum intensity is required, the intravenous administration of highly soluble methylprednisolone sodium succinate is indicated.

Multiple Sclerosis: In treatment of acute exacerbations of multiple sclerosis, daily doses of 200 mg of prednisolone for a week followed by 80 mg every other day for 1 month have been shown to be effective (4 mg of methylprednisolone is equivalent to 5 mg of prednisolone).

HOW SUPPLIED: Sterile methylprednisolone acetate suspension, USP, 40 mg/mL, is available in a 5 mL or a 10 mL multiple dose vial, individually packaged.

Sterile methylprednisolone acetate suspension, USP, 80 mg/mL, is available in a 5 mL multiple dose vial, individually packaged.

SHAKE WELL BEFORE EACH USE. PROTECT FROM FREEZING.

Store at controlled room temperature 15° - 30° C (59° - 86° F).

CAUTION: Federal law prohibits dispensing without prescription.

Literature revised: December 1993

Product Nos.: 1069-05, 1069-10, 1070-05

Mfd. by Steris Laboratories, Inc.
Phoenix, Arizona 85043 USA

Figure 8.7 A package insert (back).

Chart 8.3
(cont.)

4. Name of the patient

5. Name of the prescribing physician

6. All directions for use given on the prescription

7. Any necessary **auxiliary labels**, containing patient precautions. These labels, attached at the pharmacist's discretion, provide additional usage or precautionary information for the patient (e.g., Take with meals. Do not operate heavy machinery while taking this product. For rectal use only.). See Figure 8.8. For Schedule II, III, and IV controlled substances, the auxiliary label "TRANSFER WARNING" is required.

8. Generic or brand name of the medication

9. Strength of the medication

10. Name of the drug manufacturer

11. Quantity of the drug

12. **Expiration date** of the drug, or date after which the drug should not be used due to possible loss of potency or efficacy

13. Initials of the licensed pharmacist

14. Number of refills allowed or the phrase "No Refills"

Labels for Schedule II controlled substances must contain the fill date. Labels for Schedule III, IV, or V drugs must show the date of initial filling. Labels for all prescriptions for controlled substances should include the pharmacy name and address, the serial number of the prescription, the name of the patient, the name of the prescriber, and directions for use and cautionary statements. Labels for Schedule II, III, and IV drugs should contain the cautionary statement, "Caution: Federal law prohibits the transfer of this drug to any person other than the person for whom it was prescribed."

BILLING AND CHECKING THE PRESCRIPTION

It is important for the pharmacy technician to obtain from the customer all necessary insurance information, including any co-pay amount, when the prescription is dropped off. Once the prescription has been filled and the label prepared, the billing can be done. Billing policies and procedures differ from pharmacy to pharmacy and from customer to customer. In some cases, the customer pays for his or her prescription at the time he or she receives it. The customer may or may not then be reimbursed by an insurer for the cost of the prescription. In other cases, billing involves **third-party administration (TBA)**, or billing by the pharmacist to the third party, the customer's insurer (see below). After the price of the prescription is calculated, based on existing pricing schedules, the prescription is ready for review by the pharmacist.

It is extremely important that the pharmacist check every prescription to make sure that it is correct. The pharmacist reviews the prescription form, the patient profile, the drug and drug quantity used, the accuracy of the label, and the price. After this review, the pharmacist initials the label. In doing so, the pharmacist assumes responsibility for the correctness of the prescription.

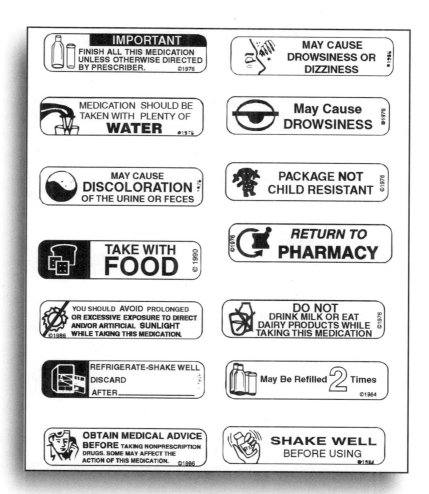

Figure 8.8 Some common auxiliary labels. Copyright © Pharmex 1998, Division of Automatic Business Products Company, Inc. 1-888-PHARMEX

However, the pharmacist does not necessarily assume, by this action, sole responsibility. Technicians have in the past been held legally responsible for dispensing and labeling mistakes, especially in situations in which the dispensing error was due to negligence on the part of the technician (such as, for example, improperly overriding a computerized adverse interaction warning).

THIRD-PARTY ADMINISTRATION

Many pharmacy customers have prescription drug insurance, and billing must be done to a third party. If the customer has such insurance, then he or she may carry a prescription card containing information such as the following: the name of the insured person, the insurance carrier, a group number, a cardholder identification number, information on dependents covered, an expiration date, and the amount of the co-payment. The technician must request this information and either enter it into the computer system or, if the pharmacy uses a manual system for third-party billing, enter it onto a form, generally a **universal claim form (UCF)**. Billing of the third party may be handled in a variety of ways. The bill may be transferred to the third party electronically, via modem, or placed on a computer diskette that is then mailed to the insurer. In other cases, the computer may generate a bill that is mailed to the third party, or a manually prepared bill, usually one on a UCF, may be sent to the insurer.

PURCHASING, RECEIVING, AND INVENTORY CONTROL

The purposes of purchasing and inventory control are to obtain pharmaceutical materials in a timely manner and to establish and maintain appropriate levels of materials in stock. Purchasing, receiving, and inventory processes should be as uncomplicated as possible so as not to disrupt or to interfere with the other activities of the pharmacy.

Selection of pharmaceutical products is accomplished by a variety of methods. In an institutional setting, for example, the **pharmacy and therapeutics committee (P & T)** determines which agents are to be maintained in stock. This committee prepares a list of agents accepted for use in the institution. Such a list is called a **formulary**. A formulary lists, for each product, the product name, dosage form, concentration, and package size.

Purchasing

Purchasing, the ordering of products for use or sale by the pharmacy or institution, is usually carried out in either of two ways. In **independent purchasing**, the pharmacist or technician works alone or with a purchasing agent and deals directly with pharmaceutical companies regarding matters such as price. In **group purchasing**, a number of institutions or pharmacies work together to negotiate discounts for high-volume purchases and other benefits. Some independent purchasing exists in almost all pharmacy settings because some products are not available through group purchasing and some settings have unique needs for specialty products.

Several purchasing methods or systems are used in pharmacies. **Direct purchasing** requires completion of a **purchase order**, generally a preprinted form with a unique number on which the product name(s), amount(s), and price(s) are entered. If the pharmacy makes use of a purchasing agent, then a **purchase requisition** is sent to that agent. The order is then transmitted directly to the manufacturer. An advantage of direct purchasing is the lack of add-on fees. A disadvantage is the commitment on the part of the pharmacy of time and staff. **Wholesaler purchasing** enables the pharmacy to use a single source to purchase numerous products from numerous manufacturers. Advantages to wholesaler purchasing include reduced turnaround time for orders, lower inventory and lower associated costs, and reduced time and staff commitment. Disadvantages include higher purchase cost, supply difficulties, the loss of the control provided by in-house purchase orders, and unavailability of some medicinals. **Prime vendor purchasing** involves an agreement made by an institution or pharmacy for a specified percentage or dollar volume of purchases. Such a system offers the advantages of competitive service fees, electronic order entry, and emergency delivery services. **Just-in-time (JIT)** purchasing involves frequent purchasing in quantities that just meet supply needs until the next ordering time. JIT reduces the quantity of each product on the shelves and thus reduces the amount of money tied up in inventory. However, such a system can only be used when supplies are readily available and needs can be accurately predicted.

Receiving

The series of procedures carried out when products that have been ordered arrive at the pharmacy or institution is known as **receiving**. It is important for institutions and pharmacies to have a system of checks and balances for purchasing and receiving. In other words, full control should not reside with a single person, and the person ordering should not be the same as the person receiving. The pharmaceutical products received must be carefully checked against the purchase order or requisition. The shipment should be compared for name of product, quantity, product strength, and product package size. Products damaged in shipment or improperly shipped must be reported immediately. Stringent laws regulate the return of pharmaceuticals to manufacturers. In the case of a damaged or incorrect shipment, the manufacturer should be notified immediately and authorization should be secured for the return of the defective shipment.

Pharmaceuticals in a shipment should be checked for expiration dates. Each pharmacy has a policy for acceptable product expiration dates. A typical requirement might be that products have expiration dates of at least 6 months from the date of receipt.

After products are received and checked, they are then placed in a proper storage location. The expiration dates of stored products are periodically checked, and expired products are removed. An accepted method for stocking pharmaceuticals is to place the units of product with the shortest expiration dates in positions where they will be the first units selected for use.

Pharmacy technicians handle and prepare medications more frequently than pharmacists do and are therefore in a better position to identify potential sources of error related to packaging and storage. A common error is the selection of the wrong pharmaceutical because two products look alike or have names that sound alike. A good work habit is to read each label three times and to avoid basing product identification on size, color, package shape, or label design.

Occasionally, a pharmaceutical product will be unavailable or temporarily unavailable form a supplier. It then becomes necessary to borrow or purchase a small quantity from another institution or pharmacy. A detailed procedure for control of and accountability with regard to loaned or borrowed products is necessary.

Two types of pharmaceuticals require special consideration: controlled substances and investigational drugs. The Controlled Substances Act defines ordering and inventory requirements. Purchase of Schedule II controlled substances must be authorized by a pharmacist and executed on a DEA form. A physical inventory of Schedule II substances is required every two years. **Investigational drugs**—ones that are being used in clinical trials and have not yet been approved by the FDA for use in the general population—require special ordering and handling procedures.

Inventory Management

The entire stock of products on hand at a given time in an institution or business is known as **inventory**. Several important issues with regard to inventory include how much inventory should be maintained, when inventory levels should be adjusted, and where inventory should be stored. Factors that bear upon decisions regarding these issues include floor space allocation, design and arrangement of shelves, and demands upon available refrigerator or freezer space.

Keeping excess inventory in stock has a number of associated costs, including the capital that is tied up in the inventory, waste due to product expiration, and increased likelihood of theft or contamination. In an ideal system, pharmaceuticals would arrive shortly before they were needed. Today, a variety of methods may be used for inventory management. In some systems, the dispenser of a product determines when a product needs to be reordered and enters it into an order book. Other systems make use of inventory cards or papers on which an ongoing use and purchase history is kept. Some systems make use of predetermined minimum and maximum product levels based upon historical use. In still other systems, purchasing is based upon calculation of the most economical order quantity or value. Computerized inventory control systems make it possible for purchase orders to be generated automatically under predetermined conditions. One goal of computerized inventory control is to reduce the time and staff required for inventory management. Ideally, such a system would require only periodic review and adjustment.

A physical inventory is taken when no perpetual inventory system is in place. In most pharmacies, the inventory, or counting of items in stock, is done once or twice annually. An inventory value is used to determine average inventory and turnover rate. The average inventory allows a pharmacy to determine the number of times that pharmaceuticals are repurchased in a specific period of time, usually annually.

$$\text{Average inventory} = \frac{\text{Beginning inventory} + \text{Ending inventory}}{2}$$

Turnover rate is the number of times the entire stock is used and replaced each year.

$$\text{Turnover rate} = \frac{\text{Annual dollar purchases}}{2}$$

chapter summary

Pharmacy technicians assume a number of responsibilities related to both over-the-counter and legend drugs. The precise responsibilities a technician may assume depend upon the laws and regulations of the state in which he or she is working. Usually, a technician can take written prescriptions from walk-in customers but cannot take new prescriptions by telephone and reduce them to writing. The parts of a prescription include prescriber information, the date, patient information, the symbol Rx, the inscription (the medication or medications prescribed and the amounts of these), the subscription (instructions to the pharmacist), the signa (directions to the patient), additional instructions, and the signature. After the prescription is checked, it is entered into the patient profile. If no patient profile already exists, a new one, with all necessary information, is created. Patient profiles may be in hardcopy or computerized form and include identifying information, insurance/billing information, medical history, medication/prescription history, and prescription preferences for each patient. Some pharmacy computer systems contain automatic warnings about possible allergic or other adverse reactions.

After the patient profile is created or updated, the prescription may be filled. Filling the prescription may involve any of a number of tasks, including retrieving drugs, supplies, containers, or equipment; setting up equipment; weighing and measuring; compounding; filling containers; and preparing labels. Container labels must contain a unique prescription number, the name of the patient, the date of the prescription, directions for use, the name and strength of the medication, the manufacturer of the medication, the quantity of the drug, the expiration date, the initials of the pharmacist, the number of refills, and auxiliary labels. After the label is prepared, a price for the prescription is calculated based upon existing tables, or schedules, in the pharmacy. Then the pharmacist checks the prescription form, the patient profile, the drug and drug quantity used, the accuracy of the label, and the price. Billing often must be done to a third party, the customer's insurer. The process of conducting such billing is called third-party administration. In addition to carrying out dispensing and billing functions, technicians are often involved in purchasing, receiving, and inventory functions.

chapter review

Knowledge Inventory

1. Technicians' duties with regard to over-the-counter drugs typically include
   a. stocking them
   b. taking inventory of them
   c. removing expired drugs from the shelves
   d. all of the above

2. In a prescription, the signa is
   a. the signature of the prescribing physician
   b. the initials of the pharmacist
   c. directions for the patient to follow
   d. instructions to the pharmacist on dispensing the medication

3. The symbol **R** stands for the Latin word *recipe* and means
   a. give
   b. take
   c. prepare
   d. mix

4. A signature on a prescription for a Schedule II controlled substance
   a. may be stamped
   b. must be handwritten
   c. must include the DEA number
   d. may be that of the prescriber or his or her agent

5. In most states, a generic drug may be substituted for a brand name or proprietary drug provided that
   a. the generic drug is cheaper
   b. the generic drug has undergone clinical trials
   c. the generic drug is therapeutically equivalent to the brand name or proprietary drug
   d. the generic drug is nontoxic

6. Pharmacy personnel can check to see if a DEA number has been falsified by
   a. looking up the number in the *Orange Book*
   b. performing a mathematical calculation
   c. checking the number in *Facts and Comparisons*
   d. using a code to translate the number into an alphabetical form—the name of the prescriber

7. An important purpose of the medication/prescription history on the patient profile is to
   a. identify potential adverse drug interactions
   b. verify the authenticity of the current prescription
   c. provide information on existing conditions, known allergies, and history of adverse drug interactions
   d. provide the information used in the pharmacy's record of the controlled substances that it has dispensed

8. A computer application program that allows one to enter, retrieve, and query records is known as a
   a. vertically integrated application
   b. operating system
   c. menu-driven application
   d. database management system

9. Child-resistant containers are required by the
   a. Controlled Substances Act
   b. Federal Anti-Tampering Act
   c. Durham-Humphrey Amendment to the Food, Drug, and Cosmetic Act
   d. Poison Prevention Packaging Act

10. In a manual third-party administration system, billing is typically done by means of a
   a. computer-generated form
   b. purchase order
   c. purchase requisition
   d. universal claim form

Pharmacy in Practice

1. For each of the prescriptions below, answer the following questions:
   a. Is any essential item missing from the prescription? If so, what is this item?
   b. What medication is prescribed, in what strength, and in what amount?
   c. What special instructions, if any, are provided in the subscription?
   d. What directions are given for the patient to follow?

MT. HOPE MEDICAL PARK
MY TOWN, USA   555-3591

\# _127352_   DEA \#_____

PT. NAME _Fred Figule_   DATE_____

ADDRESS _____

R̸   Hydrocortisone 20mg tabs
     Take A.M. 5 tabs day 1
              3   "   2
              2   "   3
              1 tab " 4 and 5

REFILLS ___ TIMES   (NO REFILL UNLESS INDICATED)

_____ M.D. _L. Demanio_ M.D.
DISPENSE AS WRITTEN   SUBSTITUTE PERMITTED

MT. HOPE MEDICAL PARK
MY TOWN, USA   555-3591

\# _42573_   DEA \#_____

PT. NAME _H. R. Robbins_   DATE _11-24-99_

ADDRESS _____

R̸   Tylenol / codeine No 4
     Take 1 PRN pain Q4-6H

REFILLS ___ TIMES   (NO REFILL UNLESS INDICATED)

_____ M.D. _J. Jolter_ M.D.
DISPENSE AS WRITTEN   SUBSTITUTE PERMITTED

MT. HOPE MEDICAL PARK
MY TOWN, USA   555-3591

\#_____   DEA \#_____

PT. NAME _Abby Gee_   DATE _9-10-99_

ADDRESS _____

R̸   Losec 20mg
     Take 1cap before eating QD
                              \#30

REFILLS ___ TIMES   (NO REFILL UNLESS INDICATED)

_C. Jones_____ M.D. _____ M.D.
DISPENSE AS WRITTEN   SUBSTITUTE PERMITTED

2. Review the patient profile given below. Then answer the following questions:
   a. What essential information is missing from this profile? What questions should you ask of the customer to complete the profile?
   b. What allergies and drug reactions does the patient have?
   c. What known medical conditions does the patient have?
   d. What prescription and OTC medications is the patient currently taking?
   e. Should the customer's prescription be filled in a child-resistant container?
   f. Does the customer have prescription insurance? If so, in whose name is this insurance held?

PATIENT PROFILE

Patient Name

Frames   _Ted_   _R._
Last   First   Middle Initial

111 Black Road
Street or PO Box
Gaston   _SC_   _29052_
City   State   Zip

Phone	Date of Birth				Social Security No.
(803) 784 7989	07	28	38	☒ Male ☐ Female	249 00 0012
	Month	Day	Year		

☒ Yes, I would like medication dispensed in a child-resistant container.
☐ No, I do not want medication dispensed in a child-resistant container.

Medication Insurance   Card Holder Name _Ted Frames_
☒ Yes ☐ No   ☒ Card Holder   ☐ Child   ☐ Disabled Dependent
                ☐ Spouse   ☐ Dependent Parent   ☐ Full Time Student

MEDICAL HISTORY

HEALTH

		ALLERGIES AND DRUG REACTIONS
☐ Angina	☐ Epilepsy	☐ No known drug allergies or reactions
☐ Anemia	☐ Glaucoma	
☒ Arthritis	☒ Heart Condition	☒ Aspirin
☐ Asthma	☐ Kidney Disease	☐ Cephalosporins
☐ Blood Clotting Disorders	☐ Liver Disease	☐ Codeine
☐ High Blood Pressure	☐ Lung Disease	☐ Erythromycin
☐ Breast Feeding	☐ Parkinson's Disease	☐ Penicillin
☐ Cancer	☐ Pregnancy	☒ Sulfa Drugs
☐ Diabetes	☐ Ulcers	☐ Tetracyclines
Other Conditions _____		☐ Xanthines
_____		Other Allergies/Reactions _____

Prescription Medication Being Taken
Feldene 20mg
Iseptin 80mg

OTC Medication Currently Being Taken
Nasalcrom

Would You Like Generic Medication Where Possible? ☒ Yes ☐ No

Comments _____

Health information changes periodically. Please notify the pharmacy of any new medications, allergies, drug reactions, or health conditions.
Ted Frames _____ Signature _9-9-99_ Date ☒ I do not wish to provide this information.

167-B

3. Create a diagram of a typical computer system. Label the following parts: the keyboard, the mouse, the central processing unit, the floppy disk drive, the monitor, the printer, and the modem.

4. Determine which of the following is a valid DEA number:

   1234563
   2749122

5. Prepare a label for each prescription given in activity 1, above.

Extemporaneous Compounding

9

Until the emergence of modern, large-scale pharmaceutical manufacturing in the nineteenth century, all medications were prepared (compounded) by individuals from raw pharmaceutical ingredients. In our time, compounding remains an important part of pharmacy practice, and in many states, pharmacy technicians assist in or carry out compounding tasks. Proper compounding requires an intimate knowledge of pharmaceutical equipment and of the techniques for using that equipment properly to weigh, measure, reduce, and combine ingredients.

Learning Objectives

- Define the term *extemporaneous compounding* and describe common situations in which compounding is required
- Enumerate and describe the equipment used for the weighing, measuring, and compounding of pharmaceuticals
- Use the proper technique for weighing pharmaceutical ingredients
- Use the proper technique for measuring liquid volumes
- Explain the common methods used for comminution and blending of pharmaceutical ingredients
- Explain the use of the geometric dilution method
- Explain the processes by which solutions, suspensions, ointments, creams, powders, suppositories, and capsules are prepared

TERMS TO KNOW

Class III prescription balance Two-pan balance used for weighing small amounts of material

Compounding slab, or ointment slab Plate of ground glass used for mixing compounds

Equilibrium The zero point of a balance scale

Extemporaneous compounding The production of medication on demand in an appropriate quantity and dosage form from pharmaceutical ingredients

Forceps Instruments for grasping small objects

Graduate A glass or polypropylene flask used for measuring liquids

Levigation Reduction of particle size of a solid combined with a nonsoluble but miscible liquid

Master formula sheet The ingredients and instructions (i.e., the recipe) for compounding a preparation

THE NEED FOR EXTEMPORANEOUS COMPOUNDING

Extemporaneous compounding is the production of medication on demand in an appropriate quantity and dosage form from pharmaceutical ingredients. In the past, compounding accounted for much of a pharmacist's job. With the emergence of widespread industrial pharmaceutical manufacturing, the need for extemporaneous compounding has decreased, but not to the vanishing point. In fact, on many occasions the pharmacist and his or her assistant, the technician, are called upon to practice this ancient art. Some examples of situations that require extemporaneous compounding include:

1. The prescription calls for unit doses smaller than those that are commercially available, as is sometimes the case with pediatric medications. For example, a prescription might call for 15 mg per unit dose of a medication available only in tablets containing 30 mg of the active ingredient. The pharmacist might thus have to pulverize, or triturate, the tablets, mix the resultant powder with a suitable diluent, and then use the diluted powder to fill 15 mg capsules.

2. A medication normally available in a solid dosage form might have to be prepared in another dosage form, such as a liquid or a suppository, for administration to a patient who cannot or will not swallow the solid form.

3. A medication with an unpleasant taste might have to be prepared in a tasty, masking syrup base to ensure compliance by a pediatric patient.

4. A medication may be available only in commercial forms containing preservatives, colorings, or other materials to

Meniscus The concave (or in some cases, convex) shape of the top of a liquid in a narrow container such as a graduate

Mortar and pestle A device used for grinding and mixing pharmaceutical ingredients, consisting of a bowl (the mortar) and a club-shaped instrument (the pestle)

Parchment paper Special nonabsorbent paper used as a surface on which to do compounding

Pipette A long, thin, calibrated hollow tube used for measurement of small liquid volumes

Punch method A technique for filling capsules

Spatulas Stainless steel, plastic, or hard rubber instruments used for transferring solid pharmaceutical ingredients from one place to another and for various compounding tasks

Spatulation Mixing with a spatula

Trituration Grinding to a fine particle size

Weighing papers Papers used on balance trays to protect the trays from contact with pharmaceutical ingredients

which a patient is allergic, and so an alternative without the unwanted ingredients might need to be prepared.

5. The strength or dosage form called for in the prescription may not be in stock or readily available.

6. A dosage form other than those commercially available may be desired in order to customize the rate of delivery, rate of onset, site of action, or other pharmacokinetic properties of the drug.

7. A non-commercially available medication must be prepared for a veterinary application.

This chapter deals with the extemporaneous compounding of **nonsterile products**, ones compounded without using special aseptic techniques.

EQUIPMENT FOR WEIGHING, MEASURING, AND COMPOUNDING

To carry out a compounding operation, a pharmacist or pharmacy technician makes use of a number of conventional instruments and supplies, as follows:

1. A **Class III prescription balance**, formerly known as a **Class A prescription balance**, is required equipment in every pharmacy (see Figure 9.1). The Class III

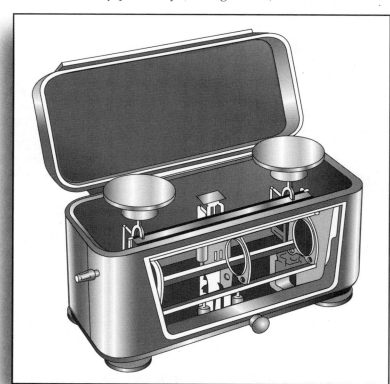

Figure 9.1 Class III prescription balance.

prescription balance is a two-pan balance that can be used for weighing small amounts of material (120 GM or less) and that has a **sensitivity requirement (SR)** of 6 mg. This means that a 6 mg weight will move the indicator on the balance one degree.

2. A **counter balance**, which also has two pans, is used for weighing larger amounts of material, up to about 5 kg (see Figure 9.2). It has a sensitivity requirement of 100 mg. Because of its lesser sensitivity, a counter balance is not used in prescription compounding but rather for tasks such as measuring bulk products, for instance, Epsom salts.

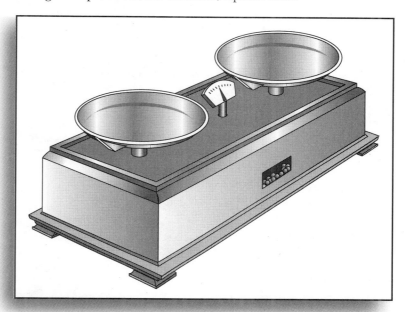

Figure 9.2 Counter balance.

3. Balance measurements are made using sets of standardized pharmaceutical **weights**. Typical weight sets contain both **metric weights** and **apothecaries' weights** (for information about the metric and apothecary measurement systems, see chapter 7). Weights are generally made of polished brass and may be coated with a noncorrosive material such as nickel or chromium. Typical metric sets may contain gram weights of 1, 2, 5, 10, 20, 50, and 100 g, which are conically shaped, with a handle and flattened top. Fractional gram weights (10, 20, 50, 100, 200, and 500 mg, for example) are also available. These are made of aluminum and are usually flat, with one raised edge (see Figure 9.3) to facilitate picking up the weight using forceps. Avoirdupois weights (again, see chapter 7) of 1/32, 1/16, 1/8, 1/4, 1/2, 1, 2, 4, and 8 oz. may also be used. Weights come in a container in which they should be stored when not in use. Care should be taken not to touch or drop a weight or otherwise expose it to damage or contamination.

4. **Forceps** are instruments for grasping small objects. They are provided with weight sets to use for picking up weights and transferring them to and from balances in order to avoid transferring moisture or oil to the weights (see Figure 9.4), thereby changing their weight. Weights should not be transferred using the hands and fingers.

5. **Spatulas** are stainless steel, plastic, or hard rubber instruments used for transferring solid pharmaceutical ingredients to weighing pans and for

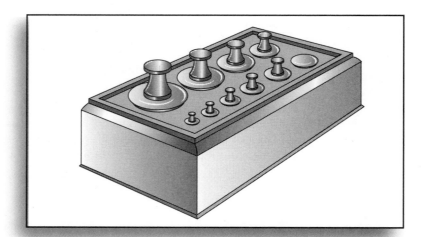

Figure 9.3 Gram and fractional gram metrical weights.

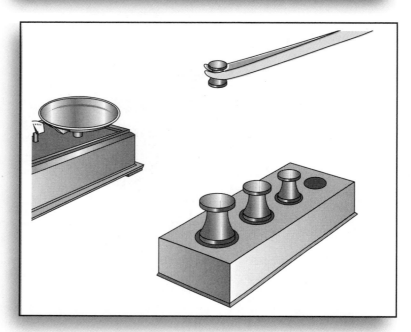

Figure 9.4 Weight being transferred using forceps.

various compounding tasks such as preparing ointments and creams or loosening material from the surfaces of a mortar and pestle (see Figure 9.5). Hard rubber spatulas are used when corrosive materials such as iodine and mercuric salts are handled.

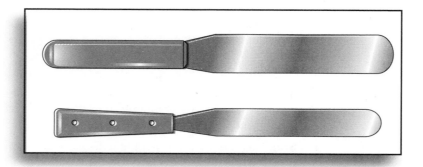

Figure 9.5 Spatulas.

6. **Weighing papers** are placed on balances to avoid contact between pharmaceutical ingredients and the balance tray. Typically, glassine paper is used. Glassine paper is a thin paper coated with nonabsorbent paraffin wax.

7. A **compounding slab**, also known as an **ointment slab**, is a plate made of ground glass that has a flat, hard, nonabsorbent surface ideal for mixing compounds.

8. In lieu of a compounding or ointment slab, compounding may be performed on special nonabsorbent **parchment paper** that is then disposed of after the compounding operation is finished.

9. A **mortar and pestle** are used for grinding and mixing pharmaceutical ingredients (see Figure 9.6). These devices come in glass, porcelain, and Wedgwood varieties. Paradoxically, the coarser the surface of the mortar and pestle, the finer the trituration, or grinding, that can be done. As a result, a coarse-grained **porcelain** or **Wedgwood mortar and pestle** set is used for trituration of crystals, granules, and powders, whereas a **glass mortar and pestle**, with its smooth surface, is preferred for mixing of liquids and semisolid dosage forms. A glass mortar and pestle also has the advantages of being nonporous and nonstaining.

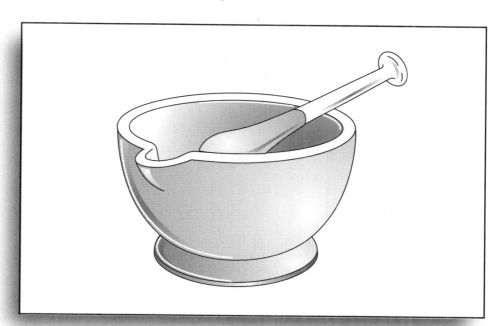

Figure 9.6 Mortar and pestle.

10. **Graduates** are glass or polypropylene flasks used for measuring liquids. They come in two varieties (see Figure 9.7). **Conical graduates** have wide tops and wide bases and taper from the top to the bottom. **Cylindrical graduates**, which are more accurate, have the shape of a uniform column. Both kinds of graduates are available in a wide variety of sizes, ranging from 5 mL to more than 1000 mL. Cylindrical graduates are generally calibrated in metric units (cubic centimeters), whereas conical graduates may be calibrated in both metric and apothecary units or using either one of these two systems.

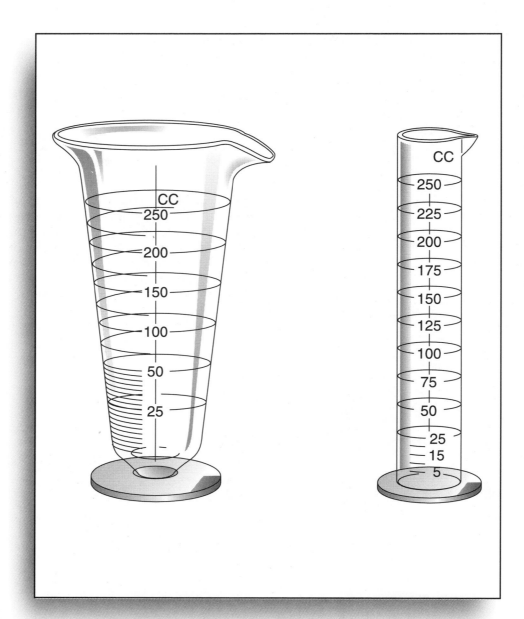

Figure 9.7 Conical (left) and cylindrical (right) graduates.

11. A **pipette** is a long, thin, calibrated hollow tube used for measurement of volumes of liquid less than 1.5 mL. A pipette filler is a device used instead of the mouth for drawing a dangerous solution, such as an acid, into the pipette.

Of course, in addition to the equipment described above, the compounding of a medication requires the necessary ingredients. Figure 9.8 shows an example of a **master formula sheet**, also known as a pharmacy compounding log, listing the ingredients and directions for manufacturing a preparation called "Magic Mouthwash."

MASTER FORMULA SHEET

PRODUCT_____   MTC LOT NUMBER_____

_____

LABEL: Date MFG:
MAGIC MOUTHWASH

Take 1 teaspoon 3 times   STRENGTH:
daily. Swish and
swallow.   QUANTITY MFG:

	MANUFACTURER'S LOT NUMBER	INGREDIENTS	AMOUNT NEEDED	WEIGHED OR MEASURED BY	CHECKED BY
1		Decadron or hydrocortisone	4.5 mg 120.0 mg		
2		Nystatin (Mycostatin)	2,000,000 units		
3		tetracycline	1g		
4		diphenhydramine (Benadryl)	qs to 120mL		
5					
6					
7					
8					

DIRECTIONS FOR MANUFACTURING

1. Draw up, by syringe, 4.5 mg Decadron or 120 mg of hydrocortisone or equivalent steroid.
2. Crush Nystatin tablets and mix with 5 mL sterile water or measure 2,000,000 units of liquid.
3. Measure 1 G of liquid Tetracycline or dissolve tablets or capsules in 5 mL sterile water.
4. Add each ingredient to liquid container and qs with Diphenhydramine to 120 mL.
5. Attach label.

Manufactured by_____
Approved by_____
Date_____

_____

Auxiliary Labeling: SHAKE WELL

_____

Figure 9.8 Master formula sheet.

TECHNIQUE FOR WEIGHING

Chart 9.1 lists the steps for weighing pharmaceutical ingredients:

Chart 9.1	WEIGHING PHARMACEUTICAL INGREDIENTS

1. Place the Class III prescription balance on a secure, level surface, at waist height, where it cannot be easily jarred. Make sure that the balance is locked. Remember, a prescription balance is a delicate instrument and must be handled with caution. The area where the balance is placed should be well lighted and free from drafts, dust, corrosive vapors, or high humidity that might affect the ingredients or the measurements.

2. Unlock the balance and level it to zero (**equilibrium**), front-to-back and back-to-front, using the **leveling screws** at its base. Once this is done, the balance is ready to use. Lock the balance once again, before transferring weight to it.

3. Place weighing papers on the two pans of the balance. These papers should be of roughly the same size and weight. The paper on the left-hand pan of the balance should be folded diagonally, or the edges of the paper should be folded upward, to hold the substance to be weighed. Do not place any materials on the weighing pans without using weighing papers. (Always make sure the balance is locked to prevent accidental damage to the balance, except when it is unlocked, temporarily, to check a measurement. After checking a measurement, the balance should be locked again immediately.)

4. Avoid spilling materials onto the balance. If any materials are spilled on the balance, wipe them off immediately. Do not place materials onto the balance while it is unlocked, as doing so may force the pan down suddenly and cause damage to the instrument.

5. Add the desired weight to the right-hand pan, using forceps to transfer the weight from the weight container.

6. Place an approximate amount of the material to be weighed to the left-hand pan, using a spatula to transfer it.

7. Slowly release the beam using the unlocking device at the front of the balance.

8. If the amount of the substance being weighed is too great or too small, lock the balance again and add or remove material using a spatula.

9. Slowly release the beam using the unlocking device and check for equilibrium.

10. Once a nearly precise amount of material has been transferred to the pan, a very small adjustment upward can be made by placing a small amount of material on the spatula, holding the spatula over the left pan, and lightly tapping the spatula with the forefinger to knock a bit of the substance onto the pan. This is done with the balance unlocked and the balance beam free to move.

TECHNIQUE FOR MEASURING LIQUID VOLUMES

Chart 9.2 lists the steps for measuring liquid volumes:

Chart 9.2

MEASURING LIQUID VOLUMES

1. Choose a graduate with a capacity that equals or very slightly exceeds the total volume of the liquid to be measured. Doing so, for reasons too complex for explanation here, reduces the percentage of error in the measurement. In no case should the volume to be measured be less than 20 percent of the total capacity of the graduate. For example, 10 mL of liquid should not be measured in a graduate exceeding 50 mL in capacity. Again, the closer the total capacity of the graduate to the volume to be measured, the more accurate the measurement will be.

2. Bear in mind that the more narrow the column of liquid in the graduate, the less substantial any reading error will be. Thus a pipette is preferable, for very small volume measurement, to a cylindrical graduate, and a cylindrical graduate is preferable, for larger measurements, to a conical graduate.

3. Pour the liquid to be measured slowly into the graduate, watching the level of the liquid in the graduate as you do so. If the liquid is viscous, or thick, attempt to pour it toward the center of the graduate to avoid having some of the liquid cling to the sides.

4. Wait for liquid clinging to the sides of the graduate to settle before taking a measurement.

5. Measure the level of the liquid at eye level. Bear in mind that most commonly the upper surface of the liquid will be a **meniscus**, or moon-shaped body, that is slightly **concave**, or bowed inward toward the center (see Figure 9.9). In other words, the level of the liquid will be slightly higher at the edges. Therefore, do not measure the level by looking down on the graduate. Instead, measure by placing the eyes at the level of the liquid. Read the level of the liquid at the *bottom* of the meniscus.

6. When pouring the liquid out of the graduate, allow ample time for all of the liquid to drain. Bear in mind that depending on the viscosity of the liquid, more or less will cling to the sides of the graduate. For a particularly viscous liquid, some compensation or adjustment for this clinging may have to be made.

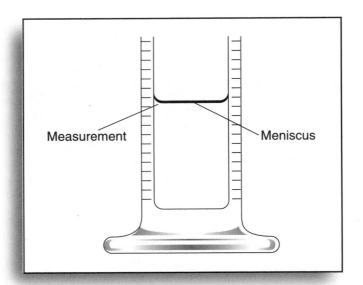

Figure 9.9 Liquid in a narrow column usually forms a concave meniscus. Measurements should be taken at the bottom of the concavity.

Measurement

Meniscus

COMMINUTION AND BLENDING OF DRUGS

Comminution is the act of reducing a substance to small, fine particles. **Blending** is the act of combining two substances. Techniques for comminution and blending include trituration, levigation, pulverization by intervention, spatulation, sifting, and tumbling. **Trituration** is the process of rubbing, grinding, or pulverizing a substance to create fine particles, generally by means of a mortar and pestle. A rapid motion with minimal pressure provides the best results. Other forms of comminution include levigation and pulverization by intervention. **Levigation** is typically used when reducing the particle size of a solid during the preparation of an ointment. A paste is formed of a solid material and a tiny amount of a liquid levigating agent, such as castor oil or mineral oil, that is **miscible**, or mixable, with the solid but in which the solid is not soluble. The paste is then triturated to reduce the particle size and added to the ointment base. The levigating agent becomes part of the final product.

Pulverization by intervention is the process of reducing the size of particles in a solid with the aid of an additional material in which the substance is soluble—a volatile solvent such as camphor and alcohol or iodine and ether. The solvent is added. The mixture is triturated. The solvent is then permitted to evaporate and so does not become part of the final product. **Spatulation** is the process of combining substances by means of a spatula, generally on an ointment tile. **Sifting**, like the sifting of flour in baking, can be used to blend or combine powders. Powders can also be combined by **tumbling**—placing the powders into a bag or container and shaking it.

Using a Mortar and Pestle

As was indicated earlier in this chapter, a porcelain mortar and pestle set is used to produce fine triturations. A glass mortar and pestle, which is nonporous and nonstaining, is used for simple mixing of ingredients.

Often a mortar and pestle are used to combine more than one drug. To combine drugs in a mortar and pestle, you can use the **geometric dilution method**. Place the most potent ingredient, which will most likely be the ingredient that occurs in the smallest amount, into the mortar first. Then add an equal amount of the next most potent ingredient and mix well. Continue in this manner, adding, each time, an amount equal to the amount in the mortar, until successively larger amounts of all the ingredients are added. Then add any excess amount of any ingredient and mix well.

Some Examples of Compounding

Thorough instruction in the complex art of extemporaneous compounding is beyond the scope of this book. Refer to the standard reference work on the subject, *Remington's Pharmaceutical Sciences: The Science and Practice of Pharmacy*. 18th ed. Easton, PA: MacK Publishing, 1990, and to the World Wide Web sites of the International Academy of Compounding Pharmacists at http://www.compassnet.com/~iacp/index.htm, and Secundum Artem: Current and Practical Compounding Information for the Pharmacist at http://www.paddocklabs.com/secundum/secarndx.html. In practice, a pharmacy technician will, if the laws of the state allow, assist in compounding only after instruction by a pharmacist in specific techniques for specific preparations, and compounding will be done in accordance with instructions in a master formula sheet (see Figure 9.9). Of course, any compounding tasks undertaken by the technician must, in any case, be supervised and checked by the pharmacist. That said, the following are some examples of compounding tasks:

Preparation of Solutions

A **solution** is a liquid dosage form in which active ingredients are dissolved in a liquid vehicle. The vehicle that makes up the greater part of a solution is known as a **solvent**. An ingredient dissolved in a solution is known as a **solute.** Solutions may be aqueous, alcoholic, or hydroalcoholic. Solutions are prepared by dissolving the solute in the liquid solvent or by combining or diluting existing solutions. Careful measurement is, of course, important for solutions, as it is for all extemporaneous compounding. Colorings or flavoring agents may be added to solutions.

When mixing solids and liquids, it is important to remember that reducing the particle size of the solid through trituration or gently heating the liquid (if the liquid is stable, or nonvolatile) will generally make the solid dissolve faster, more uniformly, and with less **precipitation**, or clinging together of the solute into particles of unacceptably large size. When mixing two liquids, a possible precipitation of solutes within the liquids can sometimes be avoided by making each portion as dilute as possible before mixing the liquids together.

Preparation of Suspensions

In a **suspension**, as opposed to a solution, the active ingredient is not dissolved in the liquid vehicle but rather is dispersed throughout it. An obvious problem with suspensions is the tendency of the active ingredient to settle. To avoid settling of the insoluble drug, a suspending agent is sometimes added. Such suspending agents include tragacanth, acacia, carboxymethylcellulose (CMC), bentonite, and Cab-O-Sil. The point at which the suspending agent is added in the mixing procedure can be crucial. Therefore, the technician must always remember to add the ingredients in the proper order, according to the master formula sheet. Regardless of their apparent stability, all suspensions should be dispensed with an auxiliary label reading "Shake Well."

Preparation of Ointments and Creams

Ointments, or **unguents**, and **creams** are semisolid dosage forms meant for topical application. Many commercially unavailable pediatric suspensions can be extemporaneously prepared in the pharmacy from adult tablets or capsules. In addition, dermatological therapies may call for combining existing ointments or creams. Most ointments and creams are prepared via mechanical incorporation of materials via levigation or via mixing in a mortar and pestle. Levigation involves forming a paste containing a small amount of liquid, generally using a spatula and an ointment slab, prior to addition to the base of the ointment or cream. In some cases, the dry ingredients of an ointment or cream may have to be triturated, or reduced to a fine powder, in a mortar and pestle before being added to the ointment or cream base. When placing a powder into an ointment, it is important to add the powder in small amounts, constantly working the mixture with the spatula or pestle to reduce particle size and to obtain a smooth, nongritty product. When an ointment slab and spatula are used, the edge of the spatula should press against the slab to provide a shearing force, which allows for a smoother product.

Preparation of Powders

Spatulation, or blending with a spatula, is used for small amounts of powder having a uniform and desired particle size and density. **Trituration** is used when a potent drug is mixed with a diluent. At first equal amounts of the potent drug and the diluent are triturated with a mortar and pestle. When these are thoroughly mixed, more of the diluent is added, equal to the amount already in the mortar. This process is continued until all of the diluent is incorporated. **Tumbling** is used to combine powders that have little or no toxic potential. The powders to be combined are placed in a bag or in a wide-mouthed container and shaken well.

Preparation of Suppositories

Suppositories are solid dosage forms that are inserted into bodily orifices, generally the rectum or the vagina or, less commonly, the urethra. They are composed of one or more active ingredients placed into a base, such as cocoa butter, hydrogenated vegetable oils, or glycerinated gelatin, that melts or dissolves when exposed to body heat and fluids. The preparation of suppositories involves melting the base material, adding the active ingredient(s), pouring the resultant liquid into a mold, and then chilling the mold immediately to solidify the suppository before the suspended ingredients have time to settle.

Preparation and Filling of Capsules

A **capsule** is a solid dosage form consisting of a gelatin shell that encloses the medicinal preparation, which may be a powder, granules, a liquid, or some combination thereof. Extemporaneous compounding of ingredients for capsules is often done to provide unusual dosage forms, such as dosage forms containing less of an active ingredient than is readily available in commercial tablets or capsules. When hand filling a capsule with powder, a pharmacist generally uses the **punch method**. First, the number of capsules to be filled is counted out. Then, the powder is placed on a clean surface of paper, porcelain, or glass and formed into a cake with a spatula. The cake should be approximately 1/4 to 1/3 the height of the capsule body. The body of the capsule is then punched into the cake repeatedly until the capsule is full. The cap is then placed snugly over the body. Granules are generally poured into the capsule body from a piece of paper. Sometimes, hand-operated capsule filling machines are used.

Labeling, Record Keeping, and Cleanup

After the compounding operation, the product must be labeled with a prescription label containing all information required by the governing laws and regulations of the state in which the compounding is done. For more information on proper labeling, see chapter 8. The ingredients of the compound and the amounts of these ingredients should be clearly stated on the label, and in lieu of an expiration date from a manufacturer, the date of the compounding should also appear on the label. A careful record of the compounding operation, including ingredients and amounts of ingredients used, the preparer of the compound, and the name of the supervising pharmacist should be kept. Master formula sheets, such as the one shown in Figure 9.8, p. 177, provide a means for keeping such a record.

Once the compounding operation is finished, equipment and the work area should be thoroughly cleaned, and ingredients should be returned to their proper places in storage. The prescription balance, when not in use, should be covered, and weights must be placed back in their original container.

chapter summary

Extemporaneous compounding, once the major source of medicines, is still used today to prepare medications in strengths, combinations, or dosage forms not commercially available. Instruments for extemporaneous compounding include the Class III prescription balance, weights, forceps, spatulas, weighing papers, the compounding or ointment slab, parchment paper, the mortar and pestle, graduates, and pipettes. Mortars and pestles come in glass, Wedgwood, and porcelain varieties. Graduates come in conical and cylindrical shapes, the latter being the more accurate.

When weighing pharmaceutical ingredients, one must take precautions to ensure that no damage is done to the delicate prescription balance, which is kept locked except when a measurement is taken. With the balance locked, the desired weight is placed onto the right pan of the balance. Then, amounts of the substance to be weighed are placed onto the left pan, and the balance is unlocked to check for equilibrium. The balance is then relocked, and substance is added or removed. Repeat this process until the balance has a reading of zero, indicating an equilibrium between the weight and the drug substance. When measuring liquid volumes, choose a graduate as close as possible in capacity to the volume of liquid to be measured and measure at eye level from the bottom of the meniscus, the concavity at the top of the column of liquid. When combining dry ingredients, one generally uses the geometric dilution method.

Extemporaneous compounding is an art to be learned under the tutelage of an experienced pharmacist and to be practiced according to formulas given on master formula sheets. Procedures vary for preparing the many kinds of extemporaneous compounds, such as solutions, suspensions, ointments, creams, powders, suppositories, and capsules.

chapter review

Knowledge Inventory

1. A large amount of material, such as 2 kg of Epsom salts, would be weighed using a
   a. Class III prescription balance
   b. Class A prescription balance
   c. counter balance
   d. any of the above

2. Two pharmaceutical ingredients are combined, one a solid and the other a soluble, volatile liquid. The mixture is pulverized to reduce the particle size of the solid, and the liquid is allowed to evaporate in a process known as
   a. levigation
   b. trituration
   c. spatulation
   d. pulverization by intervention

3. An alternative to the ointment slab is
    a. weighing paper
    b. parchment paper
    c. a graduate
    d. a pipette

4. A prescription balance is unlocked, temporarily, when the technician
    a. adds weighing papers to the trays
    b. adds pharmaceutical ingredients to the trays
    c. moves the balance from one place to another
    d. checks a measurement

5. When measuring the amount of liquid in a graduate, one should place the eyes at the level of the liquid and measure the level of the meniscus from the
    a. top
    b. bottom
    c. back
    d. front

6. When using the geometric dilution method, the most potent ingredient, usually the one that occurs in the smallest amount, is placed into the mortar
    a. half at the beginning and half at the end
    b. in stages throughout the compounding process
    c. last
    d. first

7. An ingredient dissolved in a solution is known as a
    a. suspension
    b. precipitate
    c. solute
    d. solvent

8. A suppository mold is chilled immediately after filling to
    a. solidify the compound before its volatile components evaporate
    b. reduce the possibility of spoilage
    c. prevent contamination of the compound
    d. solidify the compound before suspended ingredients have time to settle

9. The punch method is used for filling
    a. hypodermics
    b. capsules
    c. graduates
    d. unit dose containers

10. An appropriate auxiliary label for a suspension is
    a. Take with food.
    b. For topical use only. Do not swallow.
    c. Shake well before using.
    d. May cause drowsiness.

Pharmacy in Practice

1. Practice using a Class III prescription balance and a mortar and pestle to prepare the following amounts of ingredients:
   a. 2.75 g of ground cinnamon
   b. 8.5 g of sugar
   c. 75 g of ground nutmeg
   d. 1.5 g of allspice
   e. 2.5 g of triturated anise seed or clove

   Combine the ingredients and use the punch method to fill capsules with this "pumpkin pie spice" compound.

2. Prepare the following simple syrup:

   Sucrose   850 g
   Water qs ad 1000 mL

   a. Measure 500 mL tap water.
   b. Place water in pan and bring to boil.
   c. Measure sucrose (granular sugar).
   d. Add sucrose to boiling water.
   e. Let pan cool slightly.
   f. Pour into liter bottle.
   g. Label: Simple syrup, USP
      Expires in 6 months
      Exp:
      *Keep in refrigerator

3. Visit the Web site for Secundum Artem: Current and Practical Compounding Information for the Pharmacist at http://www.paddocklabs.com/secundum/secarndx.html. Read one of the articles posted on this site and based upon that article, write, in your own words, directions for compounding ointments, topical antibiotics, oral suspensions, suppositories, emulsions, troches, capsules, or gels.

Human Relations and Communications

In addition to being an important part of the healthcare system, the community or retail pharmacy is also a place of business, and the technician must take on customer service responsibilities similar to those appropriate in any retail setting. This chapter begins by noting a shift that has occurred, recently, in the orientation of retail merchandisers away from the mass merchandising model and back to the customer service model. It then explains some important aspects of providing first-rate customer service.

Learning Objectives

- Explain the role of the pharmacy technician as a member of the customer care team in a retail pharmacy
- State the primary rule of retail merchandising and explain its corollaries
- Explain the appropriate responses to rude behavior on the part of others in a workplace situation
- Define discrimination and harassment and explain the proper procedures for dealing with these
- Provide guidelines for proper use of the telephone in a retail pharmacy

TERMS TO KNOW

Appearance The overall look that an employee presents on the job

Attitude The overall emotional stance that a worker adopts toward his or her job duties, customers, employer, and coworkers

Clinical pharmacy Those aspects of pharmacy that are directly related to therapeutics; in particular, the provision by the pharmacist of information and counseling regarding medications

Discrimination Preferential treatment or mistreatment

Harassment Any action that renders the work environment inhospitable, especially the act of subjecting a coworker or subordinate to unwanted sexual advances, banter, or innuendo

Personal service Attention to the individual needs of customers

Primary rule of merchandising The idea that at all times, an employee in a merchandising operation is representing the company to the customer

PERSONAL SERVICE IN THE CONTEMPORARY COMMUNITY PHARMACY

As you read in chapter 1, since the Millis Report in 1975, the pharmacy profession has undergone an extensive self-analysis and reevaluation of its duties and goals. The upshot of this reexamination of the profession has been an increased emphasis on **clinical pharmacy**, the provision by the pharmacist of information and counseling regarding medications. It is now almost universally recognized that the pharmacist is far more than a dispenser of drugs, that he or she has the following equally important duties:

1. to make certain that a given medication will not be harmful to a patient given that patient's medical and prescription history

2. to identify any known allergies, drug interactions, or other contraindications for a given prescription

3. to ensure that a patient understands what medication he or she is taking, why he or she is taking it, how it should be taken, and when it should be taken

Just as the pharmacist increasingly plays a clinical role, so the pharmacy technician increasingly is expected to be much more than simply an operator of cash registers, a stock person, and an all-around pharmacy gofer. Instead, the technician is viewed, today, as an important part of the customer service team within the pharmacy. In the 1960s and 1970s, at the height of the mass merchandising era, customers grew used to large, impersonal supermarkets, department stores, and pharmacy superstores, with their numbered rows of merchandise and automated, bar-coded checkout stations. In the 1980s, retail merchandisers began to realize that the mass merchandising model adopted in the 1960s was terribly flawed. Customers missed the days of **personal service**—attention to individual customer needs—associated with the small, independent neighborhood retail operations of the past. For this reason, many of the large department store chains reorganized their operations to create separate small operational entities, known as boutiques, within their larger stores. They also began extensive training programs to improve the quality of customer service. In pharmacy, as well, a new and welcome emphasis on personal service has returned.

One mass marketing research firm recently conducted an experiment involving bank tellers. In the experiment, one group of tellers was instructed to lightly touch customers on the hand or wrist at some point during each teller transaction. A second control group was instructed to carry out transactions as usual, without this "personal touch." Exit surveys of customer satisfaction were then conducted, with dramatic results. Though largely unaware that they had been touched during their teller transactions, those customers who had been touched reported a 40 percent higher satisfaction rate with the overall quality of service of their banks. The lesson to be learned from this research is not that one should make a habit of touching customers. Indeed, touching should probably be avoided, in most cases, especially when the customer is of a different gender. However, it is clear that a little personal attention goes a long way. A courteous tone of voice, a smile, a bit of assistance finding merchandise or holding a door can go a long way toward making customers think of the pharmacy in which you work as a pleasant place in which to shop.

Attitude and Appearance

Attitude is the overall emotional stance a worker adopts toward his or her job duties, customers, employer, and coworkers. **Appearance** is the overall look an employee has on the job, including his or her dress and grooming. Pharmacy technicians often conduct their jobs unobtrusively—behind the scenes, as it were—stocking items in the pharmacy area, retrieving stock for compounding operations, maintaining records, filling bottles, cleaning up, and so on. It's easy, when one's immediate task is not customer-oriented, to forget the **primary rule of retail merchandising**, which is this:

> **At all times, you are representing your company to the customer.**

This rule has a number of corollaries, as follows:

1. **Always dress and groom yourself neatly.** Customers hope for the highest degree of cleanliness and professionalism from their pharmacy. After all, they are entrusting their health or the health of their loved ones to the operation for which you work. A pharmacy employee with unkempt hair or a uniform smock thrown over a pair of jeans makes a bad impression. The customer may not directly register these facts and yet goes away with a vague impression that the pharmacy is not a professional operation.

2. **Always keep one eye on your work and another on your customers.** Modern community pharmacies are often large, complex places. When customers enter, the first thing they often do is stand in the middle of the floor, looking around, a bit confused, for the part of the store where the product they seek is to be found. A good pharmacy employee thus

continually scans the area around him or her, looking for customers who are lost, confused, or need help. (Consider the following example: Imagine that you are in a diner and want some ketchup for your french fries. Three or four times, a waiter passes your table, but each time, the waiter is concentrating on his or her immediate concern: taking a meal or a check to another table, for example. In such a situation, you rapidly become frustrated and, perhaps, angry. The same principle—keep your eye on the customer—applies to any retail operation.)

3. **Know the layout of your pharmacy and the locations of merchandise.** Few things are as frustrating to a customer as asking for help and getting an insufficient or inaccurate response. Often a customer is uncertain about what he or she is looking for or whom to ask for help. Once you spot that uncertain look on a customer's face, ask, in a courteous tone of voice, "May I help you?" Then, after the customer's response, you may have to ask some clarifying questions. If, for example, the customer is looking for aspirin, he or she may need to know not only where over-the-counter analgesic products are located in the store but also may need some help locating an analgesic specific to his or her needs—a liquid form for children, for example, or an enteric-coated form for persons whose stomachs cannot tolerate conventional analgesic dosage forms. If possible, escort the customer to the place where the merchandise is located and help him or her to find it.

4. **Respect the customer's privacy and sense of decorum.** Pharmacies sell many products related to private bodily functions and conditions—condoms and other contraceptives, feminine hygiene and menstrual products, suppositories, hemorrhoid remedies, enemas, adult diapers, catheters, bed pans, scabicides, and so on. Often customers find asking about such products embarrassing and have to get up the nerve to make a request for assistance. If you find discussing such matters embarrassing, get over it. As a pharmacy employee, you are part of the healthcare profession, and you must adopt a helpful, no-nonsense, professional attitude toward the body and its functions. Responding to an inquiry about such a product with promptness, courtesy, respect, and a certain degree of nonchalance often relieves your customer's embarrassment and demonstrates your professionalism. Speak in a clear voice, but not so loudly that other customers or employees will be privy to your private interchange with the customer.

5. **Smile.** The goodwill you communicate will come back to you.

6. **Use common courtesies.** In every interaction with a customer, use courteous words and phrases. Begin and end interactions, even the briefest ones, with ceremonial courtesies such as "Good afternoon" and "Have a nice day." In between, practice courteous speech, as demonstrated in these examples:

Poor: What do you want?

Better: May I help you?

Poor: It's over there.

Better: That's in aisle three. Follow me, and I'll show you.

Poor: It's $8.39.

Better: That will be $8.39 please.

7. **Explain necessary interactions to the customer.** If, for example, you are stationed at a pharmacy window and need information for the customer's patient profile, let the customer know why you need the information. Tell the customer, for example, "I need some information for your prescription profile so that we can serve you better. May I ask you a few questions? Thank you. What is your full name and address?"

8. **Be sensitive to language differences and difficulties.** Often pharmacies are located in areas catering to a diverse customer base. If you cannot understand a customer because of a language difference, do not speak louder or in an exaggeratedly slow and punctuated manner. If necessary, apologize courteously for your language deficiency and find another store employee who can communicate in the customer's native tongue.

9. **Follow the policies and procedures of your pharmacy.** Many pharmacies, especially within large retail chains, have policies and procedures manuals covering a wide range of activities. Make sure you are thoroughly familiar with these policies and procedures and abide by them in your routine interactions.

10. **Avoid dispensing medical or pharmaceutical advice.** Remember that you are not trained or licensed to advise customers with regard to medications and their use. Use common sense to determine whether a given query from a customer exceeds the bounds of common knowledge. As a rule of thumb, questions involving the proper administration, uses, or effects of a medication, whether prescription or over-the-counter, should be referred to a pharmacist. Do not be afraid of admitting your lack of expertise. Customers will appreciate that you are concerned enough to make sure they receive accurate information. When a question deals with the effects or administration of a medication, ask the customer to wait for a moment while you get someone who can provide a professional answer to the question. In some instances technicians may provide medication-related information when providing refills and when directed to do so by a pharmacist. Of course, a technician should use common sense with regard to providing customers with information. In the case of over-the-counter medications, sometimes customers simply need basic information that is readily available on the OTC packaging. For example, a customer might ask what an analgesic is, when an enteric-coated analgesic is appropriate, which alternative brands are available, and other such routine questions. Such questions can be safely answered without referring the customer to the pharmacist.

Interprofessional Relations

In the course of their duties, pharmacy technicians encounter, personally or on the telephone, many other professionals and paraprofessionals, including pharmacists, doctors, nurses, administrators, store managers, sales representatives, insurance personnel, and other technicians. Health care is a demanding industry, often requiring long hours and involving stressful, emergency situations. As a result, practitioners in the industry often suffer from fatigue and stress. Sometimes, this stress shows itself in unintentionally rude behavior. As a matter of course, busy healthcare professionals sometimes, unfortunately, speak to subordinates as though they were not whole, complete human beings but rather part of the machine that must be kept turning to get the job done. Remember that the degree to which you maintain your courtesy and respect, even in the face of rudeness, is a measure of your professionalism. Return rudeness with kindness, and you will often find that, immediately or over time, the quality of your interactions improve. If you answer the telephone and someone barks a command at you, demonstrate your professionalism by attending to the content of the message and not to its tone. Always refer to physicians using the title "Doctor." Refer to a supervising pharmacist, as well, as "Doctor," as a sign of respect for his or her professional attainment in having achieved the Pharmacy Doctorate degree. Refer to other supervisors using appropriate courtesy titles such as "Sir" or "Madam." When customers hear the technician refer to the pharmacist as "Doctor," this raises customers' level of respect not only for the pharmacist but also for the technician, who is the doctor's assistant. A degree of formality is always in order until you are requested to use more informal modes of address.

OTHER ASPECTS OF PROFESSIONALISM: HARASSMENT AND DISPUTES

As with any job, you should bear in mind that **discrimination** (preferential treatment or mistreatment) and **harassment** (mistreatment, sexual or otherwise) are not only unethical but against the law. If you find yourself the object of discrimination or harassment, first try to resolve the issue with the person or persons involved. Do your best to maintain your composure and to express your discomfort calmly and rationally. If discrimination or harassment persists, you may need to discuss the matter with a supervisor and make inquiries regarding the discrimination and harassment laws and procedures in your state. All businesses, pharmacies included, are required by law to post information related to workplace discrimination and harassment. Bear in mind that in the past, sexual harassment was defined as unwanted physical contact or as the act of making sexual conduct a condition for advancement, preferential treatment, or other work-related outcomes. Recently, however, the Supreme Court redefined sexual harassment more generally as the creation of an unpleasant or uncomfortable work environment through sexual action, innuendo, or related means. Know, therefore, that you do not have to put up with off-color jokes if you do not wish to hear them, and be aware that you must not contribute in any way to creating an environment that is uncomfortable for your coworkers. One person's innocent remark, made in a spirit of fun, can be another person's grounds for a legal action. Generally speaking, romantic or sexual involvements with coworkers, and especially with coworkers in supervisory or subordinate positions, is inadvisable.

Disputes involving duties, hours, pay, and other matters are common occurrences in occupations of all kinds. If possible, try to resolve work-related disputes through rational, calm discussion with the parties involved. Most large pharmacies, including chain stores and institutional pharmacies, will have personnel policy manuals detailing procedures for resolving disputes.

Guidelines for Telephone Use

Customers and health-care professionals often contact pharmacies by telephone. The following are some guidelines for using the telephone properly:

1. Always begin and end the conversation with a conventional courtesy, such as "Good morning" and "Thank you for calling."

2. When you answer the phone, identify yourself and the pharmacy, as follows:

    "Good morning. This is Arden Community Pharmacy. My name is Andrea. How may I help you?"

3. If the caller is calling in a prescription, you may need to turn over the phone to a licensed pharmacist. In most states technicians are not allowed by law to take prescriptions over the telephone. However, you should confirm the regulations for the state in which you are employed.

4. If the caller has questions about the administration or effects of a medication or about a medical condition, adverse reaction, or adverse interaction, refer the call to a licensed pharmacist.

5. Make sure that any information you provide is accurate. Giving incorrect directions to a customer in need of a prescription can be a life-threatening mistake.

6. Depending on the regulations in your state and the procedures of your pharmacy, you may be authorized to handle prescription transfers or to provide information related to prescription refills. Follow the procedures outlined by your supervising pharmacist.

7. If a customer is calling about a medical emergency or a prescription error, refer the call to your supervising pharmacist.

chapter summary

In recent years, many community pharmacies have made a concerted attempt to return to the spirit, if not the physical reality, of the small, customer-oriented neighborhood pharmacy of the past. An important part of this trend is an increased emphasis on personal service—attention to the needs of individual customers. A customer orientation on the part of the technician is in order at all times. Customer orientation involves dressing and grooming oneself neatly, maintaining a constant lookout for customers in need of assistance, knowing the layout of the store and the locations of its merchandise, respecting the customer's sense of privacy and decorum, smiling and using courteous language, providing explanations as necessary to customers, being sensitive to language differences, following established policies and procedures, and referring requests for medical or pharmaceutical advice to competent professionals. At all times, it is important to maintain courteous, respectful relationships with other professionals and paraprofessionals. A pharmacy is a professional workplace. Therefore, a no-tolerance policy with regard to discrimination and harassment is in order. Common courtesy should be used in all telephone communications and conversations regarding prescriptions, medical or pharmaceutical emergencies, medication administration and effects, and adverse reactions, and adverse interactions should be referred to a supervising pharmacist.

chapter review

Knowledge Inventory

1. The provision by the pharmacist of information and counseling regarding medications is the primary concern of
   a. contemporary pharmacy
   b. pharmacology
   c. pharmacognosy
   d. clinical pharmacy

2. In the 1980s, retail merchandisers began to rethink their previous
   a. personal service merchandising model
   b. mass merchandising model
   c. customer service model
   d. retail service model

3. The emotional stance that a worker adopts toward his or her job duties is called
   a. tone
   b. mood
   c. attitude
   d. appearance

4. The primary rule of retail merchandising is
   a. Always dress and groom yourself neatly.
   b. Respect the customer's privacy and sense of decorum.
   c. Explain necessary interactions to the customer.
   d. At all times, you are representing your company to the customer.

5. *Decorum* means
   a. proper or polite behavior, or behavior that is in good taste
   b. dissatisfaction with services provided
   c. lack of understanding of the options available
   d. ability to negotiate for goods and services

6. A pharmacy technician should never
   a. waste time walking a customer across the store to show him or her the location of an item on the shelves
   b. dispense advice regarding the use of a medication
   c. attempt to speak to a customer in the customer's native language
   d. take a written prescription from a customer

7. When asking a customer for information for the patient profile, the pharmacy technician should explain
   a. how and when the prescription should be administered
   b. why the pharmacy needs this information
   c. the parts of the label of the prescription
   d. the differences between the payment policies of various third-party insurance providers

8. Preferential treatment or mistreatment based upon race, gender, age, or other criteria is known as
   a. harassment
   b. discrimination
   c. innuendo
   d. decorum

9. When answering a drugstore telephone, a person should identify himself or herself and the name of the
   a. supervising pharmacist
   b. pharmacy
   c. customer
   d. prescribing physician

10. When customers first enter a pharmacy, the first thing they typically do is
    a. look around to orient themselves
    b. head for the cashier
    c. head for the Rx area
    d. seek out a store employee to ask for information

Pharmacy in Practice

1. Identify four students to play the following roles involving typical pharmacy scenarios: a customer calling to find out when a prescription will be ready, a physician calling in a prescription, a pharmacy technician, and a supervising pharmacist. Act out for other students in the class some typical telephone calls to the pharmacy. After each call, have other students in the class critique what was said and done by the technician taking the telephone call.

2. Accurate communication in a pharmacy is essential. Try this experiment: Have one student in the class choose a sentence at random from this chapter and write the sentence down on a piece of paper. Then have the student whisper the sentence into the ear of another student sitting next to him or her. Have this student whisper the sentence into the ear of another

student, and so on, until the sentence has made the round of all the students in the class. Compare the final version of the sentence with the original version. Discuss what causes sentences to be miscommunicated and what steps can be taken to avoid such miscommunication.

3. Conduct a role-play activity with other students in which a person who is obviously embarrassed asks a store employee for an over-the-counter product related to bodily functions. After each scenario is played out, critique the technician's response. Discuss the kinds of problems that can arise in such situations and how they might be avoided.

4. Working in a small group, recall your own experiences visiting drugstores or pharmacies. Make a list of problems you have encountered in pharmacies (examples: slow service, having no comfortable place in which to wait while a prescriptions is being filled, difficulty in finding an item, etc). As a group, brainstorm some ways to solve such problems and to improve customer service.

5. Imagine you are a drugstore manager who operates a 24-hour pharmacy in a big-city, urban neighborhood with the following demographics:

10 % Vietnamese-speaking customers

26 % Spanish-speaking customers

16 % Korean-speaking customers

32 % English-speaking customers

16 % customers who speak other languages (Thai, Laotian, Hmong, Russian, Latvian, Polish, etc.)

With other students, brainstorm a list of steps you might need to take to meet the needs of the customers whom you serve.

6. With other students in a small group, brainstorm a list of positive experiences you have had in retail merchandising establishments of all kinds. Based on this list, draw up a list of recommendations for making a customer's experience in a retail establishment a positive one.

Hospital and Institutional Pharmacy Practice

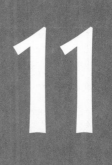

11

Many of the functions carried out by community or retail pharmacies are also carried out in hospital or institutional settings. However, such settings do have some unique functions and procedures. Of particular importance to pharmacy operations in hospital and institutional settings are use of aseptic technique, preparation of parenterals, proper handling of hazardous agents, and understanding unit-dose, floorstock, and repackaging systems. This chapter treats each of these subjects.

Learning Objectives

- Understand the origins and purpose of the hospital formulary
- List a few common universal precautions to avoid contamination
- Describe proper procedures for handling and disposal of hazardous agents
- Explain the germ theory of disease—the role of pathogenic organisms in causing disease
- Distinguish among viruses, bacteria, fungi, and protozoa
- Describe proper aseptic technique, including the use of laminar, horizontal, and vertical flow hoods
- Describe the equipment and procedures used in preparing parenterals
- Describe unit-dose and floorstock distribution systems
- Explain the proper procedure for repackaging of medications
- Describe the types of materials stored in a drug information center

TERMS TO KNOW

Antineoplastic drug Drug that attacks and destroys newly formed cells, used in the treatment of cancer

Asepsis Absence of disease-causing microorganisms

Aseptic technique Manipulation of sterile products and sterile devices in such a way as to maintain their sterility

Bacteria One-celled organisms, some of which are disease-causing, that are spherical (cocci), rodlike (bacilli), or spiral (spirilla) in shape

Cytotoxic materials Ones that are poisonous to cells

Drug usage evaluation Ongoing study of drug usage patterns and costs within a hospital or other institution

Formulary The official list of medications approved for use in an institution

THE FUNCTIONS OF THE HOSPITAL OR INSTITUTIONAL PHARMACY

As you learned in chapter 1, pharmacists and pharmacy technicians work in a wide variety of settings beyond the community pharmacy. One of the most common of these settings is the hospital or institutional pharmacy. Of course, some similarities exist between the functions of a hospital pharmacy and those of a community pharmacy. Some functions carried out by both kinds of pharmacy include:

1. maintaining drug treatment records

2. ordering and stocking medications and medical supplies

3. repackaging medications

4. dispensing medications

5. providing information about the proper use of medications

6. collecting and evaluating information about adverse drug reactions and interactions

7. preparing medications in various dosage forms for dispensing

Some functions either unique to or most commonly performed in a hospital or institutional setting are as follows:

1. preparing and maintaining a **formulary**, or list of drugs used by the hospital or institution, and conducting drug usage evaluations

2. following proper procedures, known as **universal precautions**, to guard against infection by disease-causing microorganisms, or pathogens, in blood or bodily fluids

3. preparing, using aseptic techniques, sterile parenteral solutions, such as bolus or intravenous solutions (IVs), for various purposes, such as delivery of medications or nutrition. Pharmacists and technicians in other work settings, such as home health care, also prepare such solutions.

4. following proper procedures to ensure that hazardous agents, such as drugs and other chemicals, are handled and disposed of properly

5. filling medication orders (as opposed to prescriptions) and preparing, on a routine basis, 24-hour supplies of patient medications in unit-dose form. A **unit dose** is an amount and dosage form appropriate for a single administration to a patient.

6. stocking nursing stations with medications and supplies

7. delivering medications to patients' rooms

8. maintaining an institutional drug information center and providing drug information to the other healthcare professionals in the institution

9. educating and counseling patients about their drug therapies, including both inpatient and outpatient counseling (An **inpatient** is one who stays in the institution overnight for some period of time. An **outpatient** is one who comes to the institution for treatment but then returns home.)

10. participating in clinical drug investigations and research

11. providing in-service drug-related education

12. auditing for quality assurance

13. providing expert consultations in such areas as **pediatric pharmacology** (the effects of drugs on babies and children) and **pharmacokinetics** (the absorption, distribution, and elimination of drugs by the body)

THE HOSPITAL FORMULARY

Since ancient times, one of the functions of the healer was to compile a list of medications (such as plants and mineral substances) that are **efficacious**, or useful, for treating particular conditions. Such a list is known as a formulary. One of the earliest known formularies was listed in the *Papyrus Ebers,* a scroll from ancient Egypt. Today, in a hospital or other institution, the **formulary** is the official list of medications approved for use in that institution. The formulary is generally established and periodically reviewed by the hospital Pharmacy and Therapeutics Committee and represents a consensus within the institution concerning what medications are appropriate for treatment of the institution's patients. Considerations in preparing and maintaining a formulary include the latest technical information regarding the risks and benefits of a drug; information about the costs, risks, and benefits of new drugs; ongoing **drug usage evaluations** providing information about drug usage patterns and costs within the institution; and ongoing new drug research within the institution.

UNIVERSAL PRECAUTIONS

Healthcare workers run the risk of contamination by **pathogens**, or disease-causing organisms, carried in blood and other **bodily fluids** such as saliva, semen, gastrointestinal fluid, lymphatic fluid, sebum, mucous, or excrement. Examples of diseases that can be spread by means of bodily fluids include **acquired immunodeficiency syndrome (AIDS)** and **hepatitis B**. Procedures followed in hospitals, doctors' offices, long-term care facilities, and other healthcare settings to prevent infection due to exposure to blood or other bodily fluids are known as **universal precautions**. The name *universal precautions* is a bit of a misnomer because every institution establishes its own precautions to prevent such infection. The following, however, are some common general guidelines:

1. Universal precautions apply to all people within the institution.

2. Universal precautions apply to all contact or potential contact with blood, other bodily fluids, or body substances.

3. Disposable latex gloves must be worn when contact with blood or other bodily fluids is anticipated or possible.

4. Hands must be washed thoroughly after removing the latex gloves.

5. Blood-soaked or contaminated materials such as gloves, towels, or bandages must be disposed of in a wastebasket lined with a plastic bag.

6. Properly trained custodial personnel must be called if cleanup or removal of contaminated waste is necessary.

7. Contaminated materials such as needles, syringes, swabs, and catheters must be placed into red plastic biohazardous materials containers that are labeled as such and properly disposed of, following institutional procedures (which generally involve incineration).

8. A first-aid kit must be kept on hand in any area in which contact with blood or other bodily fluids is possible. The kit should contain, at minimum, the following items:

   –a box of disposable latex gloves

   –antiseptic/disinfectant

   –a bottle of bleach, which will be diluted at time of use to create a solution containing 1 part bleach to 10 parts water, for use in cleaning up blood spills

   –disposable towels

   –sterile gauze for covering large wounds

   –medical tape

   –adhesive bandages for covering small wounds

   –a plastic bag or container for contaminated waste disposal

   –alcohol

DISEASE, STERILIZATION, AND ASEPTIC TECHNIQUE

Hospitals and other institutions make use of sterile preparations. To understand what, exactly, a sterile preparation is, one needs to know something of microbiology and the germ theory of disease. Therefore, these subjects are discussed in the following paragraphs before the subjects of sterilization and aseptic technique are treated.

The Development of the Germ Theory of Disease

In ancient days, people had no understanding of the causes of illness and disease, and so they attributed them to evil or malign spiritual influences. Knowledge of the actual causes of disease progressed slowly, over the centuries. In the seventeenth century, the Dutch merchant Anton van Leeuwenhoek made the first crude microscope. In 1673, he wrote the first of a series of letters to the Royal Society of London describing the "animalcules" that he observed through his microscope, which we would today call microorganisms. While van Leeuwenhoek observed microbes, the Englishman Robert Hooke used a microscope to observe thin slices of cork, which is composed of the walls of dead plant cells. Hooke called the pores between the walls "little cells." His discovery of this structure marked the beginning of a cell theory.

Until the second half of the nineteenth century, it was generally believed that some forms of life could arise spontaneously from matter. This process was known as **spontaneous generation**. People thought that toads, snakes, and mice could be born from moist soil, that flies could emerge from manure, and that maggots could arise from decaying flesh. In 1668, the Italian physician Francesco Redi demonstrated that maggots could not arise spontaneously from decaying meat by conducting a simple experiment in which jars containing meat were left open, sealed, or covered with a fine net. Redi showed that maggots appeared only when the jars were left open, allowing flies to enter to lay eggs.

In 1798, Edward Jenner discovered the principle of immunization against disease. He noticed that milkmaids who had caught cowpox from cows were then immune to contracting smallpox from humans. By infecting healthy persons with cowpox, Jenner successfully inoculated them against smallpox. However, since microorganisms had not yet been identified as disease-causing agents, the reasons behind the success of Jenner's immunizations were not understood.

In 1861, Louis Pasteur demonstrated that microorganisms are present in the air and that they can contaminate seemingly sterile solutions, but that the air itself does not give rise, spontaneously, to microbial life. Pasteur filled several short-necked flasks with beef broth and boiled ham. Some flasks were left open and allowed to cool. In a few days, these flasks were contaminated with microbes. The other flasks, sealed after boiling, remained free of microorganisms. In Pasteur's time, wine making was a hit and miss affair. One year, the wine would be sweet. The next year, it would be sour. No uniform method had been discovered to ensure the same quality year after year. While experimenting along the lines employed in his broth experiment, Pasteur discovered that if grape juice were heated to a certain temperature, cooled, and then treated with a certain yeast, the wine would be consistent year after year. This procedure established the basis for pasteurization and for the development of aseptic technique.

The realization that yeasts play a crucial role in fermentation led people to link the activity of microorganisms with physical and chemical changes in organic materials. This discovery alerted scientists to the possibility that microorganisms might affect plants and animals. The idea that microorganisms cause diseases came to be known as the **germ theory of disease**. Pasteur, the originator of the theory, designed experiments to prove it. In one experiment, he successfully immunized chickens against chicken cholera.

Joseph Lister, an English surgeon, built upon Pasteur's work and applied it to human medicine. Lister knew that carbolic acid (phenol) kills bacteria, one type of microorganism, so he began soaking surgical dressings in a mild carbolic acid solution. This practice reduced surgical infections and was widely and quickly adopted. In 1876, Robert Koch defined a series of steps, known as Koch's postulates, that could be taken to prove that a certain disease was caused by a specific microorganism. Koch discovered rod-shaped bacteria in cattle that had died from anthrax. He cultured the bacteria in artificial media, then infected healthy animals with the bacteria. When these animals became sick and died, Koch isolated the bacteria in their blood, compared them to the bacteria originally isolated, and found them to be the same.

Microorganisms and Disease

Since the days of Pasteur, Lister, and Koch, thousands of **pathogenic**, or disease-causing, microorganisms have been identified. Not all microorganisms are disease-causing. Some, in fact, perform essential functions, such as creating byproducts that are used as medicines, fermenting wine, fixing nitrogen in the soil, or helping the body to break down various food substances. However, some organisms of each of the following types are pathogenic.

1. **Viruses** are very small microorganisms, each of which consists of little more than a bit of genetic material enclosed by a casing of protein. Viruses need a living host in which to reproduce, and they cause a wide variety of diseases, including colds, mumps, measles, chicken pox, influenza, and AIDS.

2. **Bacteria** are small, one-celled microorganisms that exist in three main forms: spherical (cocci), rod-shaped (bacilli), and spiral (spirilla). A wide variety of illnesses, such as salmonella poisoning, strep throat, whooping cough, undulant fever, botulism, diphtheria, syphilis, rheumatic fever, meningitis, scarlet fever, pinkeye, boils, bubonic plague, pneumonia, typhoid, leprosy, pimples, and anthrax infection, are caused by bacteria. See Figure 11.1.

3. **Fungi**, organisms such as molds, mildews, mushrooms, rusts, and smuts, are parasites on living organisms or feed upon dead organic material and

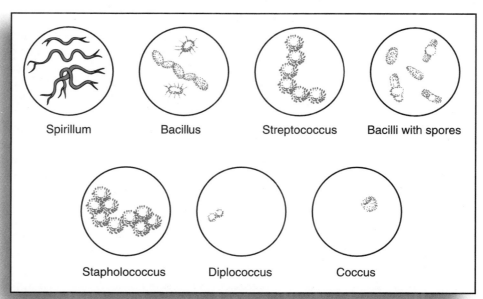

Figure 11.1 Bacterial shapes.

reproduce by means of spores. Spores and some fungi are microscopic and travel through the air. Some are associated with disease conditions such as athlete's foot and ringworm.

4. **Protozoa** are microscopic animals made up of a single cell or of a group of more or less identical cells; they live in water or as parasites inside other creatures. Examples of protozoa include paramecia and amoebae. Amoebic dysentery, malaria, and sleeping sickness are examples of illnesses caused by protozoa.

Asepsis and Sterilization

Asepsis is the absence of disease-causing microorganisms. The condition of asepsis is brought about by **sterilization**, any process that destroys the microorganisms in a substance. The scientific control of harmful microorganisms began only about one hundred years ago. Prior to that time, it was not uncommon for epidemics or pandemics caused by microorganisms (e.g., smallpox or cholera) to kill thousands or millions of people. For example, the native population of the Americas was decimated by European diseases such as smallpox and syphilis. Prior to the modern era, in some hospitals, 25 percent of delivering mothers died of infections carried by the hands and instruments of attending nurses and physicians. During the American Civil War, surgeons sometimes cleaned their scalpels on their boot soles between incisions.

Usually, if we want to sterilize an object, we do not bother to identify the species of microbes on it. Instead, we launch an attack calculated to be strong enough to kill the most resistant microbial life forms that could be present. The most common method for killing microbes is **heat sterilization**. Heat is available, effective, economical, and easily controlled. One way to kill microorganisms is by boiling. Boiling kills vegetative forms, many viruses, and fungi in about 10 minutes. Much more time is required to kill some organisms, such as spores and the Hepatitis viruses. When moist heat of 121°C or 270°F under pressure of 15 pounds per square inch (psi) is applied to instruments, solutions, powders, etc., most known organisms—including spores and viruses—will be killed in about 15 minutes.

Dry heat, such as direct flaming, also destroys all microorganisms. Dry heat is impractical for many substances but is practical as a means for disposal of contaminated objects, which are often incinerated. For proper sterilization using hot, dry air, a temperature of 170°C must be maintained for nearly two hours. Note that a higher temperature is necessary for dry heat, since a heated liquid more readily transfers heat to a cool object.

Mechanical sterilization is achieved by means of filtration, which is the passage of a liquid or gas through a screen-like material with pores small enough to block microorganisms. This method of sterilization is used for heat-sensitive materials such as culture media (used for growing colonies of bacteria or other microorganisms), enzymes, vaccines, and antibiotic solutions. Filter pore sizes are 0.22μ for bacteria and 0.01μ for viruses and some large proteins.

Gas sterilization makes use of the gas *ethylene oxide* and is used for objects that are liable, or subject to, destruction by heat. Gas sterilization requires special equipment and aeration of materials after application of the gas.

Chemical sterilization is the destruction of microorganisms on inanimate objects by chemical means. Few chemicals produce complete sterility, but many reduce microbial numbers to safe levels. A chemical applied to an object or topically to the body for sterilization purposes is known as a **disinfectant**. Alcohol, bleach, iodine, and Mercurochrome are often used as disinfectants.

Contamination

The most important thing to remember about aseptics is that harmful microorganisms, especially bacteria, are everywhere in large numbers. For example, the Harvard biologist E.O. Wilson estimates that as many as 30 billion bacteria are to be found in a single cubic gram of soil. It is extremely easy to introduce bacteria or other contaminants onto a sterile object or device or into a sterile solution. Contamination in a pharmacy occurs by three primary means:

1. **Touch.** Millions of bacteria live on our skin, in our hair, and under our nails. Proper scrubbing to reduce the numbers of bacteria on the hands prior to handling sterile materials is very important.

2. **Air.** Microorganisms are commonly found in the air, in dust particles, and in moisture droplets. It is important to prepare sterile materials in a special area in which the numbers of possible contaminants are maintained at a low level.

3. **Water.** Tap water is not free of microorganisms, and moisture droplets in the air, especially after a sneeze, often contain harmful microbes. It is important not to contaminate sterile materials by exposure to droplets of tap water or other sources of contaminated moisture.

Aseptic Technique

Aseptic technique is the manipulation of sterile products and sterile devices in such a way as not to introduce **pathogens**, or disease-causing microorganisms. **Sterile products** include fluids stored in vials, ampules, prefilled syringes, and other containers. **Sterile devices** include syringes, needles, and IV sets. Aseptic technique is used for the preparation of **parenteral admixtures**, combinations of fluids and/or medications or nutrients, that are administered using bolus (push) or other intravenous methods. Aseptic technique is treated in this chapter because of the frequency with which parenterals are prepared in hospital and other institutional settings. Chart 11.1 summarizes the steps for preparing parenterals using aseptic technique, and the sections that follow explain the procedure in more detail.

Chart 11.1	ASCEPTIC TECHNIQUE

1. Prepare yourself by removing all jewelry and changing into clean clothes with low particulate generation. Wear a cap and mask.
2. Thoroughly scrub, up to the elbows.
3. Clean the hood.
4. Place only essential materials under the hood—no paper, pens, labels, etc. Remove the syringe from its container and discard the waste.
5. Scrub again and glove.
6. Swab or spray needle penetration closures on vials, injection ports, and other materials.
7. Prepare the sterile product by withdrawing medication from vials or ampules and introducing it into the IV container.

Chart 11.1
(cont.)

8. Complete a quality check of the product for container integrity and leaks, solution cloudiness, particulates, color of solution, and proper preparation of product.
9. Present the product, containers and devices used, and the label to a pharmacist for verification of the product preparation.

Equipment Used in Aseptic Technique

When preparing a product in a sterile environment, it is necessary to use an instrument known as a **laminar flow hood**. Such an instrument produces parallel layers of highly filtered air that flow across a work area enclosed on all but one side. Two types of flow hoods are horizontal and vertical.

In a **horizontal flow hood** (see Figure 11.2), air from the room is pulled into the back of the hood where it is prefiltered with an air conditioner-like filter to remove large particles. The air then passes through a high efficiency particulate air (HEPA) filter, where 99.97% of all particles 0.3 μ or larger are removed. The air flows from the back of the hood, across the work surface, and out into the room. It is necessary to work at least six inches into the hood due to the mixing of filtered air and room air at the front of the hood.

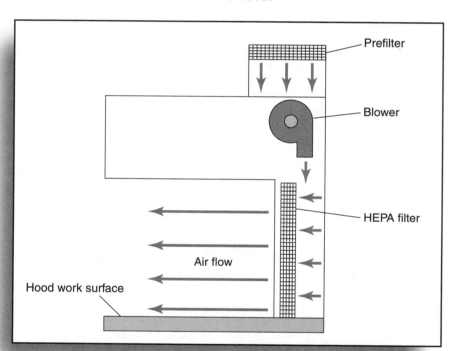

Figure 11.2 Horizontal flow hood.

In a **vertical flow hood** (see Figure 11.3), the air flows from the top of the hood down, through a prefilter and a HEPA filter, and onto the work area. The air is then recirculated through another HEPA filter and out into the room. The front of the hood is partially blocked by a glass shield. This type of hood, because of the extra protection that it provides, is used to prepare dangerous substances, such as parenteral chemotherapy solutions used for treating cancers.

At the start of each shift, the laminar flow hood should be given a good cleaning with an agent that acts both as a detergent (for cleaning) and as a

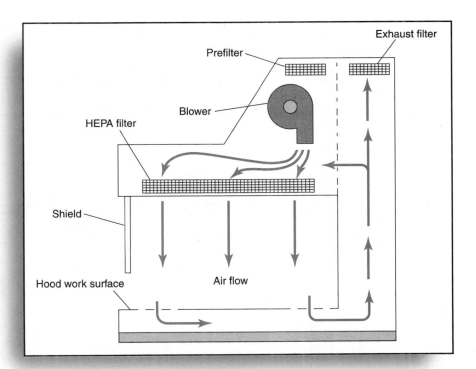

Figure 11.3 Vertical flow hood.

germicide, fungicide, and virucide. A good agent for cleaning the hood is a 2 percent Amphyl solution. The hood should be cleaned several times during a shift, or as needed (for example, after a spill), with 70 percent alcohol. The clear Plexiglas sides should be cleaned with warm, soapy water instead of alcohol. The hood should be cleaned in such a way as to work contamination from the back out toward the room. The cleaning motion should be a back-and-forth movement, with each stroke further out than the previous stroke. The parts of the hood should be cleaned in this order: top, back, sides (top to bottom), and work area or bench (back to front using side-to-side strokes).

PREPARING PARENTERALS

Parenterals, including intravenous push (bolus) and intravenous infusion (IV) dosage forms should be prepared in laminar flow hoods using aseptic techniques. Preparation should always be done under the supervision of a licensed pharmacist.

Equipment Used in Parenteral Preparation

Syringes, used for intravenous push and in the preparation of infusions, are made of glass or plastic. Glass syringes, which are more expensive, are used with medications that are absorbed by plastic. Plastic syringes, besides being less expensive, also have the advantages of being disposable and of coming from the manufacturer sterile and in a sterile package. Figure 11.4 shows the parts of a syringe. Figure 11.5 shows three types of syringes: the hypodermic, the insulin syringe, and the tuberculin syringe.

The needle of a syringe consists of two parts, the **cannula**, or shaft, and the **hub**, the part that attaches to the syringe (see Figure 11.6). Needles are made of stainless steel or aluminum. Needle lengths range from 3/8 of an inch to 6 inches

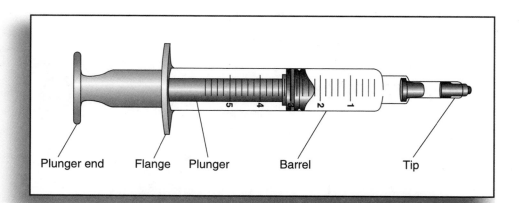

Figure 11.4 Parts of a syringe.

Plunger end   Flange   Plunger   Barrel   Tip

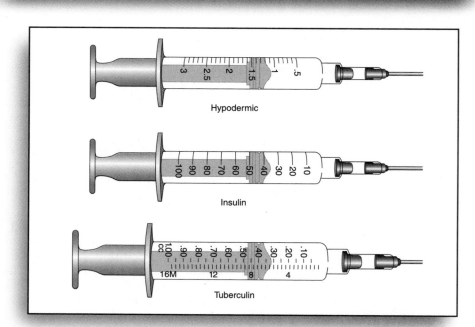

Figure 11.5 Types of syringes.

Hypodermic

Insulin

Tuberculin

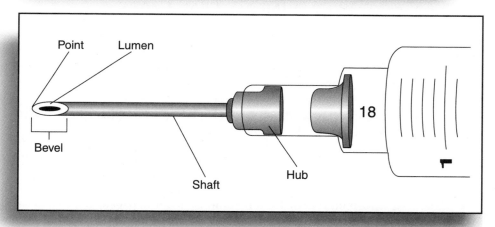

Figure 11.6 Parts of a needle.

Point   Lumen

Bevel

Shaft   Hub

18

and come in gauges ranging from 30 (highest) to 13 (lowest). The higher the **gauge**, the smaller the **lumen**, or bore, of the needle. Commonly used gauges in pharmacy range from 18 to 22.

Filters are devices used to remove contaminants such as glass, paint, fibers, and rubber cores. Filters will not remove virus particles or toxins. Filter sizes are as follows:

5.0 micrometers (microns): Random Path Membrane (RPM) filter, removes large particulate matter

0.45 micrometers: in-line filter for IV suspension drug

0.22 micrometers: filter that removes bacteria and produces a sterile solution

IV Sets

IV sets are devices used to deliver fluids, intravenously, to patients (see Figure 11.7). Nurses generally have the responsibility for attaching IV tubing to the fluid container, establishing and maintaining flow rate, and overall regulation of the system.

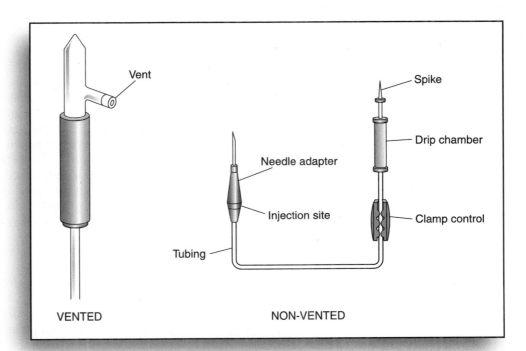

Figure 11.7
Administration set and parts.

Pharmacy personnel should also have a knowledge of intravenous sets. Changes in regulations have forced pharmacy workers to assess aspects of IV systems, including infusion sets. Pharmacists need a complete understanding of IV sets and their operation for the following reasons:

1. Pharmacists may be required to select sets optimal for prevention of incompatibilities in certain drug-drug or drug-fluid combinations.

2. Pharmacists and other pharmacy personnel serving on CPR teams may need to calculate doses and drip rates for medications as well as to prepare IV infusions, attach sets, and prime tubing.

3. Pharmacy personnel may become involved in administration of IV meds to patients, including checking and changing lines according to established guidelines.

4. Pharmacy personnel may have to provide in-service training for nurses to familiarize them with the proper use of IV sets.

5. Pharmacy personnel use IV sets when transferring fluids from container to container under a laminar flow hood.

IV sets are individually wrapped and then sterilized using either radiation or ethylene oxide. These practices guarantee that the fluid pathway is sterile and non-pyrogenic. However, in an operating room, it is desirable that the entire IV unit be sterile. Such a unit is supplied in packaging that ensures the maintenance of sterility, generally in packages with peel-off top cardboard and sealed plastic wrap. Some packaging has a clear wrap for viewing the contents, while other packaging does not have clear wrapping but instead a diagram of the enclosed set printed on the outside of the packaging.

A damaged package cannot ensure sterility, although all protectors are in place. It is best to discard sets that are found to be not original, opened, or in damaged packages.

Sets do not carry expiration dates. Sets do carry the legend for medical devices: "Federal law restricts this device to sale by or on the order of a physician."

Flanges (y-sites) and other rigid parts of an IV set are molded from tough plastic. Most of the length of the tubing is molded from a pliable polyvinyl chloride (PVC). PVC sets should not be used for nitroglycerin, which is absorbed by the tubing, nor for IV fat emulsions, which may leach materials out of the tubing. Therefore, other types of plastic sets are used for such infusions.

The length of sets varies from 6-inch extensions up to 110–120-inch sets used in surgery. The priming of tubing depends on its length, from 3 mL for the short extension up to 15 mL for longer sets. The tubing's interior lumen generally contains particles that flush out when fluid is run through the set. Use of final filtration, a filter in the set, has reduced the need for flushing the line with the IV fluid before attaching the set to the patient.

Standard sets have a lumen diameter of 0.28 cm. By varying the size of the lumen diameter, different flow rates can be achieved. Regulation of flow rates is especially critical in neonates and infants but may also be useful in limiting fluid flow to any patient.

The **spike** is a rigid, sharpened plastic piece used proximal to the IV fluid container. The spike is covered with a protective unit to maintain sterility and is removed only when ready for insertion into the IV container. The spike generally has a rigid area to grip while it is inserted into the IV container (see Figure 11.8).

If an **air vent** is present on a set, it is located below the spike. The air vent points downward and has a bacterial filter covering. The vent allows air to enter the bottle as fluid flows out. Some glass bottles do not have an air tube. For these, a vented set is necessary.

A transparent, hollow chamber, the **drip chamber**, is located below the set's spike. Drops of fluid fall into the chamber from an opening at the uppermost end, closest to the spike. The opening is generally one of two sizes. An opening that provides 10, 15, or 20 drops per mL is commonly used for adults. An opening that provides 60 drops per mL is used for pediatric patients. The drip chamber serves to prevent air bubbles from entering the tubing. Air bubbles generally rise to the top of the fluid if they do form and will not enter the patient. The chamber allows the attending nurse or pharmacy worker to set the flow rate by counting the drops.

The person administering the fluid starts the flow by filling the chamber with fluid from an attached inverted IV container (see Figure 11.9). The chamber sides

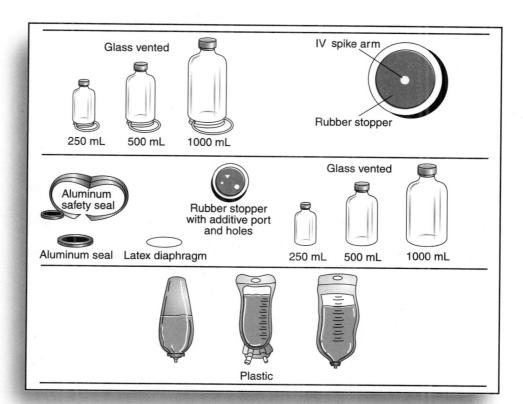

Figure 11.8 Types of IV containers.

are squeezed and released. Then fluid flows into the chamber. The procedure is repeated until an indicated level is reached or approximately half the chamber is filled. The entering drops are then counted for 15 seconds. Adjustments are made until the approximate number of drops desired is obtained. The rate should be checked five times, at 30-second intervals, and again for a last count of 1 full minute.

Clamps allow for adjusting the rate of the flow and for shutting down the flow. Clamps may be located at any position along the flexible tubing. Usually a clamp moves freely, allowing the location of the clamp to be changed to one that is convenient for the administrator.

Clamp accuracy is affected by **creep**, which is a tendency of some clamps to return, slowly, to a more open position with increased fluid flow. Accuracy is also affected by the phenomenon known as cold flow—the tendency of PVC tubing to return to its previous position. Tubing clamps are open during packaging and shipping. As a result, the tube tends to expand when the clamp constricts it. If, on the other hand, the tubing clamp has previously constricted the tubing, then as it is adjusted open, it tends to constrict with the reduced fluid flow, moving in the direction of its original position.

A **slide clamp** has an increasingly narrow channel that constricts IV tubing as it is pressed further into the narrowed area. Slide clamps do not allow for accurate adjustment of flow rate but may be used to shut off flow while a more accurate clamp is regulated.

A **screw clamp** consists of a thumbscrew that is tightened or loosened to speed or slow the flow.

A **roller clamp** is a small roller that is pushed along an incline. The roller, when moved down the incline, constricts the tubing and reduces the fluid flow. Moving the roller up the incline, in contrast, increases the flow.

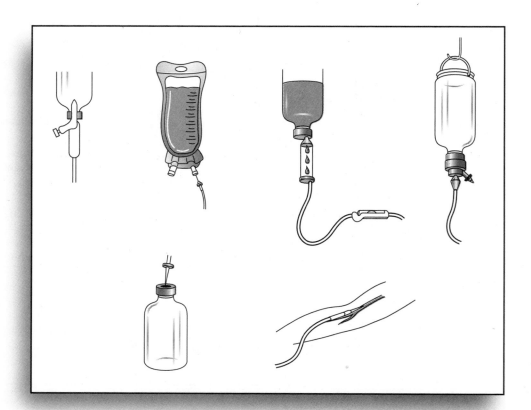

Figure 11.9 Attaching the IV set to the IV container.

A **needle adapter** is usually located at the distal end of the IV set, close to the patient. A needle or **catheter** may be attached to the adapter. The adapter has a standard taper to fit all needles or catheters and is covered by a sterile cover prior to removal for connection.

A set may have a built-in, **in-line filter**, the purpose of which is to provide a final filtration of the fluid prior to its entering the patient. Final filtration should protect the patient against particulate, bacteria, air emboli, and phlebitis. A 0.22 micrometer filter is optimal. A 5 micrometer filter removes particles that block pulmonary microcirculation but will not ensure sterility.

A **y-site** is an injection port found on most sets. The "Y" is a rigid plastic piece with one arm terminating in a resealable port. The port, once disinfected with alcohol, is ready for the insertion of a needle and the injection of medication.

Parenteral Preparation Guidelines

Begin any parenteral preparation by washing your hands thoroughly using a germicidal agent such as chlorhexidine gluconate or povidone-iodine. Wear gloves during the procedure. Make sure the laminar flow hood has been running for at least 30 minutes before beginning the preparation. Laminar air flow hoods are normally kept running. Should the hood be turned off for installation, repair, maintenance, or relocation, it should be operated at least 15 to 30 minutes before being used to prepare sterile products. It is the responsibility of the institution to ensure proper positioning of the hood away from high traffic areas, doorways, air vents, or other locations that could produce air currents contaminating the hood working area. Eating, drinking, talking, or coughing are prohibited in the laminar air flow hood. Follow these guidelines to ensure proper parenteral preparation:

1. **Before making the product, thoroughly clean all interior working surfaces.** Also make sure that the inside of the hood has been thoroughly cleaned with disinfectant. All jewelry should be removed from the hands and wrists before scrubbing and while making a sterile product. To ensure topical antimicrobial action of chlorhexidine, iodine, or other acceptable scrubs, use 3 to 5 mL with a vigorous scrub of the hands, nails, wrists, and forearms for at least 30 seconds.

2. **Gather all the necessary materials for the operation and check these to make sure they are not expired and are free from particulate.** Only essential objects/materials necessary for product preparation should be placed in the flow hood. If you are using plastic solution containers, check these for leaks by squeezing them. Work in the center of the work area within the laminar flow hood, making sure that nothing obstructs the flow of air from the HEPA filter over the preparation area. Nothing should pass behind a sterile object and the HEPA filter in a horizontal flow hood or above a sterile object in a vertical flow hood.

3. **Follow proper procedure for handling sterile devices and medication containers to ensure an accurate microbial-free product.** Remember that the plunger and tip of the syringe are sterile and must not be touched. For greatest accuracy, use the smallest syringe that can hold the desired amount of solution. In any case, the syringe should not be larger than twice the volume to be measured. A syringe is considered accurate to one-half the smallest measurement mark on its barrel. Figure 11.10 illustrates how to accurately read dose measurement. To get an accurate dose, observe closely the calibrations on the syringe barrel. Count the number of marks between labeled measurement units. If there are ten marks, each mark measures off one-tenth of the unit. If there are five marks, each mark measures two-tenths of the unit. The volume of solution drawn into a syringe is measured at the point of contact between the rubber piston and the side of the syringe barrel. The measurement is *not read* at the tip of the piston.

4. **Remove medication from a vial by first swabbing the rubber stopper with an alcohol swab using firm strokes, of the same direction, or by spraying with 70% alcohol.** The needle bevel tip should penetrate the rubber closure at an angle, which is then straightened to 90° so that as additional pressure is applied to the syringe, the bevel heel enters the closure

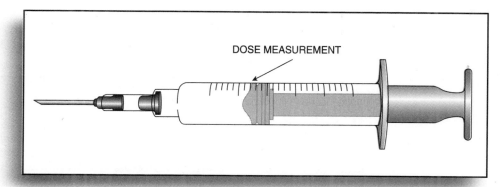

Figure 11.10 Syringe dose measurement.

DOSE MEASUREMENT

at the same point as the tip. This technique prevents coring or introducing a small chunk of the rubber closure into the solution.

5. **Vials are closed systems; therefore, the amount of air introduced should be equal to the volume of fluid removed.** An exception to this guideline is the withdrawal of cytotoxic drugs from vials where a volume of air less than the solution volume is introduced, producing a vacuum and preventing an aspirate when the needle is withdrawn from the rubber closure. Reconstituting a powder by introducing a diluent produces a positive pressure inside the vial.

The glass ampule offers another challenge. The contents in the top of the ampule must be moved into the body by swirling the ampule in an upright position, inverting it quickly, and then turning it back upright, or by tapping the top with a finger (see Figure 11.11). Clean the neck with an alcohol swab; then grasp the ampule between the thumb and index finger at the neck with the swab still in place. Use a quick motion to snap off the top. Do not break in the direction of the HEPA filer. Tilt the ampule, place the needle bevel of a filter needle or tip of a filter straw in the corner near the opening, and withdraw the medication. Then replace the needle or straw with a standard needle to push the drug from the syringe. A standard needle could be used to withdraw the drug from the ampule; it is then replaced with a filter device before the drug is pushed out of the syringe.

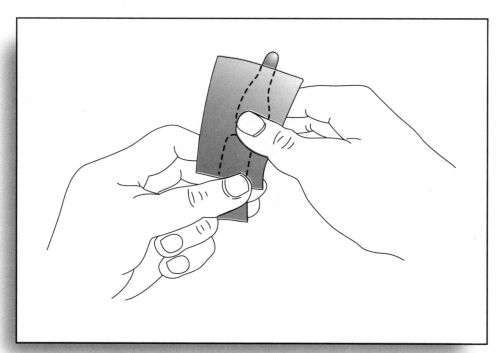

Figure 11.11 Opening an ampule.

IV Solutions

The two main types of IV solutions are **small volume parenterals (SVPs)** of 100 mL or less and **large volume parenterals (LVPs)** of more than 100 mL. Small volume parenterals are typically used for delivering medications at a controlled infusion rate. Large volume parenterals are used to replenish fluids, to provide

electrolytes (essential minerals), and to provide nutrients such as vitamins and glucose. In some cases, a patient is incapable of eating or unwilling to eat and so must be fed intravenously. The provision of the entire nutritional needs of a patient by such means is known as **total parenteral nutrition (TPN)**. In some cases, an infusion is prepared specifically to deliver a medication. In other cases, a medication is **piggybacked** on a running IV. A piggyback involves the preparation of a small amount of solution, usually 50 to 100 mL, in a minibag or bottle. Some IV piggybacks are prepared in 250 mL solution because they contain an additive that is irritating and thus requires a larger volume of solution. The piggybacked solution is infused into the tubing of the running IV, usually over a short period of time, from half an hour to 1 hour. In some cases, syringes are used instead of piggyback containers to deliver medication into a running IV.

Figure 11.12 shows some typical physician's orders for intravenous infusions. Table 11.1 shows some commonly used IV fluids and electrolytes. Table 11.2

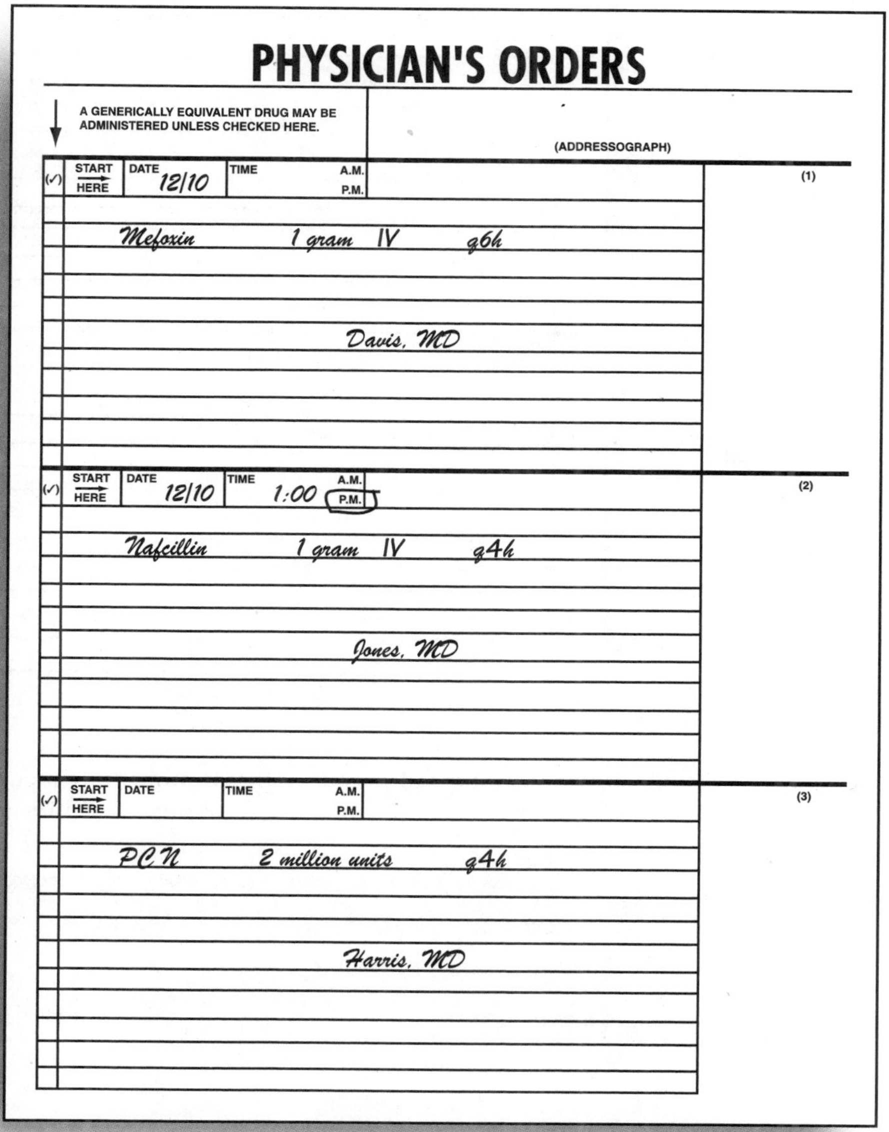

Figure 11.12 Physician's orders for IV infusions. (1 of 2)

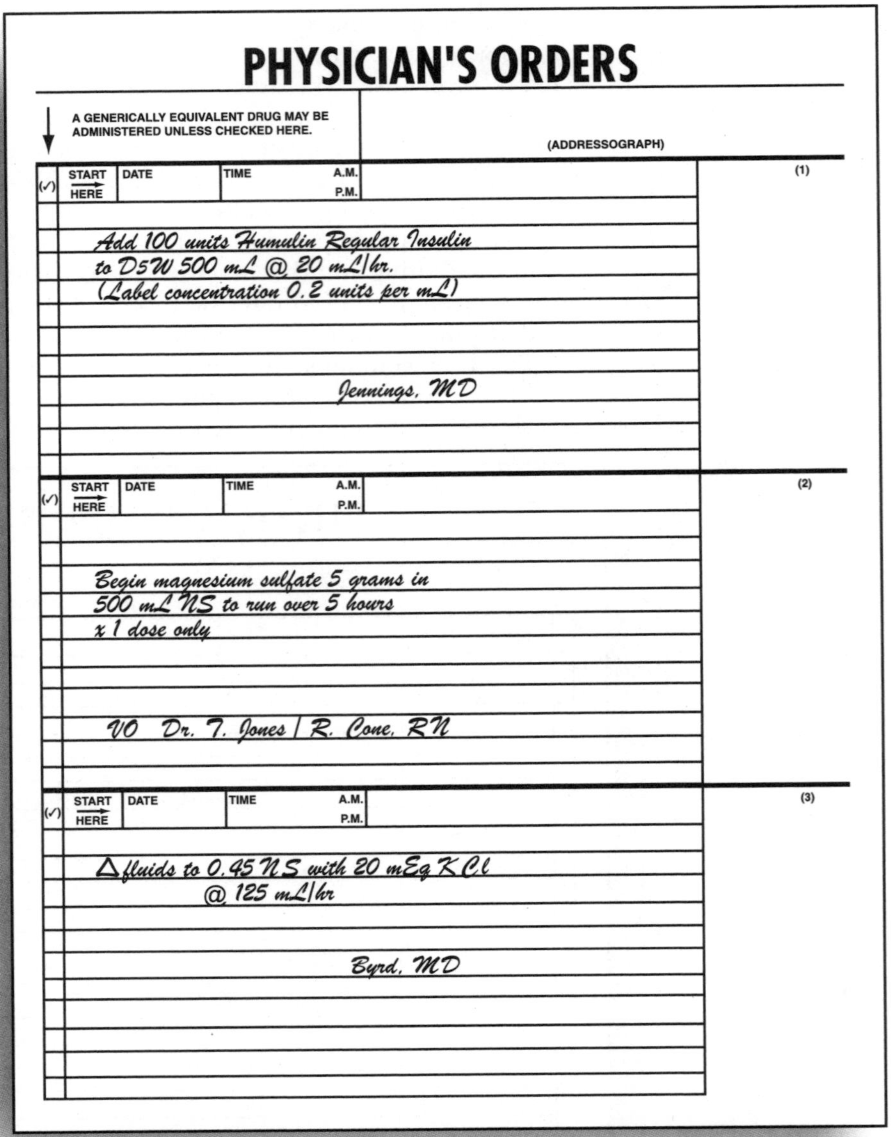

PHYSICIAN'S ORDERS

A GENERICALLY EQUIVALENT DRUG MAY BE
ADMINISTERED UNLESS CHECKED HERE.

(ADDRESSOGRAPH)

(✓)	START HERE	DATE	TIME	A.M. P.M.		(1)

*Add 100 units Humulin Regular Insulin
to D5W 500 mL @ 20 mL/hr.
(Label concentration 0.2 units per mL)*

Jennings, MD

(✓)	START HERE	DATE	TIME	A.M. P.M.		(2)

*Begin magnesium sulfate 5 grams in
500 mL NS to run over 5 hours
x 1 dose only*

VO   Dr. T. Jones / R. Cone, RN

(✓)	START HERE	DATE	TIME	A.M. P.M.		(3)

*Δ fluids to 0.45 NS with 20 mEq KCl
@ 125 mL/hr*

Byrd, MD

Figure 11.12 Physician's orders for IV infusions. (2 of 2)

describes some typical protocols for administering medications via piggybacked minibags. Figure 11.13 shows a typical order form for adult parenteral nutrition.

Table 11.1

COMMONLY USED FLUIDS, ELECTROLYTES, AND ADDITIVES

COMMONLY USED IV FLUIDS

Name of Fluid	Abbreviation
5% dextrose in water	D5W
5% dextrose and normal saline	D5NS
5% dextrose and 0.45% normal saline	D5/0.45NS (1/2 normal saline)

Name of Fluid	Abbreviation
normal saline	NS
0.45% normal saline	0.45NS
5% dextrose and lactated Ringer's	D5RL
lactated Ringer's	RL
10% dextrose in water	D10W
sterile water for injection	SW for Injection
sterile water for irrigation	SW for Irrigation
normal saline for irrigation	NS for Irrigation
2.5% dextrose in water	D2.5W
2.5% dextrose and 0.45% normal saline	D2.5/0.45NS

Commonly Used IV Electrolytes

Electrolyte	Abbreviation
potassium chloride	KCl
potassium phosphate	K phos
magnesium sulfate	$MgSO_4$
potassium acetate	K acet
sodium phosphate	Na phos
sodium chloride	NaCl

Commonly Used Additives

Additive	Abbreviation
multivitamin for injection	MVI
trace elements (combinations of essential trace elements such as chromium, manganese, copper, etc.)	TE
zinc (a trace element)	Zn
selenium (a trace element)	Se

Table 11.2

MINIBAG ADMINISTRATION PROTOCOL

Note: Prepare each agent in D_5W unless advised otherwise.

Agent	Volume	Infusion Rate	EXP	IVS (IV SPECIAL)
acyclovir (Zovirax)	≤ 1 g; 50 mL "Do not refrigerate"	60 min	24 hr RT	NO
Aldomet (methlydopa)	≤ 500 mg; 100 mL	60 min 24 hrs	24 hr RT	YES
amikacin	≤ 500 mg; 100 mL > 500 mg; 250 mL	60 min	24 hr RT	NO
aminocaproic acid (Amicar)	≤ 2 g; 50 mL > 2 g; 100 mL > 5 g; 250 mL	30 min 30 min 30 min	24 hr RT	NO
aminophylline bolus	≤ 250 mg; 50 mL > 250 mg; 100 mL	30 min 30–60 min	24 hr RT	NO

Table **11.2** (cont.)

Agent	Volume	Infusion Rate	EXP	IVS (IV SPECIAL)
ampicillin*	≤ 1.5 g; 50 mL NS	60 min	8 hr RT	NO
	> 1.5 g; 100 mL NS	60 min	72 hr REF	
ampicillin/sulbactam*	≤ 1.5 g; 50 mL NS	60 min	8 hr RT	NO
(Unasyn)	> 1.5 g; 100 mL	60 min	72 hr REF	
aztreonam	≤ 1 g; 50 mL	60 min	48 hr RT	NO
(Azactam)	> 1 g; 100 mL	60 min	7 day REF	
cefamandole	≤ 2 g; 50 mL	60 min	24 hr RT	NO
(Mandol)	> 2 g; 100 mL	60 min	96 hr REF	
cefazolin	≤ 2 g; 50 mL	60 min	24 hr RT	YES
(Ancef, Kefzol)	> 2 g; 100 mL	60 min	96 hr RT	
cefonicid	≤ 2 g; 50 mL	30 min	24 hr RT	NO
(Monocid)	> 2 g; 100 mL	30 min	72 hr REF	
cefoperazone	≤ 3 g; 50 mL	30 min	24 hr RT	NO
(Cefobid)	> 3 g; 100 mL	30 min	120 hr REF	
cefotaxime	≤ 2 g; 50 mL	30 min	24 hr RT	YES
(Claforan)	> 2 g; 100 mL	30 min	120 hr REF	
ceftazidime	≤ 2 g; 50 mL	60 min	24 hr RT	NO
(Fortaz, Tazidime)	> 2 g; 100 mL		7 day REF	
cefotetan	≤ 1 g; 50 mL	60 min	24 hr RT	NO
(Cefotan)	> 1 g; 100 mL	60 min	96 hr REF	
ceftizoxime	≤ 2 g; 50 mL	30 min	24 hr RT	NO
(Cefizox)	> 2 g; 100 mL	30 min	48 hr REF	
ceftriaxone	≤ 2 g; 50 mL	30 min	72 hr RT	NO
(Rocephin)	> 2 g; 100 mL	30 min	10 day REF	
cefoxitin	≤ 2 g; 50 mL	30 min	24 hr RT	NO
(Mefoxin)	> 2 g; 100 mL	30 min	48 hr REF	
cefuroxime	≤ 750 mg; 50 mL	60 min	24 hr RT	NO
(Zinacef)	> 750 mg; 100 mL	60 min	48 hr REF	
cephalothin	≤ 2 g; 50 mL	30 min	24 hr RT	YES
(Keflin)	> 2 g; 100 mL	30 min	96 hr REF	
chloramphenicol	≤ 2 g; 50 mL	30 min	24 hr RT	YES
(Chloromycetin)	> 2 g; 100 mL	30 min	30 day REF	
cimetidine	≤ 300 mg; 50 mL	30 min	48 hr RT	NO
(Tagamet)	> 300 mg; 100 mL	30 min	7 day REF	
clindamycin	≤ 300 mg; 50 mL	30 min	16 day RT	
(Cleocin)	> 300 mg; 100 mL	30 min	30 day REF	
doxycycline	≤ 200 mg; 200 mL	60 min	24 hr RT	NO
(Vibramycin)	> 200 mg; 250 mL	1.5 hr	72 hr REF	
erythromycin*	≤ 1 g; 100 mL NS	60 min	8 hr RT	NO
lactobionate	> 1 g; 250 mL NS	1.5 hr		
famotidine	≤ 40 mg; 100 mL	30 min	96 hr RT	YES
(Pepcid)				
gentamicin	≤ 120 mg; 50 mL	30 min	96 hr RT	YES
(Garamycin)	> 120 mg; 100 mL	30 min	30 day REF	
imipenem-cilastin*	≤ 500 mg; 100 mL NS	60 min	10 hr RT	NO
(Primaxin)	> 500 mg; 250 mL NS	60 min	48 hr REF	

*Denotes normal saline use only.

Agent	Volume	Infusion Rate	EXP	IVS (IV SPECIAL)
methicillin (Staphcillin)	≤ 1 g; 50 mL	60 min	8 hr RT	YES
	> 1 g; 100 mL	60 min	96 hr REF	
mezlocillin	≤ 2 g; 50 mL	30 min	48 hr RT	NO
	> 2 g; 100 mL	30 min	7 day REF	
nafcillin	≤ 1 g; 50 mL	60 min	24 hr RT	NO
	> 1 g; 100 mL	60 min	96 hr REF	
oxacillin*	≤ 2 g; 50 mL NS	60 min	96 hr RT	NO
	> 2 g; 100 mL NS	60 min	7 day REF	
penicillin	≤ 3 mu; 50 mL	30 min	24 hr RT	YES
IVS pentamidine (Pentam)	≤ 300 mg; 100 mL	60 min	24 hr RT	NO
	> 300 mg; 250 mL	60 min		
piperacillin (Pipracil)	≤ 4 g; 50 mL	30 min	24 hr RT	NO
	> 4 g; 100 mL	30 min	7 day REF	
potassium Cl	> 40 mEq; 100 mL	60 min	24 hr RT	NO
ranitidine (Zantac)	≤ 50 mg; 50 mL	30 min	48 hr RT	NO
	> 50 mg; 100 mL	30 min	10 day REF	
ticarcillin (Ticar)	≤ 3 g; 50 mL	60 min	24 hr RT	NO
	> 3 g; 100 mL	60 min	72 hr REF	
Timentin	≤ 3.1 g; 50 mL	60 min	24 hr RT	NO
	> 3.1 g; 100 mL	60 min	72 hr REF	
tobramycin (Nebcin)	≤ 120 mg; 50 mL	30 min	24 hr RT	NO
	> 120 mg; 100 mL	30 min	96 hr REF	
vancomycin	≤ 250 mg; 50 mL	60 min	96 hr RT	YES
	> 250 mg; 100 mL	60 min		
	> 1 g; 250 mL	60 min		
Septra	Each 5 mL amp in each 75 mL	60–90 min	2 hr RT	NO
	Each 5 mL amp in each 125 mL "Do not refrigerate"	60–90 min	6 hr RT	
furosemide (Lasix)	Do not exceed 4 mg/min Protect from light		24 hr RT	NO
Flagyl	500 mg RTU	60 min	Manuf.	NO
Any other dose of Flagyl	"Do not refrigerate"	60 min	24 hr RT	

*Denotes normal saline use only.

Adult Parenteral Nutrition Order Form
Mt. Hope Hospital
My Town, SC

Date: _____ Time: _____ PM _____ AM

☐ Consult Nutritional Support Service (Beeper 0349)

☐ Conduct Indirect Calorimetry Test

Central Formula (per liter)		**Peripheral Formula (per liter)**	
Amino Acids	40 g	Amino Acids	25 g
Dextrose	17.5% (600 Kcals)	Dextrose	6% (200 Kcals)
Fat 20%	125 mL (250 Kcals)	Fat 20%	200 mL (400 Kcals)
Standard Electrolytes*		Standard Electrolytes*	
Trace Elements-4 1 mL/Day		Trace Elements-4 1 mL/Day	
Multivitamins-12 10 mL/Day		Multivitamins-12 10 mL/Day	
		Osmolarity: 740 mOsm/L	

Total Volume _____ mL/Day   Total Volume _____ mL/Day

*Standard Electrolytes (per liter) Na: 50 mEq, Ca: 7.5 mEq, Cl: 45 mEq, Acetate: 45 mEq, Phos: 9 mM

Special Formulation (Indicate Total Daily Requirements)   **Guidelines**   **General Rule**

1. Amino Acids _____ g/Day   0.5–2.5 g/Kg/Day   1 g/Kg/Day
   Type _____

2. Total Nonprotein
   Calories _____ Kcals/Day*   10–40 Kcals/Kg/Day 25
   Kcals/Kg/Day

   Dextrose _____%   0–100%   65%
   Fat _____%   0–65%   35%
   100%

3. Total Volume _____ mL/Day   Minimum Volume: 1 Kcal/1.0 mL
*Substrate must equal 100%.

Special Formulation—Electrolytes (check one)

☐ Standard Electrolytes/Liter   ☐ Standard Electrolytes plus
                                             Additional Electrolytes

☐ Standard Electrolytes/Liter—No Potassium   ☐ Custom Electrolytes

Sodium Acetate	_____ mEq/Day	Potassium Acetate	_____ mEq/Day
Sodium Chloride	_____ mEq/Day	Potassium Chloride	_____ mEq/Day
Sodium Phosphate	_____ mEq/Day	Potassium Phosphate	_____ mEq/Day
Magnesium Sulfate	_____ mEq/Day	Calcium Gluconate	_____ mEq/Day

Multivitamins-12 (10 mL) per _____   Other _____
Trace Elements-4 (1 mL) per _____   Other _____

HUMAN REGULAR INSULIN _____ Units/Day

Phytonadione (Vit. K) 10 mg IM per _____

OTHER _____

Special Instructions _____
_____

M.D.   Pharmacy Must Receive TPN Orders by 12 Noon
76016153

(Front)

Figure 11.13 Order for adult parenteral nutrition. (1 of 2)

MVI-12 10 mLs* contains: (indicates adult RDA)

1. Ascorbic Acid	100.0 mg	(45mg)
2. Vitamin A	3,300.0 IU	(4,000–5,000 IU)
3. Vitamin D	200.0 IU	(4,000–5,000 IU)
4. Thiamine	3.0 mg	(1.0–1.5 mg)
5. Riboflavin	3.6 mg	(1.1–1.8 mg)
6. Pyridoxine	4.0 mg	(1.6–2.0 mg)
7. Niacin	40.0 mg	(12–20 mg)
8. Pantothenic Acid	15.0 mg	(5–10 mg)
9. Vitamin E	10.0 IU	(12–15 IU)
10. Biotin	60.0 mg	(150–300 mcg)
11. Folic Acid	400.0 mcg	(400 mcg)
12. Vitamin B$_{12}$	5.0 mcg	(3 mcg)

*Provides 100% of AMA guidelines for parenteral vitamin supplementation.

Trace Elements 1 mL contains: (AMA daily recommendations)

1. Zinc 5.0 mg (2.5–4 mg)   3. Manganese 0.5 mg (0.15–0.8 mg)
2. Copper 1.0 mg (0.5–1.5 mg)   4. Chromium 10.0 mcg (10–15 mcg)

Pharmacy Use

INSTRUCTIONS FOR USING ORDER FORM

1. Check N.S.S. CONSULT or INDIRECT CALORIMETRY (Metabolic Cart) if desired.

2. Order STANDARD CENTRAL or STANDARD PERIPHERAL FORMULAS by total mLs per day. Nutritional components listed on form as per liter. Standard formulas include MVI, TE, and standard electrolytes.

3. Use SPECIAL FORMULATION section for any orders other than standard formulas including addition of electrolytes and other than standard lytes.

4. AMINO ACIDS ordered in mLs per day. If a change in rate is desired, place a new order for acid products (i.e., renal, hepatic, or HBC).

5. TOTAL NONPROTEIN CALORIES ordered as kcals per day. Specify percentage of total calories to be supplied by dextrose and percentage to come from lipids.

6. TOTAL VOLUME ordered in mLs per day. If a change in rate is desired, a new order form needs to be filled out to ensure the change is acknowledged by the IV pharmacy.

7. If either STANDARD LYTES or STANDARD LYTES—NO POTASSIUM are desired, check the appropriate box.

8. If CUSTOM ELECTROLYTES are desired, check the box and order total mEq per day. If STANDARD ELECTROLYTES PLUS ADDITIONAL ELECTROLYTES are desired, check the appropriate box and specify additional electrolytes in mEq/day.

   Use standard electrolytes (per liter) listed under standard formulas as a guide. Note: 4.0 mEq of Na phosphate or 4.4 mEq K phosphate provides 3 mM phosphate.

9. MULTIVITAMINS and TRACE ELEMENTS should be ordered per day.

10. Specify INSULIN (in units/day) and VITAMIN K if desired; then outline any SPECIAL INSTRUCTIONS if applicable.

ALL TPN ORDERS RECEIVED IN THE PHARMACY BY 12:00 NOON WILL BE HUNG BETWEEN 6:00 P.M. AND 10:00 P.M. THE SAME DAY.

(Back)

Figure 11.13 Order for adult parenteral nutrition. (2 of 2)

Preparing a Label for an IV Admixture

When making an IV admixture, one must prepare a label for it. The label should contain the following information:

1. patient's name and identification/account number
2. room number
3. fluid and amount
4. drug name and strength (if appropriate)
5. infusion period
6. flow rate (example: 100 mL/hr or infuse over 30 min)
7. expiration date and time
8. additional information as required by the institution or by state or federal guidelines, including auxiliary labeling, storage requirements, and device-specific information

Figure 11.14 shows examples of labels prepared for a minibag and for a large volume parenteral.

```
┌─────────────────────────────────────────────────────────────┐
│ ┌ ─ ─ ─ ─ ─ ─ ─ ─ ─ ─ ─ ─ ─ ─ ─ ─ ─ ─ ─ ─ ─ ─ ─ ─ ─ ─ ─ ─ ┐ │
│                                                               │
│   PATIENT NAME                      ROOM NUMBER               │
│   IDENTIFICATION NUMBER                 DATE                  │
│   FLUID VOLUME                                                │
│   DRUG DOSE                                                   │
│   DRUG DOSE                                                   │
│   INFUSION RATE (for minibags)                                │
│   SCHEDULE (times due)              RATE (for LVPs)           │
│                                                               │
│   EXPIRATION DATE & TIME                                      │
│                                                               │
│ └ ─ ─ ─ ─ ─ ─ ─ ─ ─ ─ ─ ─ ─ ─ ─ ─ ─ ─ ─ ─ ─ ─ ─ ─ ─ ─ ─ ─ ┘ │
│  Minibag example                                              │
│ ┌ ─ ─ ─ ─ ─ ─ ─ ─ ─ ─ ─ ─ ─ ─ ─ ─ ─ ─ ─ ─ ─ ─ ─ ─ ─ ─ ─ ─ ┐ │
│                                                               │
│   John Brown                        815-2                     │
│   04596875                          10/10/xx                  │
│   D5W     50 mL                                               │
│   Tagamet    300 mg                                           │
│                                                               │
│   Infuse over 30 minutes                                      │
│   Q8H 1p 9p 5a                                                │
│                                                               │
│   EXP: 10/17/xx    5p                                         │
│                                                               │
│ └ ─ ─ ─ ─ ─ ─ ─ ─ ─ ─ ─ ─ ─ ─ ─ ─ ─ ─ ─ ─ ─ ─ ─ ─ ─ ─ ─ ─ ┘ │
│  LVP example                                                  │
│ ┌ ─ ─ ─ ─ ─ ─ ─ ─ ─ ─ ─ ─ ─ ─ ─ ─ ─ ─ ─ ─ ─ ─ ─ ─ ─ ─ ─ ─ ┐ │
│                                                               │
│   John Brown                        815-2                     │
│   04596875                          10/10/xx                  │
│   D5/0.45NS     1000 mL                                       │
│   Potassium Chloride   20 mEq                                 │
│   MVI-12    10 mL                                             │
│                                                               │
│   Q13H 6p 7a/11                     75mL/HR                   │
│                                                               │
│   EXP: 10/11/xx    5p                                         │
│                                                               │
│ └ ─ ─ ─ ─ ─ ─ ─ ─ ─ ─ ─ ─ ─ ─ ─ ─ ─ ─ ─ ─ ─ ─ ─ ─ ─ ─ ─ ─ ┘ │
└─────────────────────────────────────────────────────────────┘
```

Figure 11.14 Minibag label and large volume parenteral label.

HANDLING AND DISPOSAL OF HAZARDOUS AGENTS

In all pharmacy settings, but particularly in hospital and other institutional settings, workers bear the risk of coming into contact with hazardous medications and other chemicals. Many kinds of dangerous drugs and chemicals are encountered in pharmacy, including **corrosive materials** (ones that can dissolve or eat away at bodily tissues) and **cytotoxic materials** (ones that are poisonous to cells), as is the case with **antineoplastic drugs** (used in the treatment of cancer). Table 11.3 lists some commonly used cytotoxic and hazardous drugs.

Table 11.3

COMMONLY USED CYTOTOXIC AND HAZARDOUS DRUGS

Asparaginase	Dacarbazine	Hydroxyurea	Mitotane
Bleomycin	Dactinomycin	Idarubicin	Mitoxantrone
Busulfan	Daunorubicin	Ifosfamide	Plicamycin
Carboplatin	Doxorubicin	Lomustine	Procarbazine
Carmustine	Estramustine	Mechlorethamine	Streptozocin
Chlorambucil	Etoposide	Melphalan	Thioguanine
Cisplatin	Floxuridine	Mercaptopurine	Thiotepa
Cyclophosphamide	Fluorouracil	Methotrexate	Vinblastine
Cytarabine	Ganciclovir	Mitomycin	Vincristine

Three **routes of exposure** to hazardous substances include:

1. **trauma**, or injury. For example, a technician using a syringe to add a drug substance to an IV bag might accidentally prick himself or herself with the needle.

2. **inhalation**, or breathing in, of the hazardous substance. For example, a technician might drop and break a bottle containing a volatile acid.

3. **direct skin contact**. For example, a technician might accidentally spill a medication on himself or herself when pouring it from a large container into a smaller container or flask.

All personnel in an institution should have proper training in procedures involving cytotoxic and other hazardous drugs. Such training should cover proper handling, storage, preparation, disposal, and cleanup. Any pharmacy worker who is pregnant, breast feeding, or trying to conceive should notify her supervisor so that extra precautions can be taken to minimize contact with hazardous substances.

Receipt and Storage of Hazardous Agents

Hazardous drugs should be delivered directly to the storage area, checked, and, if necessary, refrigerated. The person checking the shipment should wear gloves. Damaged packages should be inspected in an insulated area, such as a vertical air flow hood (see below). Broken vials of unreconstituted drugs should be treated as drug spills. Protective clothing should be worn when disposing of damaged packages.

A list of cytotoxic and otherwise hazardous drugs should be compiled and posted in appropriate locations in the workplace. Storage areas, such as drug cartons, shelves, bins, counters, and trays should carry appropriate warning labels and should be designed in such a way as to minimize the possibility of falling and breakage. Access to storage areas and work areas for hazardous materials should be limited to specified trained personnel. Hazardous drugs requiring refrigeration should be stored separately from other drugs. Refrigeration storage bins should prevent breakage and contain leakage.

Protective Clothing

Disposable, lint-free, nonabsorbent, closed-front gowns with cuffed sleeves should be worn, along with double gloves, one glove under and one over the sleeve. Hands should be washed before and after gloving. After exposure to cytotoxic or hazardous drugs, no protective clothing should be worn outside the area where the exposure occurred. Caution should be taken, including warning others, so as not to contaminate other persons or objects. Gloves should be turned inside out as they are taken off.

Technique for Handling Hazardous Agents

Rapid movements should be minimized to prevent air flow disturbances. Completed preparations should be wiped with alcohol before being removed from the hood and placed in a sealable container. All contaminated materials should be placed in leakproof, puncture-resistant containers and then placed in larger containers for disposal. Needles should be discarded without being clipped in two. When handling such materials, proper aseptic technique should be followed. All syringes and IV containers should be labeled according to institutional guidelines. Syringes used should be large enough that they will not be full when the full drug dose is drawn into them. Vials should not be vented unless one is using a filter device. When adding diluent to a vial, one should do so slowly, allowing pressure in the vial and the syringe to equalize. When opening an ampule, one should tap the drug from the top of the ampule, wrap a pad around the ampule, and hold the ampule away from the face before breaking off the top (refer to Figure 11.11).

Disposal of Hazardous Agents

Disposal of hazardous materials must be in appropriate, properly labeled containers. When filled, such containers must be sealed and picked up by appropriate personnel. All hazardous waste, such as chemicals, must be separated from other trash and should be handled only by persons designated and trained for this purpose. Disposal must be in compliance with institutional policies and with local, state, and federal regulations.

Spills

All spills must be dealt with immediately. Proper attire should be worn, including gowns, double gloves, goggles, and a mask or respirator. Soaked items and glass should be transferred to a disposal container. When cleaning up the spill, one should start from the edge of the spill and work inward, using absorbent sheets, spill pads, or pillows for liquids and damp cloths or towels for solids. For spills inside an air flow hood, see below.

Procedures in Case of Exposure

Any body area exposed should be flooded with water and thoroughly cleansed with soap and water. Normal saline for irrigation should be used to cleanse the eyes. The exposed person should be sent or escorted to the employee health or emergency room. If the substance comes in contact with the skin, wash the skin thoroughly with soap and water and seek appropriate medical attention. If the substance comes in contact with the eyes, flush the affected eye with large amounts of water, or use an eye flush kit and seek appropriate medical attention. Remove contaminated garments and/or gloves, and wash hands after removing the gloves. Dispose of contaminated garments appropriately in biohazard materials containers.

Nonparenteral Hazardous Dosage Forms

Tablets and capsule forms of hazardous nonparenterals should not be placed in any automated counting or packaging machine. During routine handling of these drugs, workers should wear one pair of gloves of good quality and thickness. The counting and pouring of these drugs should be done carefully, and contaminated equipment should be cleaned with detergent and rinsed. Compounding with any of these drugs should be done in a protected area away from drafts and traffic. The worker should wear a gown and respirator in addition to gloves. When one is crushing a hazardous drug in a unit-of-use package, the package should be placed in a small, sealable plastic bag and crushed with a spoon or pestle, using caution not to break the plastic bag. For additional information on cytotoxic drug preparation, consult ASHP's video called *Safe Handling of Cytotoxic and Hazardous Drugs*.

MEDICATION ORDERS AND UNIT DOSE DISTRIBUTION

In a hospital or other institution, the pharmacy receives prescriptions in the form of **medication orders**. Figure 11.15 shows some examples of such medication orders.

PHYSICIAN'S ORDERS

A GENERICALLY EQUIVALENT DRUG MAY BE ADMINISTERED UNLESS CHECKED HERE.

(ADDRESSOGRAPH)

(1)

START HERE | DATE 10/16/99 | TIME 1500 | A.M. P.M.

Doe, Jane
588123
1035 10 East

Continue home meds:

1) Capoten 12.5 mg po q 12
2) Nystatin cream to affected area   tid
3) Digoxin 0.125 mg   po   qd
4) Nafcillin 1 g IV q6h
5) Enteric-coated aspirin X gr po qd

Smith, MD

(2)

START HERE | DATE 10/16/99 | TIME 1300 | A.M. P.M.

Ruth, Barbara
5984545
825 8 West

Start following meds ASAP:

1) Hydralazine 10 mg IV q6h
2) Emetecon IM q2-3h prn nausea
3) D5 1/2 NS 20 KCl at 50 mL/hr
4) Vital signs q shift
5) npo after 12 M.

Blood, MD

Figure 11.15 Medication orders (1 of 4).

NAME	ROOM #	ADMIT TIME
John H. Jones	235	
Nalfon 300 mg q8h		
Benadryl Cough Syrup 5 mL hs		
Mucomyst 10% 10 mL on call		
Billy Martin	821	
MOM 30 mL prn hs		
Lithium Carbonate 30 mg tid		
ASA 10 gr q4h		
Hilda Hornblower	822	
Vistaril 25 mg q4h		
Tagamet 300 mg tid		
Acetaminophen 60 mg q6h		
Vera Long	121	
Elixophyllin 250 mg bid give 1 now		
Ascorbic acid daily		
Lufyllin 400 mg q6h		
John Henry	432	
Garamycin 20 mg IM tid		
Baby Powder		
ASA 5 gr q6h		
Casey Jones	333	
Mellaril 100 mg bid now		
Nitrostat		
Vasodilan 10 mg tid		
Dolly Madison	242	
Principen 500 mg bid now		
Oretic 50 mg bid		
Senokot hs and bid		
Neil Buckner	383	
Colace 150 mg A.M.		
Decadron 0.75 mg BA		
Motrin 600 mg q6h		
Darla Molari	422	
Endep 100 mg bid		
Folvite qd		
Feosol qd		
Larry Brindle	246	
Dilantin 30 mg qid now		
Dimetapp bid		
Oretic 25 mg		

Figure 11.15 Medication orders (2 of 4).

NAME	ROOM #	ADMIT TIME
Oscar Wilder	503	
Nitrostat prn		
Apresoline 50 mg tid now		
Susan Anthony	610	
Catapres 0.3 mg tid		
Coumadin 5 mg qd		
MOM 20 mL prn hs		
Raul Garcia	111	
Oretic 50 mg tid now		
K-Lor qd		
Medrol 16 mg BA		
Tom Smith	230	
Ascorbic acid qd		
Basaljel prn AC and hs		
Toradol 10 mg q4-6h		
Tim Turner	407	
10,000 Units Heparin now		
Gentamicin 60 mg tid		
Donnatal prn pc		
Rick Bono	606	
Compazine 25 mg prn		
Benylin Cough Syrup q4h		
V-Cillin K 500 mg q6h		
Marc Janzen	414	
Elixophyllin 125 mg qd now		
EES granules 280 mg q6h		
Triamterene 100 mg A.M.		
Julia Shriver	409	
Orinase 250 mg bid		
Prednisone 15 mg qd 8 A.M.		
Antivert 12.5 mg tid		
Marian Carter	520	
PPD test with syringe		
Robaxin tid		
Naprosyn 500 mg q6h		
Natalie Wang	311	
Diamox 125 mg q6h		
Dimetapp q4h		
MOM prn		

Figure 11.15 Medication orders (3 of 4).

NAME	ROOM #	ADMIT TIME
Ray Stevens	230	
Nitrostat prn		
Aldactone 100 mg tid		
Lasix 40 mg bid		
Deborath Gunther	143	
Zyloprim 100 mg tid now		
Acetaminophen elixir 60 mg q6h		
Mylicon 80 mg q pc		
George Milar	502	
Oretic 25 mg bid now		
Klotrix 10 mg qd		
Sudafed 60 mg q12h		
Kathy Sooner	402	
Dexamethasone 100 mg QSA now		
Dulcolax 5 mg qd		
Robaxin q8h		
Gloria Kramer	433	
Pen-Vee K 375 mg q6h		
Parafon Forte q6h		
MOM hs		
Wesley Adams	321	
Inderal 60 mg bid now		
MOM q pc		
Colace 150 mg hs		
Jennie Conners	401	
Nitro Patch 10 cm qd send now		
Fleet Prep Kit		
ASA 600 mg q4h		
Jeffrey Hart	213	
Ceclor 250 mg oral liquid q6h		
Baby oil		
Esidrix 75 mg bid		
Jennifer Hightower	334	
Darvon 100 mg q6h		
Mylantin 60 mL AC hs		
Motrin q6h if react to Darvon		
Serena Sarles	416	
Larodopa 500 mg qd A.M.		
Captopril 12.5 mg tid		
Tylenol 650 mg q4h		

Figure 11.15 Medication orders (4 of 4).

Hospitals and other institutions typically make use of a unit-dose system for dispensing medications. A **unit dose** is an amount of a drug prepackaged for a single administration. In other words, it is an amount of medication in a dosage form ready for administration to a particular patient at a particular time. Unit-dose preparation increases efficiency by making the drug form as ready to administer as possible rather than forcing nurses to prepare dosages from multiple dose containers. Tablets and capsules are labeled, liquids are premeasured, injections are diluted as ordered and accurately measured into syringes, parenteral admixtures are compounded, and oral powders and other dosage forms are prepared appropriately.

A unit-dose system saves time and money. It provides increased security for medications, makes charging and crediting easy, reduces medication errors, reduces nursing time, and makes administration, charging, and crediting easier. It also ensures that proper institutional and departmental policies will be followed.

Because manufacturers do not, in all instances, prepare drugs in single-dose form, and because individual medication orders may call for nonstandard dosages, preparing unit doses often involves repackaging. **Repackaging** may involve the use of a variety of equipment, such as counting trays, automated packaging machines (see Figure 12.4), and liquid filling apparatuses. Typical unit-dose packaging includes heat-sealed zip-lock bags, adhesive sealed bottles, blister packs, and heat-sealed strip packages for oral solids, and plastic or glass cups, heat-sealable aluminum cups, and plastic syringes labeled "For Oral Use Only" for liquid orals. Oral medication specials (preparations made for a particular patient), IV specials, intramuscular injections, and suppositories are examples of drug forms typically provided in unit-dose form. Ointments, creams, ear drops, and eye drops are not unit dose. These are bulk items that are not resupplied daily. They are provided only on request. When doing repackaging, one must keep a record of what is done in order to track each dose for purposes of recall and quality assurance. Such a record is known as a **repackaging control log** and contains the following information:

1. internal control or lot number

2. drug, strength, dosage form

3. manufacturer's name

4. manufacturer's lot number and expiration date

5. assigned expiration date

6. resulting concentration

7. quantity of units

8. the initials of the repackager

9. the initials of the pharmacist who has checked the repackaging

Additional information may be required, depending on institutional policy and state guidelines. An example of such a log appears in Figure 11.16.

Each day, a **medication fill list** is generated by computer. This is a complete list of all the patients' current medications. From this list, a unit-dose profile is prepared. The unit-dose profile provides the information necessary to prepare the unit doses and includes patient name and location, medication and strength, frequency or schedule of administration, and quantity, as follows:

John Doe   Room 535
Ampicillin 250 mg
q6h   5p 11p 5a 11a

REPACKAGING CONTROL LOG

DEPARTMENT OF PHARMACEUTICAL SERVICES

PHARMACY LOT NUMBER	DRUG-STRENGTH DOSAGE FORM	MANUFACTURER AND LOT NUMBER	EXP. DATE MANUF. MTC	RESULTING CONC.	QUANTITY	PREP. BY CK'D

Figure 11.16
Repackaging control log.

Joanne Riggs   Room 532
Nalfon 300 mg
q8h   8a 4p 12a

Doses are prepared, labeled, and placed in patient drawers on carts that are taken to the wards. Labels include the following information:

- nonproprietary or generic name, or the proprietary or trade name of the drug
- dosage form (if special or other than oral)
- strength of the dose and the total contents delivered (e.g., the number of tablets and their total dose)
- any special notes (e.g., "Refrigerate")

- internal expiration date
- internal control number

A fill list is needed in order to stock patient drawers in a medication cart. This list is used to check what medications are left in the drawers. If no meds are in a drawer, a 12-hour or 24-hour supply is stocked. If some meds are left in the drawer, these are subtracted from the 12-hour or 24-hour supply, and the difference is placed in the drawer. So, for example, if the fill list called for

medication	sch	DQTY POST	QTY
Tagamet 300 mg	18 h	3	2

and the drawer had 1 300 mg Tagamet tablet from the previous day, 2 tablets would be added to the drawer.

FLOOR STOCK

The floor stock system provides medications for each nursing unit. Floor stock distribution deals with those medications that are dispensed frequently on a PRN (pro re nata, or as needed) basis. It would be impractical, of course, to dispense such drugs on a unit dose basis. Typical floor stock consists of emergency medications and bulk items such as antacids, cough syrup, Tylenol elixir or drops, ointments, creams, inhalers, and narcotics. Advantages of the floor stock system are a quick turnaround time from the writing of the order to the administration of the medication and the convenience of immediate availability of medications to the nursing staff. Disadvantages include increased diversion, increased medication errors, and expense due to lost charges and revenue.

The pharmacy assumes responsibility for maintaining inventory through a floor stock replacement system. Pharmacy personnel maintain the inventory according to predetermined levels. Floor stock must be inspected regularly for proper storage, expired drugs, narcotic control, and removal of discontinued drugs. Medications administered to patients by nursing units are charged to the appropriate records by manual and/or electronic data processing systems.

As with any distribution system, checks are necessary to determine usage and levels of remaining supply. When checking floor stock, one should make sure that the stocked drugs have not expired, that excess meds are removed, that items requiring refrigeration are refrigerated, that the refrigerator temperature is correct, that all medications are stored properly, and that controlled substances are accounted for.

In many institutions, floor stock items are kept in automated dispensing machines rather than in a stock room or on shelf space on the patient care unit. Automated dispensing machines keep an electronic record of bulk, floor stock, and items utilized by each patient.

THE DRUG INFORMATION CENTER

In order to fulfill its clinical functions, a hospital or institutional pharmacy may maintain a **drug information center,** which is basically a library containing reference works, including books, periodicals, microfilm, CD-ROMs, and databases providing information about drugs and their uses. Types of references that might be kept in the drug information center are described in chapter 6 of this text.

chapter summary

Hospital and other institutional pharmacies carry out many functions of community pharmacies but also undertake a number of activities unique to or especially common in the institutional setting. These activities include, but certainly are not limited to, the preparation of a formulary, or list of drugs approved for use; training of staff in universal precautions and proper handling and disposal of hazardous agents; preparation, using sterile techniques, of parenteral admixtures; filling of medication orders using unit dose systems; stocking of nursing stations; and maintenance of a drug information center.

chapter review

Knowledge Inventory

1. A formulary is a
   a. list of approved drugs
   b. description of contents and pharmacological characteristics of manufactured drugs
   c. set of formulae for extemporaneous compounding
   d. set of formulae for preparation of common parenteral admixtures

2. Universal precautions deal with infections by disease-causing microorganisms found in
   a. tap water and other liquid sources
   b. blood and other bodily fluids
   c. emergency rooms
   d. pharmacies

3. A unit dose is
   a. a supply prepared for a hospital ward, or unit
   b. an amount and dosage form appropriate for a single administration to a single patient
   c. the average recommended dosage for an adult male
   d. the dosage recommended by the *United States Pharmacopeia*

4. The term used to describe a person confined to a hospital bed is
   a. outpatient
   b. ambulatory patient
   c. peripatetic patient
   d. inpatient

5. A pathogen causes
   a. a desired therapeutic outcome
   b. an embolism
   c. a thrombosis
   d. a disease

6. The germ theory of disease is credited to
    a. Robert Hooke
    b. Edward Jenner
    c. Anton Van Leeuwenhoek
    d. Louis Pasteur

7. People used to believe that life forms, such as microorganisms and maggots, could arise miraculously out of decayed or other matter in a process known as
    a. spontaneous combustion
    b. spontaneous generation
    c. zoomorphogenesis
    d. parthenogenesis

8. Small microorganisms that consist of little more than some genetic material surrounded by a protein case are known as
    a. bacteria
    b. protozoa
    c. viruses
    d. fungi

9. The absence of disease-causing microorganisms is known as
    a. sterilization
    b. asepsis
    c. aseptic technique
    d. mechanical sterilization

10. The provision of the entire nutritional needs of a patient by means of intravenous infusion is known as
    a. LVP
    b. PRN
    c. SVP
    d. TPN

Pharmacy in Practice

1. Use a microscope to find and draw some microorganisms in pond water and/or tap water. Sketch a drawing of the microorganisms.

2. Write out a complete description, not using abbreviations, of the medication orders given in Figure 11.15. Refer to Chapter 3, Pharmaceutical Terminology and Abbreviations, as necessary.

3. Complete the following activity to learn about commonly accepted methods for disinfecting hands and to make yourself more conscious of the hands as a likely means for transfer of disease-causing microorganisms. This exercise also demonstrates the effectiveness of various materials and length of scrubbing for reducing skin surface bacterial numbers.

    Supplies needed:

    a. Nutrient agar plates

    b. Hand soap (Group No. 1)

    c. Iodine base disinfectant (Group No. 2)
        (Other scrub soaps may be substituted for students with allergies to iodine.)

d. Alcohol wipes (Group No. 3)

e. Hand brushes

f. Sterile hand towels (optional)

g. Sterile cotton swabs

h. Sterile nutrient broth

Procedure: Students should work in groups of four. One student in each group acts as the control and should culture and swab an unwashed hand before streaking an agar plate. Each of the other three students should do *one* of the wash, scrub, or wipe techniques listed in item b, below, and then complete the steps listed in a.

a. Inoculate control plate.

   −Wet swab with sterile water or sterile nutrient broth.

   −Rub swab over hand.

   −Rub swab lightly over nutrient agar plate.

   −Be careful not to tear the agar when inoculating it.

   −This plate will serve as one control in your experiment.

b. Follow *one* of these hand washing procedures, as assigned to you by your instructor.

   −Wash your hands with soap and running water. Dry with a sterile towel.

   −Scrub your hands with a sterile hand brush and an iodine base disinfectant for an assigned time. Dry your hands with a sterile towel.

   −Clean your hands with an alcohol wipe. Air dry your hands.

   −Scrub your hands for 15 seconds.

c. Inoculate a culture plate, following the steps in a, above.

d. Label the plate with your group number, method, and time of washing.

e. Group No. 2 students should wash, scrub, or wipe hands for 30 seconds. Then inoculate a culture plate as in steps a and d, above.

f. Group No. 3 students should wash, scrub, or wipe hands for 1 minute. Then inoculate a culture plate as in steps a and d, above.

g. Allow the culture plates to incubate at room temperature or in a slightly warm environment for at least 48 hours.

h. Record the results of your test and those done by other students in your class.

Which of the hand washing techniques was most effective in decontaminating the hands? What differences did you notice in the amount of culture produced using different lengths of time for scrubbing? Explain.

4. Using the orders below and the reconstitution chart in this chapter, answer the medication questions.

(✓)	START → HERE	DATE	TIME	A.M. P.M.	PROFILED BY:	FILLED BY:	CHECKED BY:	PATIENT NAME AND I.D.
	Acyclovir 1 g q12h							
			Welby, MD					

a. What fluid is it mixed in?
b. What is the expiration time at room temperature?
c. Can it be refrigerated?

(✓)	START → HERE	DATE	TIME	A.M. P.M.	PROFILED BY:	FILLED BY:	CHECKED BY:	PATIENT NAME AND I.D.
	Vancomycin 1.5 g q8h							
			Johnson, MD					

d. What size of bag is used?
e. What is the infusion time?
f. What is the room temperature expiration?

(✓)	START → HERE	DATE	TIME	A.M. P.M.	PROFILED BY:	FILLED BY:	CHECKED BY:	PATIENT NAME AND I.D.
	Primaxin 500 mg q6h x 3 days							
			Marsh, MD					

g. What fluid is it mixed in?
h. What size of bag?
i. How many bags will be needed?

(✓)	START HERE	DATE	TIME	A.M. P.M.	PROFILED BY:	FILLED BY:	CHECKED BY:	PATIENT NAME AND I.D.
	Oxacillin 1 g x 5 days							
		Docigrio, MD						

j. What size of bag is needed?

k. What fluid?

l. If all bags are prepared today, will the last one expire before the end of therapy?

m. What is the infusion rate?

5. Unit dose filling. Directions: Complete the total Daily Quantity ordered and the Amount to (Post) Add.

		Daily Quantity	(Post) Add
1.	Ibuprofen 600 mg PO q8h 1 was left in the drawer	( )	( )
2.	Colace 100 mg Liq PO bid POS 0 were left in the drawer	( )	( )
3.	Ferrous sulfate 325 mg PO tid 2 were left in the drawer	( )	( )
4.	Doxycycline 100 mg PO q12h 0 were left in the drawer	( )	( )
5.	Prednisone 7.5 mg PO qAM 0 were left in the drawer	( )	( )
6.	Benadryl 25 mg PO qhs 0 were left in the drawer	( )	( )
7.	Amoxil 250 mg PO tid 2 were left in the drawer	( )	( )
8.	Lasix 40 mg PO qAM and PM 1 was left in the drawer	( )	( )
9.	Zantac 150 mg PO bid 1 was left in the drawer	( )	( )
10.	Dexamethasone 2 mg IV q6h IVS 2 were left in the drawer	( )	( )
11.	Heparin flush IV q8h PRN 1 was left in the drawer	( )	( )
12.	Reglan 10 mg PO ac&hs 1 was left in the drawer	( )	( )

Your Future in Pharmacy Practice 12

The past century has seen dramatic changes in the pharmacy profession, but nothing compared to the changes that we shall doubtless see in the coming years. Exciting changes are afoot, including a movement toward national certification of pharmacy technicians and the placement of technicians in new roles and responsibilities. This chapter provides useful information and skills to prepare you for becoming a pharmacy technician at the dawn of a new century.

Learning Objectives

- Explain some ways in which the job of the pharmacy technician is changing
- Describe the format and content of the Pharmacy Technician Certification Examination
- Explain the criteria for recertification for pharmacy technicians
- Enumerate a wide variety of strategies for successful adaptation to the work environment
- Make a plan for a successful job search
- Write a résumé
- Write a cover letter
- Prepare for and successfully complete an interview
- Enumerate some trends for the future of the pharmacy profession

TERMS TO KNOW

Block style A format for letters in which each item is aligned left
Certified Pharmacy Technician (CPhT) A person who has passed the national Pharmacy Technician Certification Examination and who continues to meet recertification requirements established by the PTCB
Cover letter A letter submitted with a résumé for the purpose of summarizing one's qualifications, presenting one's résumé, and soliciting a job interview
Modified block style A format for letters in which the inside address, complimentary close, and signature are aligned from the center of the letter and the rest of the letter is aligned left
Pharmacy Technician Certification Board (PTCB) The body that certifies pharmacy technicians

INCREASING YOUR EMPLOYABILITY

As you learned in chapter 1, the pharmacy technician career field is presently undergoing dramatic changes. Throughout the country, pharmacy technicians are gaining recognition for the vital role they play in providing a wide range of pharmaceutical services in a wide range of employment settings. The occupational outlook for the pharmacy paraprofessional is quite bright. Some estimates put the number of new pharmacy technicians to be employed over the coming years in the tens of thousands. In many parts of the country, technicians are now receiving official recognition from state boards of pharmacy and are being asked to register with the state. At least one state is experimenting with having technicians check the work of other technicians in institutional settings. Chain drugstores and other employers are increasingly calling for technicians to become certified by taking the national Pharmacy Technician Certification Examination. Some people and organizations within the profession, including the Pharmacy Technicians Educators Council, are calling for the development of a two-year associate degree standard for technician training. All of these developments point to an increase in the presence, responsibilities, and status of the technician within the pharmacy community.

The elevation of the career of pharmacy technician to paraprofessional status brings with it increasing demands upon the technician. Today's employers expect more (and deliver more) to their technician employees. This section provides some useful information to help you to meet these increased demands and to place your best foot forward as you enter the field.

CERTIFICATION AND THE NATIONAL CERTIFICATION EXAMINATION

Pharmacy Technician Certification Examination (PTCE) A national certification examination for pharmacy technicians, covering three broad content areas: assisting a pharmacist, medication distribution and inventory control, and operations

Professional Examination Service (PES) A nonprofit testing company that develops and administers the Pharmacy Technician Certification Examination

Résumé A brief written summary of what you have to offer to an employer

In January of 1995, the **Pharmacy Technician Certification Board (PTCB)** was created by the American Pharmaceutical Association (APhA), the American Society of Health-System Pharmacists (ASHP), the Illinois Council of Health-System Pharmacists (ICHP), and the Michigan Pharmacists Association (MPA). The mission of the PTCB is to establish and maintain criteria for certification and recertification of pharmacy technicians on a national basis. A nonprofit testing company, the **Professional Examination Service (PES)** administers the **Pharmacy Technician Certification Examination (PTCE)**, which people must pass in order to become certified and receive the title of **CPhT**, or **certified pharmacy technician**. While institutional and retail pharmacies rarely require their pharmacy technicians to be certified, employers increasingly encourage certification. Often they are willing to pay for the training pharmacy technicians must take in preparation for the certification exam and may even pay the exam fee. Of course, technicians often receive higher pay once they are certified.

The PTCE is a multiple-choice examination containing a total of 125 questions organized into three sections, each of which is weighted differently. Candidates for certification are given three hours to complete the exam. Additional points are not deducted for incorrect answers on the exam. Therefore, it pays to answer every question on the exam. Candidates must receive a score of 650 or higher to pass the exam and receive certification. They may retake the exam as many times as is necessary to achieve a passing score.

Candidates should bring with them to the examination a silent, hand-held, nonprogramable, battery-operated calculator and a supply of No. 2 pencils. No reference materials, books, papers, or other materials may be taken into the examination room. The PTCB recommends that persons taking the exam be familiar with the material in "any of the basic pharmacy technician training manuals." According to the PTCB, the exam itself was constructed, reviewed, and edited using the reference texts described in Table 12.1. Familiarity with the contents of these texts will, of course, be invaluable when taking the exam.

Table 12.1

REFERENCE TEXTS USED IN CONSTRUCTION, REVIEW, AND EDITING OF THE PHARMACY TECHNICIAN CERTIFICATION EXAMINATION

Stoklosa M., and H. Ansel. *Pharmaceutical Calculations.* 10th ed. Baltimore, MD: Williams & Wilkins, 1996.

Manual for Pharmacy Technicians. 2nd ed. Bethesda, MD: American Society of Health-System Pharmacists, 1998.

Pharmacy Certified Technician Training Manual. Lansing, MI: Michigan Pharmacists Association, 1997.

Pharmacy Technician Workbook: A Self-Instructional Approach. Bethesda, MD: American Society of Health-System Pharmacists, 1994.

Moss, Susan. *Pharmacy Technician Certification Quick Study Guide.* Washington, DC: American Pharmaceutical Association, 1995.

Drug Facts and Comparisons. 52nd ed. St. Louis, MO: Facts and Comparisons, 1997.

Nielsen, J.R. *Handbook of Federal Drug Law.* Philadelphia, PA: Lea & Febiger, 1992.

Handbook of Non-Prescription Drugs. 2 vols. 11th ed. Washington, DC: American Pharmaceutical Association, 1996.

Abood, R.R., and D. B. Brushwood. 2nd ed. *Pharmacy Practice and the Law.* Gaithersburg, MD: Aspen, 1997.

Hunt M. *Training Manual for Intravenous Admixture Personnel.* 5th ed. Chicago: Bonus Books, 1995.

Table 12.2 explains the content of the examination, as specified by the PTCB.

Table 12.2	CONTENTS OF THE PHARMACY TECHNICIAN CERTIFICATION EXAMINATION

For purposes of national voluntary certification, pharmacy technicians are defined as individuals working in a pharmacy who, under the supervision of a licensed pharmacist, assist in pharmacy activities not requiring the professional judgment of the pharmacist. The following functions and responsibilities are a subset of functions performed in pharmacy practice determined and verified throughout the national study of pharmacy practice, the Scope of Pharmacy Practice Project. The Pharmacy Technician Certification Examination samples candidates' knowledge and skill base for activities performed in the work of pharmacy technicians. Functions and responsibilities of pharmacy technicians may be specifically defined by state rules and regulations as well as job-center policies and procedures. The pharmacy technician is accountable to the supervising pharmacist, who is legally responsible by virtue of state licensure for the care and safety of patients served by the pharmacy. The pharmacy technician performs activities as the result of having certain knowledge and skills. These activities are characterized under three broad function areas:

I. Assisting the Pharmacist in Serving Patients—50% of Examination

II. Medication Distribution and Inventory Control Systems—35% of Examination

III. Operations—15% of Examination

I. Assisting the Pharmacist in Serving Patients: Includes activities related to traditional pharmacy prescription dispensing and medication distribution, and collecting and organizing information.

1. Receive prescription/medication order from patient/patient's representative, prescriber, or other healthcare professionals, including:

 – Accept new prescription /medication order from patient/patient's representative, prescriber, or other health care professionals.

 – Accept refill request from patient/patient's representative, or prescriber.

 – Accept new prescription/medication order electronically (e.g., telephone, fax, computer).

 – Accept refill request electronically (e.g., telephone, fax, computer).

 – Call prescriber for clarification of prescription/medication order refill.

2. At the direction of the pharmacist, assist in obtaining from the patient/patient's representative such information as diagnosis or desired therapeutic outcome, medication use, allergies, adverse reactions, medical history, psychosocial history, visual impairment, physical disability, socioeconomic history, and reimbursement mechanisms.

3. Assess prescription/medication order for completeness (e.g., patient's name/address), correctness (e.g., consistency with products available), authenticity, legality, and reimbursement eligibility.

Table 12.2

(cont.)

4. At the direction of the pharmacist, assist in obtaining from prescriber and/or other healthcare professionals such information as diagnosis or desired therapeutic outcome, medication use, allergies, adverse reactions, medical history, psychosocial history, visual impairment, physical disability, socioeconomic history, and reimbursement mechanisms.

5. Update the medical record/patient profile with such information as medication history, allergies, medication duplication (e.g., medication misuse), and/or drug-disease, drug-drug, drug-laboratory, and drug-nutrient interactions.

6. Process the prescription/medication order, including:

   - Enter prescription information onto patient profile.

   - Select the manufacturing source of supply of product(s) to be dispensed for prescription/medication order written in generic terminology.

   - Select the manufacturing source of supply of product(s) to be dispensed for a brand name prescription/medication order.

   - Obtain medications or devices from inventory.

   - Calibrate equipment needed to prepare or compound the prescription/medication order.

   - Compound medications for dispensing according to prescription formula or instructions.

   - Measure or count finished dosage forms for dispensing.

   - Prepare IV admixtures.

   - Record preparation of medication in various dosage forms.

   - Record preparation of controlled substances for dispensing.

   - Package the preparation.

   - Prepare and/or obtain the label(s).

   - Affix label(s) and auxiliary label(s) to container(s).

   - Assemble patient information materials.

   - Perform intermediate checks during processing of the prescription/medication order.

7. Deliver medication to patient/patient's representative, including:

   - Store medication prior to distribution.

   - Deliver medication to patient/patient's representative.

   - Place medication in unit-dose cart.

   - Deliver medication to patient-care unit.

   - Record distribution of prescription medications.

   - Record distribution of controlled substances.

8. Determine charges and obtain compensation for services.

9. Provide supplemental information, as indicated (e.g., patient package inserts, computer-generated information, videos).

10. Communicate with third-party payers to determine or verify coverage.

II. Medication Distribution and Inventory Control Systems: Includes activities related to medication and supply purchasing, inventory control, and preparation and distribution of medications according to approved policies and procedures.

1. Place orders for pharmaceuticals, durable medical equipment, devices, and supplies, including expediting of emergency orders.

2. Receive goods and verify specifications on original purchase orders.

3. Place pharmaceuticals, durable medical equipment, devices, and supplies in inventory under proper storage conditions.

4. Remove from inventory expired/discontinued/slow-moving pharmaceuticals, durable medical equipment, devices, and supplies, and document actions taken.

5. Remove from inventory recalled pharmaceuticals, durable medical equipment, devices, and supplies, and document actions taken.

6. Identify pharmaceuticals, durable medical equipment, devices, and supplies to be ordered (e.g., "want book").

7. Communicate changes in product availability (e.g., formulary changes, recalls) to pharmacy staff, patient/patient's representative, physicians, and other healthcare professionals.

8. Maintain policies and procedures to deter theft and/or drug diversion.

9. Maintain a record of controlled substances received, stored, and removed from inventory.

10. Maintain record-keeping systems for repackaging, recalls, and returns of pharmaceuticals, durable medical equipment, devices, and supplies.

11. Compound medications in anticipation of prescriptions/medication orders (e.g., bulk compounding).

12. Prepackage finished dosage forms for dispensing.

13. Collect and analyze data on the quality of pharmacy products and services.

III. Operations: Includes activities related to the administrative processes for the pharmacy practice center, including operations, human resources, facilities and equipment and information systems.

1. Coordinate communications throughout the practice center and/or service area.

2. Participate in meetings to obtain feedback regarding the performance of the practice center and/or service area.

3. Monitor the practice center and/or service area for compliance with federal, state, and local laws, regulations, and professional standards.

4. Implement and monitor policies and procedures for sanitation management, hazardous waste handling (e.g., needles), and infection control (e.g., protective clothing).

5. Perform and record routine sanitation, maintenance, and calibration of equipment.

6. Maintain a manual or computer-based information system.

Sample questions from the certification examination are available on the PTCB Web site at http://www.ptcb.org

RECERTIFICATION

Recertification is required by the PTCB every two years. To be recertified, one must earn a total of 20 hours credit in pharmacy-related continuing education, with at least one of these hours being in pharmacy law. Certified technicians receive notification of the need for recertification approximately 60 days before their certification lapses.

ADJUSTING TO THE WORK ENVIRONMENT

If you have not worked before, or if your work experience has been sporadic, then getting used to your job as a technician might seem like getting used to life in a foreign country. You will have to adjust to a new "work culture," to different behaviors, to unfamiliar customs, and even to a new "language," the technical jargon of the profession. The following chart provides some advice for making your adjustment to the job a comfortable one.

Chart 12.1

ADVICE FOR SUCCESSFUL ADAPTATION TO THE WORK ENVIRONMENT

Attitude: Do not give in to the temptation to behave in ways that are elitist or superior. Remember you are part of a healthcare team, and cooperation is extremely important.

Reliability: Health care, like teaching, is one of those industries in which standards for reliability are very high. One simply cannot show up late for work, take days off arbitrarily, without good reason, and so on. Unreliable employees in the healthcare industry do not keep their jobs for long. Therefore, make sure that your employer can always depend on you to arrive at work on time. Staying late does not make up for a tardy arrival. Remember that tardiness can play havoc with other people's work schedules and work loads. Finish your grooming and eating before you enter your work area.

Accuracy and Responsibility: In a pharmacy, one rarely has the leeway to be partially correct. An error, even a small one, can have dire consequences for a patient or customer. Develop work habits to ensure accuracy, and expect to be held responsible for what you do on the job. Work steadily and methodically. Keep your attention on the task at hand, and always double check everything you do.

Relating to Your Supervisor: Always show your supervisor a reasonable degree of deference and respect. Ask your supervisor how he or she prefers to be addressed. Be respectful of your supervisor's experience and knowledge. If tensions arise between you and your supervisor, take positive steps to lessen them. Remember that your supervisor has power over your raises, promotions, benefits, and references for future employment.

Personality: It may come as some surprise to you, but personality is one of the greatest predictors of job success. Be positive, cooperative, self-confident, and enthusiastic.

Performance: Demonstrate that you can get things done and that you put the job first.

Questioning: Sometimes people are afraid to ask questions because doing so might make them appear less intelligent or knowledgeable. Nothing could be further from the truth. When you do not know how something should be done, always ask.

Dress: Follow the dress code of the company or institution for which you work.

Receptivity: Listen to the advice of others who have been on the job longer. Accept criticism gracefully. If you make a mistake, own up to it. If you are criticized unfairly, adopt a nondefensive tone of voice and explain your view of the matter calmly and rationally.

Organizational Etiquette: Every workplace has its unique culture. Especially at first, pay close attention to the details of that culture. Pick up on the habits of interaction and communication practiced by other employees and model the best of these.

Alliances: In all organizations, two kinds of power systems exist—formal, or organizational ones, and informal ones, based upon alliances. Cultivate others on the job, but make sure that you are not seen as part of a clique. Even as a new employee, you will begin to build power through making alliances. If a problem or an opportunity arises, you will probably hear about it first through your allies on the job. If a change in the workplace affects you, advance notice may give you the time to plan a strategic response.

Reputation: Many people assume that if they work hard and are loyal, then they will be rewarded. This is often but not necessarily always true. People in management may be so involved with their own concerns that you remain little more than a face in the crowd. Being pleasant to others will help you to be noticed, as will making helpful or useful suggestions. Don't keep your professional qualifications a secret. Join professional organizations. Serve on committees within the institution. See that your name is publicized when you have won an award or achieved some other success (in, for example, institutional newsletters, community newspapers, or the newsletters of professional organizations). Give presentations at professional meetings, civic groups, churches, or synagogues. Write articles for publication in professional publications. In short, do whatever you can not to hide your light under a bushel.

Luck: Most of the big lucky breaks in life come through knowing the right people at the right time. So, by cultivating alliances, you can, more than you might expect, control your luck.

Crisis: When a crisis occurs, don't overreact. Take time, if you can, to think and then act, and do not keep the crisis a secret from your supervisor.

Learning: Pharmacy is a rapidly changing field. Accept the idea of continuing education as a way of life. You need not take formal course work every year (unless you are doing so to maintain your certification), but do make a point to read and to attend professional meetings to learn about the latest trends. Think of the job-related learning that you do as a regular "information workout," as necessary to your employment fitness as aerobic workouts are to your physical fitness.

Expertise: How can you become a person who makes things happen? Become highly knowledgeable about a specialty within your field. Become the most expert technician that you can become in that area. Then move on and master another area. Soon, others will be asking your advice, and your reputation will build.

Reflectiveness About Your Career: There will never be a time in your career to coast and relax. Good career chances can come your way at any time in life, so make a regular habit of taking the time to think about your career and where you are headed. Planning lends structure and substance to your career management.

THE JOB SEARCH

Before you can implement the excellent strategies introduced in the preceding section, you must, of course, find the right job. Many people find the prospect of job hunting overwhelming. Avoid such negative thinking. Instead, think of the job hunt as an adventure, a period of exploration that can lead to exciting new possibilities. The following chart lists some steps you can take to make the job search successful:

Chart 12.2

TEN STEPS FOR ORGANIZING A JOB SEARCH

1. **Clarify Your Career Goals.** It will be very difficult to find a job if you are not sure what you are looking for. Do you want to work in a community pharmacy? in a hospital? in a long-term care facility? in a home infusion pharmacy? If you have uncertainties about the setting in which you wish to work, arrange to interview some people who work in these settings. Also do some thinking about what you want out of the job. Are you interested in jobs with opportunities for advancement in retail management? Are you more interested in the Rx component of the job? Do you want to master the preparation of parenterals? compounding? ordering and inventory? billing? maintenance of a drug information library? Think about what you want to do. Then look for jobs that suit your ambitions. Many schools have career counselors who can help you to answer such questions. Make an appointment to visit and talk to one of these people.

2. **Write a Good Résumé.** Read the section on résumé writing in the section that follows. Make use of some of the excellent résumé writing software now available, or avail yourself of a résumé-writing service.

3. **Identify Potential Employers.** Your school may have a career placement office. Use the services of that office. Check the classified ads in newspapers. Go to a career library and look up employers in directories. Look up potential employers in telephone directories. Make use of career opportunities posted on Web sites such as Rx Trek (http://ourworld.compuserve.com/homepages/RxTrek/homepage.htm) and the site of the Pharmacy Technician Certification Board (http://www.ptcb.org). Make use of job-search Web sites such as America's Job Bank (http://www.ajb.dni.us) and Health Care Jobs Online (http://www.hcjobsonline.com).

4. **Establish a Network.** Tell everyone you know that you are looking for a job. Identify faculty, acquaintances, friends, and relatives who can assist you in your job search. Identify people within employers' organizations who can give you insight into their needs. Join professional associations. Attend meetings, and network with colleagues and potential employers.

5. **Research Potential Employers.** Find out everything that you can about a company or institution before you go for an interview. Better yet, do this work before you write the cover letter that you send with your résumé. Knowing details about a potential employer can help you to assess whether the employer is right for you and can win points in your cover letter or interview.

6. **Make Interview Appointments If Possible.** Whenever possible, make an appointment, by telephone, to come in for an interview. If such an appointment cannot be made (if, for example, you are responding to a job posting that reads, "No telephone calls, please"), then send a cover letter and résumé.

7. **Write a Strong Cover Letter.** Follow the guidelines given on p. 245.

8. **Before the Interview.** Review your research on the employer and role-play an interview situation. Get plenty of sleep and eat well on the day before the interview.

9. **During the Interview.** Follow the guidelines given on p. 247.

10. **After the Interview.** Follow up with a thank-you note and, within an appropriate time, a telephone call. Be persistent but not pushy.

Writing a Résumé

A résumé is a brief written summary of what you have to offer an employer. It is a sales tool, and the product you are selling is yourself. A résumé is an opportunity to present your work experience, your skills, and your education to an employer. The following chart outlines the general topics to be included in a chronological résumé:

Chart 12.3

THE PARTS OF A RÉSUMÉ

Heading: Give your full name, address, and telephone number. Remember to include your Zip code and area code.

Employment Objective: This is the first thing an employer wants to know. The objective should briefly describe the position you are seeking and some of the abilities you would like to be able to use on the job. Identify the requirements of the position. Then tailor the employment objective to match those requirements.

Education: Give your college, city, state, degree, major, date of graduation, and additional course work related to the job, to the profession, or to business in general. State your cumulative grade point average if it is 3.0 or higher.

Experience: In reverse chronological order, list your work experience, including on-campus and off-campus work. Do not include jobs that would be unimpressive to your employer. Be sure to include cooperative education experience. For each job, indicate your position, employer's name, the location of the employment, the dates employed, and a brief description of your duties. Always list any advancements, promotions, or supervisory responsibilities.

Skills: If you do not have a lot of relevant work experience, include a skills section that details the skills that you can bring to bear on the job. Doing so is a way of saying, "I'm really capable. I just haven't had much opportunity to show it yet."

Related Activities: Include any activities that show leadership, teamwork, or good communication skills. Include any club or organizational memberships, as well as professional or community activities.

References: State that these are "Available on request."

Make sure that your résumé follows a consistent, standard format, like that shown in Figure 12.1. Limit it to a single page. Type it, or print it on a high-quality inkjet or laser printer, using high-quality 8-1/2 x 11-inch paper. Many special résumé papers are available from stationary and office supply shops. However, ordinary opaque white paper is acceptable. Be sure to check your résumé very carefully for errors in spelling, grammar, usage, punctuation, capitalization, and form. No one wants to hire a sloppy technician.

Figure 12.1 Sample résumé.

Ronald Cashman
1700 Beltline Blvd.
My Town, SC 29169
(345) 555-3245

Objective: Position as pharmacy technician that makes use of my training in dispensing and compounding medications, ordering and inventory, patient profiling, third-party billing, and other essential functions

Education	My Town Technical College
	My Town, South Carolina
	Diploma in Health Science—Pharmacy
	Program Accredited by the American Society of
	Health-System Pharmacists
	Dean's List
Skills	Converting units of measure
	Setting up ratios and proportions for proper
	performance of pharmacy calculations
	Aseptic preparation of intravenous solutions
	Proper interpretation of prescriptions and
	physician's orders
	Proper interpretation and updating of
	prescription records
	Attention to clerical detail
	Operation of pharmacy computer systems

Employment
1997-98   Clerk
                 Arborland Pharmacy
                 Erewhon, SC

References available on request.

Writing a Cover Letter

The cover letter, or letter of application, is the first letter that you send to an employer. It is generally sent in response to a job ad or posting or prior to a cold call to a potential employer. The résumé should accompany the cover letter. Both the cover letter and the résumé should be typed or printed on the same stock, or kind, of paper, and both should be placed in a matching business envelope addressed by means of typing or printing on an inkjet or laser printer. The letter should be single-spaced, using a block or modified block style. In the block style, all items in the letter begin at the left margin. In the modified block style, the sender's address, the complimentary close, and the signature are left-aligned from the center of the paper, and all other parts of the letter begin at the left margin.

The cover letter should highlight your qualifications and call attention to your résumé. As with your résumé, proofread the cover letter carefully for errors in spelling, grammar, usage, punctuation, capitalization, and form. Address the letter, when possible, to a particular person, by name and by title, and make sure to identify the position for which you are applying. If necessary, call the employer to get the correct spelling of the recipient's name. Use the format shown in Chart 12.4 for your letter.

Chart 12.4

SUGGESTED FORMAT FOR COVER LETTERS

First Paragraph: In your initial paragraph, state why you are writing, the specific position or type of work for which you are applying, and how you learned of the opening (e.g., from the placement office, the news media, or a friend).

Second Paragraph: Explain why you are interested in the position, the organization, or the organization's products and services. State how your academic background makes you a qualified candidate for the position. If you have had some practical experience, point out your specific achievements.

Third Paragraph: Refer the reader to the enclosed résumé, a summary of your qualifications, training, and experience.

Fourth Paragraph: Indicate your desire for a personal interview and your flexibility as to the time and place. Repeat your telephone number in the letter. Close your letter with a statement or question to encourage a response, or take the initiative by indicating a day and date on which you will contact the employer to set up a convenient time for a personal meeting.

Figure 12.2 shows a sample cover letter.

February 1, 2000

James Green, Pharm.D.
Main Street Community Pharmacy
1500 Main Street
My Town, SC 29201

Dear Dr. Green:

I learned of Main Street Community Pharmacy's need for a pharmacy technician through the Placement Office at My Town Technical College. I was pleased to learn of an opening for a technician at the very pharmacy that my family has frequented for years.

I believe that my education and experience would be an asset to Main Street Community Pharmacy. This May, I will be graduating from My Town Technical College's superb pharmacy technician training program. I would welcome the opportunity to apply what I have learned to a career with your pharmacy. I bring to the job a number of assets, including a 3.4 grade point average, commitment to continuing development of my skills as a technician, a willingness to work hard, and a desire to be of service.

I am a responsible person, concerned with accuracy and accountability, someone whom you can depend upon to carry out the technician's duties reliably. I have enclosed my résumé for your consideration.

I would appreciate an opportunity to discuss the position with you. I will call next week to inquire about a meeting. Thank you for considering my application.

Sincerely,

Ronald Cashman
1700 Beltline Blvd.
My Town, SC 29169

Enc.: résumé

Figure 12.2 Sample cover letter.

Interviewing for a Job

The following chart lists some guidelines for conducting a successful job interview.

Chart 12.5

GUIDELINES FOR JOB INTERVIEWS

1. Find out the exact place and time of the interview.

2. Know the full name of the company, the address, the interviewer's full name, and the correct pronunciation of the interviewer's name. Call the employer, if necessary, to get this information.

3. Know something about the company's operations.

4. Be courteous to the receptionist, if there is one, and to other employees. Any person that you meet or speak with may be in a position to influence your employment.

5. Bring to the interview your résumé and the names, addresses, and telephone numbers of people who can provide references.

6. Arrive ten to fifteen minutes before the scheduled time for the interview.

7. Wear clothing and shoes appropriate to the job.

8. Greet the interviewer and call him or her by name. Introduce yourself at once. Shake hands only if the interviewer offers to do so. Remain standing until invited to sit down.

9. Be confident, polite, poised, and enthusiastic.

10. Look the interviewer in the eye.

11. Speak clearly, loudly enough to be understood. Be positive and concise in your comments. Do not exaggerate, but remember that an interview is not an occasion for modesty.

12. Focus on your strengths. Be prepared to enumerate these, using specific examples as evidence to support the claims you make about yourself.

13. Do not hesitate to ask about the specific duties associated with the job. Show keen interest as the interviewer tells you about these.

14. Avoid bringing up salary requirements until the employer broaches the subject.

15. Do not chew gum or smoke.

16. Do not criticize former employers, coworkers, working conditions.

17. At the close of the interview, thank the interviewer for his or her time and for the opportunity to learn about the company.

Be prepared to answer questions similar to the following:

1. Why did you apply for a job with this company?

2. What part of the job are you most interested in and why?

3. What do you know about this company?

4. What are your qualifications?

5. What did you like the most and the least about your work experience? (Note: Explaining what you liked least should be done in as positive a manner as possible. For example, you might say that you wish that the job had provided more opportunity for learning about this or that and then explain, further, that you made up the deficiency by study on your

Chart 12.5

(cont.)

own. Such an answer indicates your desire to learn and grow and does not cast your former employer in an unduly negative light.)

6. Why did you leave your previous job? (Again, avoid negative responses. Find a positive reason for leaving, such as returning to school or pursuing an opportunity.)

7. What would you like to be doing in five years? How much money would you like to be making? (Keep your answer reasonable, and show that you have ambitions consistent with the employer's needs.)

8. What are your weak points? (Again, say something positive, such as "I am an extremely conscientious person. Sometimes I worry too much about whether I have done something absolutely correctly, but that can also be a positive trait.")

9. Why do you think you are qualified for this position?

10. Would you mind working on the weekends? overtime? traveling?

11. Do you prefer working with others or by yourself? in a quiet or a noisy environment?

12. If you could have any job you wanted, what would you choose and why?

13. Tell me a little about yourself.

14. What are your hobbies and interests?

15. Why did you attend [the college that you attended]?

16. Why did you choose this major?

17. What courses did you like best? least? (Again, couch your responses to both questions in positive ways.)

18. What have you learned from your mistakes?

19. What motivates you to put forth your greatest efforts?

20. Do you plan to continue your education?

Rehearse answers to these questions before the interview. Bear in mind, when coming up with answers to such questions, the employer's point of view. Try to imagine what you would want if you were the employer, and take the initiative, during the interview, to explain to the employer how you can meet those needs.

TRENDS IN PHARMACY PRACTICE

One of the wonderful things about a career in pharmacy is that the profession changes continually. Consider how different the average community pharmacy of today is from the druggist's shop at the turn of the century, in which premanufactured medicines were novelties and rows of bottled tonics and elixirs vied for customers' attention with open barrels of hard candies. Doubtless the profession will change as much or more in the next 30 years as it did in the past one hundred, and that's a lot of change. The following are but a few of the exciting developments that lie in store:

1. **New Medicines and New Drug Development Technologies.** Every day, new medicines come to market, many involving new drug development technologies such as genetic engineering. To work in pharmacy is to be at

the front lines when new medications are introduced to combat AIDS, cancer, heart disease, cystic fibrosis, Parkinson's disease, and other scourges.

2. **New Dosage Forms and Drug Delivery Mechanisms.** New dosage forms and drug delivery mechanisms are not introduced as commonly as new drugs, but here, as well, the pace of innovation is increasing rapidly. The past few years have seen the introduction of such innovations as transdermal patches, conjunctival discs, and wearable intravenous infusion pumps. What the future holds is anyone's guess, but the one certainty is that new dosage forms and delivery mechanisms will emerge.

3. **Robotics.** Robotic machinery is already used in many institutional settings for unit-dose repackaging procedures. It is likely that in the future robotics will play a larger role in pharmacy, providing, for example, automated compounding, filling, labeling, and record keeping in a single device.

4. **Higher Professional Standards.** In the near future, the entry level degree for the pharmacist will be the Pharm.D., and the national certification movement for pharmacy technicians is growing rapidly.

5. **Continued Growth in Clinical Applications.** The clinical pharmacy movement also continues to grow. In the future, more and more of the pharmacy professional's time and energies will be given to educational and counseling functions.

6. **Increased Emphasis on Home Health Care.** The home healthcare industry is one of the most rapidly growing of all industries in the developed world. The reasons behind this growth include reduced cost, improvements in technology that make home care more practical, and the preference of individuals for remaining at home rather than in institutions. The growth of the home-care industry shows no signs of abating, and so, in the future, more pharmacists and technicians will find themselves servicing that industry.

7. **Increased Technician Responsibility and Specialization.** Some states are already experimenting with allowing trained technicians to check the work of other technicians. Expect, in the future, for technicians to be given ever more responsibility and for more and more technicians to become specialized in particular areas of service such as radiopharmaceuticals or pediatric or geriatric pharmacy.

8. **Web Pharmacies.** A very recent development with much promise is the emergence of the online pharmacy, allowing patients and healthcare professionals to access records, communicate or refill prescriptions, monitor drug regimens, order nonprescription drugs and medical supplies, and conduct many other functions via the World Wide Web.

9. **Online Reference Works.** Already, many standard reference works in pharmacy are available in CD-ROM format. See chapter 6 for examples. In the future, expect to see the most important reference works all become available in easily accessible and searchable online form via the World Wide Web.

10. **Increase in Geriatric Applications.** As the population of the United States ages, the importance of geriatric pharmacy will increase. The aging of the population will place great financial burdens on the healthcare system as a whole and on pharmacy in particular, leading inevitably to political decisions that will affect the functions of the pharmacist and the technician.

chapter summary

The occupational outlook for the pharmacy technician is promising. Increasingly, states are requiring certification or registration with the state board of pharmacy. Certification is offered through the Pharmacy Technician Certification Board (PTCB), an organization created by the American Pharmaceutical Association and other pharmacy groups in 1995. People who pass the certification examination receive the title of CPhT, or certified pharmacy technician.

Preparing to work in an institutional or community-based pharmacy requires serious thought about one's attitude, reliability, accuracy, sense of responsibility, personal appearance, organizational skills, and the ability to relate to others, particularly the supervisor. Luck plays a role, too, as does the desire to learn throughout life. After carefully planning a job search, you are ready to write a comprehensive, attractive resume and cover letter that will result in interviews and, eventually, one or more job offers.

New medicines and drugs are continually being developed. Other trends to watch for include the use of robotics in drug manufacturing and compounding, higher professional standards, an increased emphasis on home health care, increased technician responsibility, and healthcare changes brought about by the expansion of the senior population.

chapter review

Knowledge Inventory

1. The organization that certifies pharmacy technicians is the
   a. Pharmacy Technician Certification Board
   b. Committee for the Certification of Pharmacy Technicians
   c. Pharmacy Technician Review Council
   d. American Society of Pharmacy Technicians

2. The Pharmacy Technician Certification Examination is
   a. an essay examination
   b. a multiple-choice examination
   c. a true/false examination
   d. all of the above

3. When taking the Pharmacy Technician Certification Examination, the candidate is allowed to bring into the room
   a. two reference works of his or her choosing
   b. scrap paper on which to do calculations
   c. a calculator
   d. one pharmacy technician training manual

4. The person legally responsible by virtue of state licensure for the care and safety of patients served by a pharmacy is the
   a. pharmacy technician
   b. pharmacist
   c. supervising pharmacist
   d. pharmacologist

5. The Pharmacy Technician Certification Examination tests candidates on
   a. assisting the pharmacist in serving patients
   b. medication distribution and inventory control systems
   c. operations
   d. all of the above

6. A standard résumé does *not* list
   a. the job objective
   b. employment history
   c. name, address, and telephone number of the applicant
   d. names, addresses, and telephone numbers of references

7. If someone does not have a great deal of work experience, he or she can compensate for this deficiency by emphasizing the
   a. employment history section of the résumé
   b. references section of the résumé
   c. job objective section of the résumé
   d. skills section of the résumé

8. The cover letter sent with a résumé should highlight one's
   a. qualifications
   b. personality
   c. network of connections
   d. need for the job

9. The transdermal patch is an example of a recently developed
   a. dosage form
   b. drug
   c. drug delivery mechanism
   d. drug development technology

10. In the future, it is likely that most pharmacy reference works will become available via
    a. microfiche
    b. microfilm
    c. CDi, or CD interactive
    d. the World Wide Web

Pharmacy in Practice

1. Visit the Web site of the Pharmacy Technician Certification Board at http://www.ptcb.org and study the sample test questions available on that site. Print the sample questions and work with other students in small groups to answer them. To answer some of these questions, you may have to refer to reference works or to more advanced texts in pharmacology or pharmacy calculations.

2. Write, e-mail, or call the Pharmacy Technician Certification Board and order information on the PTCE.

3. Do some research and compile a list of three potential employers of pharmacy technicians in each of the following areas: community pharmacy, hospital pharmacy, long-term care, and home infusion. Each list should include the name of the employer, the address, the telephone number, and a contact person. Collect the lists prepared by students in the class to make a master list.

4. Choose one potential employer of pharmacy technicians and do some research to find more information about the employer. Write a brief report providing information that might be of interest to a potential employee of this pharmacy or institution.

5. Write a résumé and cover letter that you might use to apply for a job as a pharmacy technician.

6. Practice role-playing an interview situation with other students in your class. Use the interview questions supplied in this chapter.

appendix A

IN THE LAB

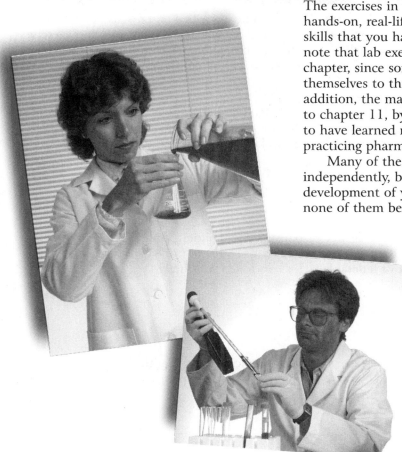

The exercises in this appendix will provide actual hands-on, real-life experience in performing the skills that you have learned in the text. You will note that lab exercises are not provided for every chapter, since some chapters do not lend themselves to this kind of hands-on practice. In addition, the majority of the exercises are related to chapter 11, by which time you will be expected to have learned most of the skills demanded of the practicing pharmacy technician.

Many of the exercises can be performed independently, but, at this stage in the development of your skills, it is advisable that none of them be attempted without the direct supervision of your instructor. Similarly, all of the forms, orders, compounds, and preparations resulting from these exercises will be subject to review by your instructor.

These exercises are intended to expand and extend your mastery of the increasingly responsible skills demanded of the pharmacy technician. As you continue on the path to your chosen profession, they can serve as a guide to the thorough and conscientious performance of your job.

Chapter 2: Pharmacy Law, Standards, and Ethics for Technicians

LAW

Legal aspects of pharmacy practice should be described and discussed among members of your class, with emphasis on the areas in the questions and exercises below. The two forms included in this exercise are representative of the kinds of forms used in dispensing and inventory control of controlled substances in hospitals.

1. Explain the difference between federal and state pharmacy laws and identify which takes precedence in case of a conflict. Identify, from your state pharmacy practice act, differences between federal and state law, if any.

2. Identify the state agency responsible for inpatient drug dispensing, outpatient dispensing, enforcement of state-controlled substances, and enforcement of federal laws for controlled substances.

3. Identify, in your state pharmacy practice act, legal authority for pharmacists, interns, residents, and technicians in providing pharmaceutical services.

4. Identify statements from your state pharmacy practice act relating to pharmacy and technician students.

5. Describe areas of pharmacy practice covered by the Food, Drug and Cosmetic Act of 1938, the Comprehensive Drug Abuse and Prevention Act of 1970 (Controlled Substances Act), and the Poison Prevention Act of 1970.

Name _____ Date _____

6. List necessary components of a label for controlled substances.

7. List the five (5) schedules of controlled substances and give two examples of each schedule.

   Schedule 1 (C-I)

   Schedule 2 (C-II)

   Schedule 3 (C-III)

   Schedule 4 (C-IV)

   Schedule 5 (C-V)

8. How often are inventories taken for controlled substances?

9. Explain security requirements for controlled substance storage.

10. Explain distribution and record keeping for controlled substances.

DRUG NAME:	STRENGTH:		ORAL	SERIAL NUMBER
				*
PREPARED BY:	CHECKED BY:	RECEIVED BY:		NURSING UNIT AND TEAM NUMBER
DATE ISSUED:	DATE RETURNED: (and quantity, if any)			QUANTITY ISSUED:

PHARMACY RECEIPT

CHARGE CODE: 04570

76002455-ORAL

Name _____ Date _____

CONTROLLED DRUG WASTE REPORT

*Instructions: Describe in detail how the drug was wasted and ask any and all witnesses to sign this report. Describe the final disposition of the drug, i.e., discarded down sink.

REPORT #1

DATE	TIME	PATIENT'S NAME	ROOM	DRUG AND STRENGTH	QUANTITY USED

REASON AND DISPOSITION _____

_____

_____

_____

NURSE	WITNESS	HEAD NURSE	NURSE COORD./SUP.

REPORT #2

DATE	TIME	PATIENT'S NAME	ROOM	DRUG AND STRENGTH	QUANTITY USED

REASON AND DISPOSITION _____

_____

_____

_____

NURSE	WITNESS	HEAD NURSE	NURSE COORD./SUP.

REPORT #3

DATE	TIME	PATIENT'S NAME	ROOM	DRUG AND STRENGTH	QUANTITY USED

REASON AND DISPOSITION _____

_____

_____

_____

NURSE	WITNESS	HEAD NURSE	NURSE COORD./SUP.

ADDITIONAL FORMS MAY BE OBTAINED FROM PHARMACY IF NEEDED.

Chapter 6: Sources of Information

This reference exercise will encourage your understanding and use of pharmacy reference sources. You should utilize pharmacy reference works to answer questions in the exercise. The completed exercise will be checked by an instructor, or a class review may be held to ensure that students have answered the questions correctly. Both reference works and periodicals will be used for this exercise.

Suggested reference works include, but are not limited to, the *United States Pharmacopeia/National Formulary* (USP/NF), *Remington's Pharmaceutical Sciences, Drug Facts and Comparisons, Patient Drug Facts, American Hospital Formulary Service Drug Information* (AHFS), *Physician's Desk Reference, American Drug Index, Goodman and Gilman's The Pharmacological Basis of Therapeutics, Merck Manual of Diagnosis and Therapy*, and Trissel's *Handbook on Injectable Drugs*.

Suggested periodicals include *American Journal of Health System Pharmacy* (AJHP), *American Druggist, Pharmacy Times*, and *Journal of Pharmacy Technology*.

Additional suggested reference information would include drug package inserts.

1. Identify tablet presented by the instructor (include name and strength). What reference was used?

2. Where can you find the signs, symptoms, and treatments of appendicitis?

3. Are Lasix (furosemide) and potassium chloride compatible in the same IV bag? What reference was used?

4. Do Percocet and Roxicet contain the same ingredients? List the main ingredients. What reference was used?

5. Where can you find the address for Parke-Davis drug company?

Name _____ Date _____

6. What reference(s) list ingredients and compounding instructions for green soap?

7. What is the molecular weight of calcium gluceptate? What reference was used?

8. Which reference book contains information on the evolution of pharmacy, ethics of pharmacy, chemical applications of pharmacy calculations, and pharmacy law?

9. List the strength of Zaroxolyn available. What reference was used?

10. What is the pediatric dose of chloramphenicol? Is it available in a liquid? What reference was used?

11. What reference would best describe pharmacology of local anesthetics?

12. What is another brand name for Motrin containing 600 mg of ibuprofen? What reference was used?

13. What is Hyserp?

14. What is the phone number of Astra Pharmaceutical Products, Inc.? What reference was used?

15. What reference(s) would give the chemical structure of paraldehyde and give information on packaging and storage?

16. What reference would explain the "controlled substance" labeling?

17. From pharmacy periodicals available with the last 3 months, list 5 drugs advertised that include package insert information.

	Periodical	Page Number	Drug
1)	_____	_____	_____
2)	_____	_____	_____
3)	_____	_____	_____
4)	_____	_____	_____
5)	_____	_____	_____

Name _____ Date _____

Chapter 7: Basic Pharmaceutical Measurements and Calculations

IV CALCULATIONS

In this exercise on IV calculations, you are to utilize appropriate methods of math calculations to arrive at correct answers. Refer to the Reconstitutions chart (pages A-34—A-35) or consult the *Handbook on Injectable Drugs* to determine appropriate answers. Numbers 3 and 4 will be answered based on the medication provided. For the last order, number 5, a label should be written and the product made.

1. An order is written for 30mEq KCl in 1L D5&1/2NS. Run IVF at 150 mL/hr.

    a. Is this a large volume?

    b. A stock bottle of KCl has 2 mEq/mL. How many mLs of KCl will be needed for this order?

    c. How long will one bag last?

    d. How many bags will be needed?

2. Order reads: Give Rocephin 0.5 g IV q24hrs.

    a. Is this a large volume or minibag?

    b. What size bag will be needed?

    c. How many mLs of Rocephin will be needed? Start with a 1 g vial that needs reconstitution.

    d. How many bags will be needed every 24 hours?

3. Label #1

```
┌─────────────────────────────────────────────────────────┐
│              Mt. Hope Pharmacy Services                   │
│                                                           │
│  Patient: COLMAN, SHERRY      ID. No. 024371   Rm. No. 541-1 │
│                                                           │
│  Prepared: 10:50AM            Date: 10/15/99              │
│                                                           │
│                 Rate: OVER 60 MIN                         │
│          SOD CHLORIDE 0.9%  100 ML                        │
│          AMPICILLIN/SULBACTUM                             │
│                                                           │
│                  *REFRIGERATE*                            │
│                                                           │
│                                                           │
│  AS: UNASYN                                               │
│  FREQ: Q6H                                                │
│                                                           │
│  Expiration: 10/18/99 10:50AM              By:            │
└─────────────────────────────────────────────────────────┘
```

a. What is the drug used for?

b. How many mLs are used to reconstitute a 3 g vial of Unasyn?

c. What is the resulting concentration?

d. How long is the expiration in the refrigerator?

e. How many bags will be sent in a 24-hour period?

4. Label #2
    KCl has 2 mEq/mL.
    Sodium bicarb has 1 mEq/mL.

```
┌─────────────────────────────────────────────────────────┐
│              Mt. Hope Pharmacy Services                   │
│                                                           │
│  Patient: BROWN, ROBERT       ID. No. 035481   Rm. No. 649-1 │
│                                                           │
│  Prepared: 1:30PM             Date: 03/25/99              │
│                                                           │
│                 Rate: 85ML/HR                             │
│          DEXTROSE 5% W1/2NS  1000 ML                      │
│          POTASSIUM CHLORIDE  30 mEq                       │
│          SODIUM BICARBONATE  20 mEq                       │
│                                                           │
│                                                           │
│  AS: IV FLUSH                                             │
│  FREQ: Q12H                                               │
│                                                           │
│  Expiration: 03/26/99 1:30PM              By:             │
└─────────────────────────────────────────────────────────┘
```

Name _____ Date _____

a. How many mLs of each will be needed?

KCl _____

sodium bicarb _____

b. How long will one bag last?

c. How many bags will be needed every 24 hours?

5. Order reads: Give Cefobid 1 g q12hrs x 3 days.

a. Prepare a label for the order.

```
┌─────────────────────────────────────────────────────────┐
│              Mt. Hope Pharmacy Services                   │
│   Patient: _____  ID. No._____  Rm. No. _____ │
│   Prepared: _____  Date:_____       │
│                                                           │
│                                                           │
│                                                           │
│                                                           │
│                                                           │
│                                                           │
│   Expiration: _____              By:               │
└─────────────────────────────────────────────────────────┘
```

b. Prepare the order.
  – Gather materials
  – Wash hands
  – Aseptic technique

Chapter 8: Dispensing, Billing, and Inventory Management

PRESCRIPTION AND LABEL REQUIREMENTS

Read carefully the prescriptions in the Prescriptions exercise and answer the questions regarding each prescription. Missing information should be identified by drawing a circle at the location where the appropriate information should appear. Complete a label for each prescription.

In the Problems section, answer the questions with the help of drug reference materials.

Prescriptions

A. Controlled Substances

1.

```
┌─────────────────────────────────────────────────────┐
│              MT. HOPE MEDICAL PARK                    │
│                MY TOWN, USA   555-3591                │
│                                                       │
│  #_____         DEA # _____    │
│  PT. NAME  Larry Walker    DATE  1/21/99              │
│  ADDRESS _____                      │
│          _____                     │
│                                                       │
│   R       Tylox                                       │
│   x       One Q4-6 hrs  Prn Pain                      │
│           #30                                         │
│                                                       │
│  REFILLS _____ TIMES  (NO REFILL UNLESS INDICATED)    │
│  _____ M.D. _____ M.D.    │
│     DISPENSE AS WRITTEN      SUBSTITUTE PERMITTED      │
└─────────────────────────────────────────────────────┘
```

a. What information is missing?

b. Write out the law that pertains to this situation.

c. Write a label.

d. Check the dose and directions for each medication.

Name _____ Date _____

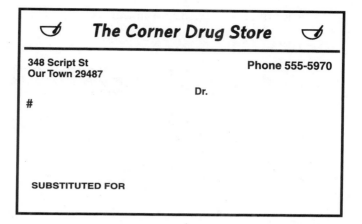

The Corner Drug Store

348 Script St
Our Town 29487

Phone 555-5970

Dr.

#

SUBSTITUTED FOR

2.

MT. HOPE MEDICAL PARK
MY TOWN, USA   555-3591

#_____   DEA # _MJ12345678_
PT. NAME _Nancy Cruth_   DATE _____
ADDRESS _____

℞   Demerol
     #45
     one daily

REFILLS _2_ TIMES (NO REFILL UNLESS INDICATED)
_____ M.D. _M. Johnson_____ M.D.
DISPENSE AS WRITTEN   SUBSTITUTE PERMITTED

a. What information is missing?

b. Write out the law that pertains to this situation.

c. Write a label.

d. Check the dose and directions for each medication.

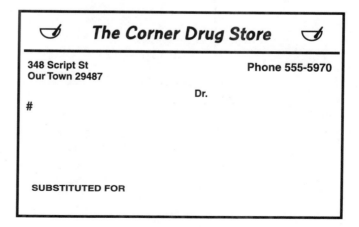

The Corner Drug Store

348 Script St
Our Town 29487

Phone 555-5970

Dr.

#

SUBSTITUTED FOR

B. Noncontrolled Substances

1.

MT. HOPE MEDICAL PARK
MY TOWN, USA 555-3591

\#_____   DEA \# _____

PT. NAME___*David Marsh*_____   DATE _____

ADDRESS _____

_____

℞   *Zantac 150 #60*
    One Q 8 hrs

REFILLS __*3*__ TIMES (NO REFILL UNLESS INDICATED)

_____ M.D.   *D. White*_____ M.D.
DISPENSE AS WRITTEN   SUBSTITUTE PERMITTED

a. What information is missing?

b. Write out the law that pertains to this situation.

c. Write a label.

d. Check the dose and directions for each medication.

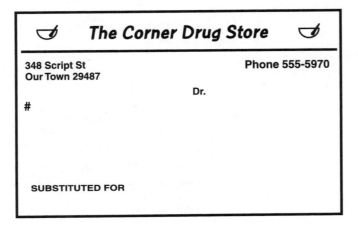

The Corner Drug Store

348 Script St   Phone 555-5970
Our Town 29487

                        Dr.

\#

SUBSTITUTED FOR

Name _____ Date _____

2.

MT. HOPE MEDICAL PARK
MY TOWN, USA 555-3591

#_____   DEA # _____

PT. NAME____David Marsh_____   DATE _____

ADDRESS _____

_____

℞ Trimox 500
     One Q 8 hrs

REFILLS _____ TIMES (NO REFILL UNLESS INDICATED)

_____ M.D. ____D. White____ M.D.
DISPENSE AS WRITTEN   SUBSTITUTE PERMITTED

a. What information is missing?

b. Write out the law that pertains to this situation.

c. Write a label.

d. Check the dose and directions for each medication.

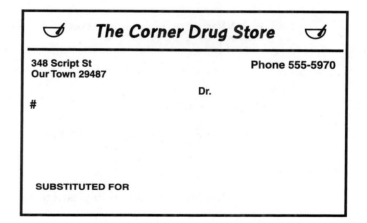

The Corner Drug Store

348 Script St
Our Town 29487   Phone 555-5970

                                 Dr.
#

SUBSTITUTED FOR

Problems

A. Mary Lawson has the following prescriptions currently on file at *The Corner Drug Store:*

Rx Number	Medication	Directions	Date Dispensed	Refills
12345	Ortho-Novum 7/7/7	Take one tablet daily	12/27/98	6
12346	Pepcid 20 mg	Take one tablet daily	1/3/99	4
12347	Darvocet-N-100	One tab q4-6hrs prn	4/16/99	2

Answer the following questions:

1. She brings in a new prescription for Ery-Tab 333. Are there any interactions with any of her current medications? If so, please describe.

2. Darvocet-N-100

   a. What is this medication?

   b. What schedule is it?

   c. What is the maximum recommended dose per day?

3. Pepcid 20 mg

   a. What class of medication is Pepcid?

   b. What are some other medications in this class?

   c. Are there any OTC products in this class? If so, name them.

Name _____ Date _____

B. Donald Wayne is an inpatient at Mt. Hope Hospital. Currently he is on the following intravenous (IV) medications:

Order #	Medication and Strength	Route	Schedule	Date Started	Status
1	Ciprofloxacin 400 mg	IV	Q12hrs	1/19/99	Active
2	Fluconazole 200 mg	IV	QD	1/19/99	Active
3	Metronidazole 500 mg	IV	Q8hrs	1/21/99	Active

Answer the following questions:

1. Metronidazole
   a. How many times a day is metronidazole given?

   b. The patient gets an order for vancomycin 1 g daily.
      Is vancomycin compatible with metronidazole at the y-site?

2. What are the brand names for each drug above?

   _____

   _____

   _____

3. How long should fluconazole be infused over?

4. Are there oral dosage forms for these IV meds? Fill in Yes or No.

   a. Ciprofloxacin   _____

   b. Fluconazole   _____

   c. Metronidazole   _____

Chapter 8, continued

OVER-THE-COUNTER PRODUCTS

Consumers are turning increasingly to products they can purchase at will, to self-administer for their health problems. There are a number of factors affecting this change. At the forefront are economic trends, increased cost of physician visits, and rising cost of prescription medications.

Although over-the-counter (OTC) medications may be purchased without a prescription, the active ingredients generally are the same as those found in higher-strength prescription versions. The FDA will approve an OTC preparation when the agency is assured the dosage strength is beneficial and yet not likely to cause harm to the general public when taken as directed.

Pharmacists are devoting a greater amount of their time recommending OTC products to their customers. OTC products are being shifted to the technician, and these products will become an increasingly important part of technician responsibilities.

In this exercise you will review the medication categories and answer for each product: Active Ingredient(s), Drug Action (how it works, what it does), and Indication for Use (what condition is the product used for).

Category:

Allergy		
Hay Fever/Allergy (Liquid)	Chlor-Trimeton®	Active Ingredient(s) -
		Drug Action -
		Indication for Use -
Hay Fever/Allergy (Caps/Tabs)	Tavist-D®	Active Ingredient(s) -
		Drug Action -
		Indication for Use -
Nasal Decongestant (Liq/Spray)	Neo-Synephrine®	Active Ingredient(s) -
		Drug Action -
		Indication for Use -
Cold/Cough		
Adult Cold Product (Tabs)	Comtrex®	Active Ingredient(s) -
		Drug Action -
		Indication for Use -

Name _____ Date _____

Long-Acting Cold Remedy	Dimetapp®	Active Ingredient(s) -
		Drug Action -
		Indication for Use -
Multi-Symptom/ Flu Preparation	TheraFlu®	Active Ingredient(s) -
		Drug Action -
		Indication for Use -
Sinus Remedy	Sudafed®	Active Ingredient(s) -
		Drug Action -
		Indication for Use -
Sore Throat Preparation	Chloraseptic®	Active Ingredient(s) -
		Drug Action -
		Indication for Use -

Gastrointestinal

Antacid (Liq)	Maalox®	Active Ingredient(s) -
		Drug Action -
		Indication for Use -
Antacid (Tabs)	Mylanta®	Active Ingredient(s) -
		Drug Action -
		Indication for Use -
Antiflatulent	Mylicon®	Active Ingredient(s) -
		Drug Action -
		Indication for Use -
Diarrhea Remedy	Imodium A-D®	Active Ingredient(s) -
		Drug Action -
		Indication for Use -

Fiber Laxative/ Supplement	Metamucil®	Active Ingredient(s) -
		Drug Action -
		Indication for Use -
Stimulant Laxative	Dulcolax®	Active Ingredient(s) -
		Drug Action -
		Indication for Use -

Oral Care

Mouthwash	Scope®	Active Ingredient(s) -
		Drug Action -
		Indication for Use -

Pain Reliever

Adult Analgesic	Advil®	Active Ingredient(s) -
		Drug Action -
		Indication for Use -
External Analgesic	Myoflex®	Active Ingredient(s) -
		Drug Action -
		Indication for Use -
Headache Remedy	Percogesic®	Active Ingredient(s) -
		Drug Action -
		Indication for Use -
Pediatric Analgesic	Tylenol®	Active Ingredient(s) -
		Drug Action -
		Indication for Use -

Personal Care

Louse Preparation	Nix®	Active Ingredient(s) -
		Drug Action -
		Indication for Use -

Name _____ Date _____

Diet Aid	Dexatrim®	Active Ingredient(s) -
		Drug Action -
		Indication for Use -
Dry Mouth Remedy	Xero-Lube®	Active Ingredient(s) -
		Drug Action -
		Indication for Use -
Eye Drops	Visine®	Active Ingredient(s) -
		Drug Action -
		Indication for Use -
Hemorrhoidal Preparation	Preparation H®	Active Ingredient(s) -
		Drug Action -
		Indication for Use -
Sleep Aid	Sominex®	Active Ingredient(s) -
		Drug Action -
		Indication for Use -
Vaginal Antifungal	Monistat® 7	Active Ingredient(s) -
		Drug Action -
		Indication for Use -
Vaginal Moisturizer	Replens®	Active Ingredient(s) -
		Drug Action -
		Indication for Use -
Skin Care		
Acne Preparation	Oxy-10®	Active Ingredient(s) -
		Drug Action -
		Indication for Use -

Anti-Itch/Rash	Cortaid®	Active Ingredient(s) -
		Drug Action -
		Indication for Use -
Athlete's Foot Preparation	Tinactin®	Active Ingredient(s) -
		Drug Action -
		Indication for Use -
Emollient and Protective Skin Product	Lubriderm®	Active Ingredient(s) -
		Drug Action -
		Indication for Use -
Jock Itch Preparation	Micatin®	Active Ingredient(s) -
		Drug Action -
		Indication for Use -
Wound Care Product	Neosporin®	Active Ingredient(s) -
		Drug Action -
		Indication for Use -

Name _____ Date _____

Chapter 9: Extemporaneous Compounding

NONSTERILE COMPOUNDING

Follow directions provided in the compounding recipes to accurately prepare mixtures of medicinal products in a pharmaceutically elegant form. This exercise provides an opportunity to experience the combining of various materials into medicinal products and product forms generally not available from a manufacturer. Several recipes are provided that may be used in this exercise. An example of a completed Pharmacy Compounding Log (or Master Formula Sheet) for the preparation "Magic Mouthwash" is shown in Figure 9.8 (p. 177). A blank form is provided for your use in compounding the other recipes. Your instructor might prefer to use a favorite recipe, or to design one not available on the following pages.

Compounding equipment used in weighing, measuring liquids, grinding, mixing, and so on, will be needed to complete this exercise.

It is suggested that students work in pairs to complete each compound, or all of the compounds, selected by the instructor. Groups may be assigned by the instructor to prepare different compounds so that all groups are not working on the same compound at the same time.

Completed products will be checked by the instructor for technique, correctness of label, correct quantities of ingredients, and appearance.

Compounding Recipes

1. Sugardyne

Betadine Ointment 15 g
Betadine Solution 6 mLs
Sugar 60 g

1) Measure all ingredients.
2) Pool sugar (*Hint* like potatoes and gravy).
3) Mix ingredients from the middle of the pool outward.

* Remember * Neatness counts *
Place in a 2 oz jar.

LABEL: Sugardyne
            Expires in 6 months
            Exp:
            * For topical use only *

2. Salicyclic Acid/Eucerin

Salicyclic acid 1 g
Hydrocortisone 1.2 g
Eucerin 60 g

1) Measure ingredients.
2) Pool Eucerin cream (* Hint* like potatoes and gravy).
3) Mix ingredients from the middle of the pool outward.

Place in a 2 oz jar.
LABEL: Salicyclic Acid/Eucerin
         Expires in 6 months
         Exp:
         * For topical use only *

3. Simple Syrup

Sucrose 850 g
Water qs ad 1000 mL

1) *Hint* Measure 500 mL tap water.
2) Place water in pan and bring to boiling.
3) Measure sucrose (granular sugar).
4) Add sucrose to boiling water.
5) Let pan cool slightly.
6) Pour into liter bottle.

LABEL: Simple syrup, USP
         Expires in 6 months
         Exp:
         * Keep in refrigerator*

4. Spironolactone Oral Suspension

Spironolactone 25 mg tablets
4 tablets
Simple syrup 50 mL
Water qs ad 100 mL

1) Crush tablets in mortar.
2) Measure simple syrup.
3) Add syrup into powdered spironolactone and mix well.
4) Add 25 mL water and mix well.
5) Pour into 4 oz bottle.
6) QS with water to total of 100 mL.
7) Shake bottle well.

LABEL: Spironolactone Oral
         Suspension
         Conc. = 1 mg/mL
         Expires in 30 days
         Exp:
         Shake well

5. Magic Mouthwash

Hydrocortisone powder 100 mg
(may use pwd or inj.)
Nystatin Suspension 100,000, 25 mL
units per mL
Benadryl Elixir qs ad 200 mL

1) Measure all ingredients.
2) Mix all ingredients in a mortar.
3) Pour into an 8 oz bottle.

LABEL: Modified Magic Mouthwash
         Expires in 230 days
         Exp:
         Shake well

6. Allopurinol Oral Suspension

Allopurinol 100 mg tablets
5 tablets
Simple syrup qs ad 100 mL

1) Crush tablets in mortar.
2) Add the simple syrup gradually and mix to uniform suspension.
3) Place in 4 oz bottle.

LABEL: Allopurinol Oral Suspension
         Conc. = 5 mg/mL
         Expires in 14 days
         Exp:
         Shake well
         Refrigerate

7. Allergy Cream

Menthol 60 mg
Triamcinolone Cream 0.1% 60 mg
Cetaphil Lotion QS 180 ml

1) Crush menthol in mortar and pestle.
2) Add 1-2 drops of alcohol to dissolve menthol.
3) Add approximately 1 oz of Cetaphil Lotion.
4) Add approximately 1/2 of triamcinolone cream.
5) Mix and pour into 8 oz bottle.
6) Mix remainder of cream and some lotion.
7) Pour into jar.
8) QS to 180 ml with Cetaphil Lotion.
9) Shake well as you add.

LABEL: Allergy Cream
         Exp:
         Shake well
         For topical use only

Name _____   Date _____

PHARMACY COMPOUNDING LOG

PRODUCT _____   PHARMACY LOT NUMBER _____

LABEL: _____

Date MFG: _____

STRENGTH: _____

QUANTITY MFG: _____

	MANUFACTURER'S LOT NUMBER	INGREDIENTS	AMOUNT NEEDED	WEIGHED OR MEASURED BY	CHECKED BY
1					
2					
3					
4					
5					
6					
7					
8					

DIRECTIONS FOR MANUFACTURING:

Manufactured by _____

Approved by _____

Date _____

_____

Auxiliary Labeling:

_____

PHARMACY COMPOUNDING LOG

PRODUCT _____   PHARMACY LOT NUMBER _____

_____

LABEL:

Date MFG: _____

STRENGTH: _____

QUANTITY MFG: _____

	MANUFACTURER'S LOT NUMBER	INGREDIENTS	AMOUNT NEEDED	WEIGHED OR MEASURED BY	CHECKED BY
1					
2					
3					
4					
5					
6					
7					
8					

DIRECTIONS FOR MANUFACTURING:

Manufactured by _____

Approved by _____

Date _____

_____

Auxiliary Labeling:

_____

Name _____ Date _____

PHARMACY COMPOUNDING LOG

PRODUCT _____   PHARMACY LOT NUMBER _____

LABEL: _____

Date MFG:

STRENGTH: _____

QUANTITY MFG: _____

	MANUFACTURER'S LOT NUMBER	INGREDIENTS	AMOUNT NEEDED	WEIGHED OR MEASURED BY	CHECKED BY
1					
2					
3					
4					
5					
6					
7					
8					

DIRECTIONS FOR MANUFACTURING:

Manufactured by _____

Approved by _____

Date _____

_____

Auxiliary Labeling:

_____

PHARMACY COMPOUNDING LOG

PRODUCT _____   PHARMACY LOT NUMBER _____

_____

LABEL: Date MFG:

_____

STRENGTH:

_____

QUANTITY MFG:

_____

	MANUFACTURER'S LOT NUMBER	INGREDIENTS	AMOUNT NEEDED	WEIGHED OR MEASURED BY	CHECKED BY
1					
2					
3					
4					
5					
6					
7					
8					

DIRECTIONS FOR MANUFACTURING:

Manufactured by _____

Approved by _____

Date _____

_____

Auxiliary Labeling:

_____

Name _____ Date _____

PHARMACY COMPOUNDING LOG

PRODUCT _____ PHARMACY LOT NUMBER _____

LABEL: _____

Date MFG: _____

STRENGTH: _____

QUANTITY MFG: _____

	MANUFACTURER'S LOT NUMBER	INGREDIENTS	AMOUNT NEEDED	WEIGHED OR MEASURED BY	CHECKED BY
1					
2					
3					
4					
5					
6					
7					
8					

DIRECTIONS FOR MANUFACTURING:

Manufactured by _____

Approved by _____

Date _____

_____

Auxiliary Labeling: _____

_____

PHARMACY COMPOUNDING LOG

PRODUCT _____   PHARMACY LOT NUMBER _____

_____

LABEL: Date MFG:

                                                    _____

                                                    STRENGTH:

                                                    _____

                                                    QUANTITY MFG:

                                                    _____

	MANUFACTURER'S LOT NUMBER	INGREDIENTS	AMOUNT NEEDED	WEIGHED OR MEASURED BY	CHECKED BY
1					
2					
3					
4					
5					
6					
7					
8					

DIRECTIONS FOR MANUFACTURING:

Manufactured by _____

Approved by _____

Date _____

_____

Auxiliary Labeling:

_____

Name _____ Date _____

PHARMACY COMPOUNDING LOG

PRODUCT _____   PHARMACY LOT NUMBER _____

_____

LABEL: Date MFG:

_____

STRENGTH:

_____

QUANTITY MFG:

_____

	MANUFACTURER'S LOT NUMBER	INGREDIENTS	AMOUNT NEEDED	WEIGHED OR MEASURED BY	CHECKED BY
1					
2					
3					
4					
5					
6					
7					
8					

DIRECTIONS FOR MANUFACTURING:

Manufactured by _____

Approved by _____

Date _____

_____

Auxiliary Labeling:

_____

Chapter 11: Hospital and Institutional Pharmacy Practice

SMALL FLUID VOLUMES (MINIBAGS)

Read each medication order carefully and answer the questions related to that order. Drug references and reconstitution charts should be consulted. (The Reconstitutions and Minibag Administration Protocol charts included with this exercise will be needed in other exercises related to chapter 11.) Prepare a label for each order. These orders may also be prepared as practice with aseptic compounding.

A.

(✓)	START HERE	DATE 1/28	TIME 10:00	A.M. P.M.	PROFILED BY:	FILLED BY:	CHECKED BY:	PATIENT NAME AND I.D.
								Robinson, Mary 1234567 Rm 159

Azactam 2g Q8hrs

70. Dr. Smith/
/K. Nurse, RN

1. Use of medication?

2. Oral dosage form (Yes or No)

3. How long to infuse over?

4. What size minibag to use?

5. Amount of diluent needed?

Mt. Hope Pharmacy Services

Patient: _____ ID. No._____ Rm. No. _____

Prepared: _____ Date:_____

Expiration: _____   By: _____

Name _____ Date _____

B.

(✓)	START HERE →	DATE 1/29	TIME 11:00	A.M. (P.M.)	PROFILED BY:	FILLED BY:	CHECKED BY:	PATIENT NAME AND I.D.
	D/C Azactam							Robinson, Mary 1234567 Rm 159
	Start Ampicillin 1g Q6hrs.							
			Smith M.D.					

1. Use of medication?

2. Oral dosage form (Yes or No)

3. How long to infuse over?

4. What size minibag to use?

5. Amount of diluent needed?

Mt. Hope Pharmacy Services

Patient: _____ ID. No. _____ Rm. No. _____

Prepared: _____ Date: _____

Expiration: _____   By: _____

RECONSTITUTIONS

MEDICATIONS	VIAL	ADD (ML)	TO MAKE
Ampicillin	10 Gram 2 Gram 1 Gram 500 mg	44.5 9.0 4.5 2.5	1 Gram/5 mL " " "
Ancef (Cefazolin)	10 Gram 1 Gram 500 mg	45.5 4.5 2.5	1 Gram/5 mL " "
Azactam (Aztreonam)	2 Gram 1 Gram 500 mg	7.4 3.8 2.5	1 Gram/5 mL " "
Cefizox (Ceftizoxime)	2 Gram 1 Gram	9.0 4.5	1 Gram/5 mL "
Cefobid (Cefoperazone)	2 Gram 1 Gram	9.0 4.5	1 Gram/5 mL "
Chloramphenicol	1 Gram	4.7	1 Gram/5 mL
Claforan (Cefotaxime)	10 Gram 1 Gram	47 4.5	1 Gram/5 mL "
Fortaz **VENT** (Ceftazidime or Tazidime)	2 Gram 1 Gram **VENT BEFORE AND AFTER**	8.7 4.4	1 Gram/5 mL "
Keflin (Cephalothin)	20 Gram 2 Gram 1 Gram	108 11.2 5.6	*1 Gram/6 mL " "
Mandol (Cefamandole)	2 Gram 1 Gram	9.0 4.5	1 Gram/5 mL "
Mefoxin (Cefoxitin)	10 Gram 2 Gram 1 Gram	45.5 9.0 4.5	1 Gram/5 mL " "
Methicillin	4 Gram 1 Gram	5.7 1.5	*1 Gram/2 mL "

Name _____ Date _____

RECONSTITUTIONS (cont.)

MEDICATIONS	VIAL	ADD (ML)	TO MAKE
Mezlin (Mezlocillin)	4 Gram 1 Gram	18.5 1.5	1 Gram/5 mL "
Monocid	1 Gram	4.5	1 Gram/5 mL
Nafcillin	10 Gram 2 Gram 1 Gram 500 mg	44.5 9.0 4.5 2.5	1 Gram/5 mL " " "
Pediatric Multivitamins **VENT**	50 mL size 10 mL size	49 9.4	
Penicillin G	* NOTE SIDE OF VIAL *		
Pentamidine	300 mg	5	300 mg/5 mL
Piperacillin	4 Gram 3 Gram	18 13.5	1 Gram/5 mL "
Rocephin (Ceftriaxone)	2 Gram 1 Gram 500 mg	9.0 4.5 2.5	1 Gram/5 mL " "
Ticar (Ticarcillin)	20 Gram 3 Gram 1 Gram	47 7 2.5	*1 Gram/3 mL " "
Unasyn (Ampicillin/ Sulbactam)	3 Gram 1.5 Gram	6.4 3.2	3 Grams/8 mL 1.5 Grams/4 mL
Vancomycin	5 Gram	100	50 mg/mL
Vibramycin	200 mg 100 mg	9.2 4.6	100 mg/5 mL "
Zinacef (Cefuroxime)	1.5 Gram 750 mg	16 8	90 mg/mL "

Name _____ Date _____

MINIBAG ADMINISTRATION PROTOCOL

Prepare each agent in D₅W unless advised otherwise

AGENT	VOLUME	INF. RATE	EXP	IVS
(IV SPECIAL) Acyclovir (Zovirax)	≤1 g; 50 mL **Do not refrigerate**	60 min	24 hr RT	NO
Aldomet (Methyldopa)	≤500 mg; 100 mL >500 mg; 250 mL	60 min 24 hrs	24 hr RT	YES
Amikacin	≤500 mg; 100 mL >500 mg; 250 mL	60 min	24 hr RT	NO
Aminocaproic Acid (Amicar)	≤2 g; 50 mL >2 g; 100 mL >5 g; 250 mL	30 min " "	24 hr RT	NO
Aminophylline Bolus	≤250 mg; 50 mL >250 mg; 100 mL	30 min 30-60 min	24 hr RT	NO
Ampicillin*	≤1.5g; 50 mL NS >1.5g; 100 mL NS	60 min "	8 hr RT 72 hr REF	NO
Ampicillin/Sulbactam* (Unasyn)	≤1.5 g; 50 mL NS >1.5 g; 100 mL NS	60 min "	8 hr RT 72 hr REF	NO
Aztreonam (Azactam)	≤1 g; 50 mL >1 g; 100 mL	60 min "	48 hr RT 7 day REF	NO
Cefamandole (Mandol)	≤2 g; 50 mL >2 g; 100 mL	60 min "	24 hr RT 96 hr REF	NO
Cefazolin (Ancef, Kefzol)	≤2 g; 50 mL >2 g; 100 mL	60 min "	24 hr RT 96 hr RT	YES
Cefonicid (Monocid)	≤2 g; 50 mL >2 g; 100 mL	30 min "	24 hr RT 72 hr REF	NO
Cefoperazone (Cefobid)	≤3 g; 50 mL >3 g; 100 mL	30 min "	24 hr RT 120 hr REF	NO
Cefotaxime (Claforan)	≤2 g; 50 mL >2 g; 100 mL	30 min "	24 hr RT 120 hr REF	YES
Ceftazidime (Fortaz, Tazidime)	≤2 g; 50 mL >2 g; 100 mL	60 min "	24 hr RT 7 day REF	NO
Cefotetan (Cefotan)	≤1 g; 50 mL >1 g; 100 mL	60 min "	24 hr RT 96 hr REF	NO

*Denotes normal saline use only.

Name _____ Date _____

AGENT	VOLUME	INF. RATE	EXP	IVS
Ceftizoxime (Cefizox)	≤2 g; 50 mL >2 g; 100 mL	30 min "	24 hr RT 48 hr REF	NO
Ceftriaxone (Rocephin)	≤2 g; 50 mL >2 g; 100 mL	30 min "	72 hr RT 10 day REF	NO
Cefoxitin (Mefoxin)	≤2 g; 50 mL >2 g; 100 mL	30 min "	24 hr RT 48 hr REF	NO
Cefuroxime (Zinacef)	≤750 mg; 50 mL >750 mg; 100 mL	60 min "	24 hr RT 48 hr REF	NO
Cephalothin (Keflin)	≤2 g; 50 mL >2 g; 100 mL	30 min "	24 hr RT 96 hr REF	YES
Chloramphenicol (Chloromycetin)	≤2 g; 50 mL >2 g; 200 mL	30 min "	24 hr RT 30 Day REF	YES
Cimetidine (Tagamet)	≤300 mg; 50 mL >300 mg; 100 mL	30 min "	48 hr RT 7 day REF	NO
Clindamycin (Cleocin)	≤300 mg; 50 mL >300 mg; 100 mL	30 min "	16 day RT 30 day REF	
Doxycycline (Vibramycin)	≤200 mg; 200 mL >200 mg; 250 mL	60 min 1.5 hr	24 hr RT 72 hr REF	NO
Erythromycin* Lactobionate	≤1 g; 100 mL NS >1 g; 250 mL NS	60 min 1.5 hr	8 hr RT	NO
Famotidine (Pepcid)	≤40 mg; 100 mL	30 min	96 hr RT	YES
Gentamicin (Garamycin)	≤120 mg; 50 mL >120 mg; 100 mL	30 min "	96 hr RT 30 day REF	YES
Imipenem-Cilastin* (Primaxin)	≤500 mg; 100 mL NS >500 mg; 250 mL NS	60 min "	10 hr RT 48 hr REF	NO
Methicillin (Staphcillin)	≤1 g; 50 mL >1 g; 100 mL	60 min "	8 hr RT 96 hr REF	YES
Mezlocillin	<2 g; 50 mL >2 g; 100 mL	30 min "	48 hr RT 7 day REF	NO
Nafcillin	≤1 g; 50 mL >1 g; 100 mL	60 min "	24 hr RT 96 hr REF	NO
Oxacillin*	≤2 g; 50 mL NS >2 g; 100 mL NS	60 min "	96 hr RT 7 day REF	NO

*Denotes normal saline use only.

Name _____ Date _____

AGENT	VOLUME	INF. RATE	EXP	IVS
Penicillin	≤3 µg; 50 mL <3 µg>5; 100 mL >5 µg; 250 mL	30 min 60 " 60 "	24 hr RT 7 day REF	YES
IVS Pentamidine (Pentam)	<300 mg; 100 mL >300 mg; 250 mL	60 min 60 "	24 hr RT	NO
Piperacillin (Piperacil)	<4 g; 50 mL >4 g; 100 mL	30 min 30 "	24 hr RT 7 day REF	NO
Potassium Cl	<40 mEq; 100 mL	60 min	24 hr	NO
Ranitidine (Zantac)	<50 mg; 50 mL >50 mg; 100 mL	30 min 30 "	48 hr RT 10 day REF	NO
Ticarcillin (Ticar)	<3 g; 50 mL >3 g; 100 mL	60 min 60 "	24 hr RT 72 hr REF	NO
Timentin	<3.1 g; 50 mL >3.1 g; 100 mL	60 min 60 "	24 hr RT 72 hr REF	NO
Tobramycin (Nebcin)	<120 mg; 50 mL >120 g; 100 mL	30 min 30 "	24 hr RT 96 hr REF	NO
Vancomycin	<250 mg; 50 mL >250 mg; 100 mL >1g; 250 mL	60 min 60 " 60 "	96 hr REF	YES
Septra	Each 5 mL amp in each 75 mL Each 5 mL amp in each 125 mL Do not refrigerate	60-90 min 60-90 min	2 hr RT 6 hr RT	NO
Furosemide (Lasix)	Do not exceed 4 mg/min Protect from light		24 hr	NO
Flagyl Any other dose of Flagyl	500 mg RTU Do not refrigerate	60 min 60 "	Manuf. 24 hr RT	NO

Name _____ Date _____

Chapter 11, continued

LARGE FLUID VOLUMES (LVP—LARGE VOLUME PARENTERALS)

Read carefully each medication order and answer the questions related to that order. Prepare a label for each medication order. These orders may also be prepared as practice with aseptic compounding.

A.

(✓)	START HERE →	DATE 1/28	TIME 8:00 A.M. (P.M.)	PROFILED BY:	FILLED BY:	CHECKED BY:	PATIENT NAME AND I.D.
		Put 20 mEq KCl in 1L D₅W at 100ml/hr Smith, MD					Robinson, Mary 1234567 Rm 159

1. What size bag will be needed?

2. What is the infusion rate?

3. How many hours will one bag last?

Mt. Hope Pharmacy Services

Patient: _____   ID. No. _____   Rm. No. _____

Prepared: _____   Date: _____

Expiration: _____   By: _____

B.

(✓)	START HERE →	DATE 1/29	TIME 9:00	A.M. ⃝ P.M.	PROFILED BY:	FILLED BY:	CHECKED BY:	PATIENT NAME AND I.D.

Change IVF to
20mEq Potassium
2 g Mag Sulfate
in 1L Normal Saline @ 100mL/hr

R. J. Smith, MD

Robinson, Mary
1234567   Rm. 159

1. What size bag will be needed?

2. What is the infusion rate?

3. How many hours will one bag last?

Mt. Hope Pharmacy Services

Patient: _____   ID. No._____   Rm. No. _____

Prepared: _____   Date:_____

Expiration: _____   By: _____

Name _____ Date _____

Chapter 11, continued

Read each of the four labels carefully and answer the questions concerning each label.

For additional aseptic compounding experience, follow the instructions in the last problem of this exercise. Prepare a label and the admixture. Demonstrate all procedures and techniques for the instructor.

Label #1

a. Is this a minibag or large-volume prep?

b. How long will this drug be infused over?

c. How many times a day will the patient get this drug?

```
            Mt. Hope Pharmacy Services
Patient: MEEKS, AGNES        ID. No. 042311        Rm. No. 589-1
Prepared: 8:00AM             Date: 12/02/99

              Rate: OVER 60 MIN
       SOD CHLORIDE 0.9%  100  ML
       IMIPENEM/CILASTATIN

            *REFRIGERATE*


AS: PRIMAXIN
FREQ: Q12H

Expiration: 12/04/99  8:00AM                 By:
```

Label #2

a. Is this a minibag or large volume?

b. What is the rate of infusion?

c. How long will one bag last?

```
            Mt. Hope Pharmacy Services
Patient: NEWTON, NANCY       ID. No. 033371       Rm. No. 510-2
Prepared: 2:45PM             Date: 12/02/99

              Rate: 50  ML/HR
       DEXTROSE 5%W1/2NS  1000  ML
       POTASSIUM CHLORIDE  60  mEq




AS: PRIMAXIN
FREQ:

Expiration: 12/03/99  2:45PM                 By:
```

Label #3

a. Is this a minibag or large volume?

b. How long will this drug be infused over?

c. How many times a day will the patient receive the medication?

```
┌────────────────────────────────────────────────┐
│          Mt. Hope Pharmacy Services            │
│ Patient:  SPALDING, MICHELE   ID. No. 053481    Rm. No. 515-2 │
│ Prepared: 6:00AM              Date: 12/02/99     │
│                                                 │
│               Rate: OVER 60 MIN                 │
│ DEXTROSE 5%  250  ML                            │
│ VANCOMYCIN HCL  1000  MG                         │
│                                                 │
│                                                 │
│ AS: VANCOMYCIN                                  │
│ FREQ: Q12H                                      │
│                                                 │
│ Expiration: 12/06/99  6:00AM          By:       │
└────────────────────────────────────────────────┘
```

Label #4

a. Is this a minibag or large volume?

b. What is the rate of infusion?

c. How long will one bag last?

```
┌────────────────────────────────────────────────┐
│          Mt. Hope Pharmacy Services            │
│ Patient:  TAYLOR, JAMES       ID. No. 066281    Rm. No. 327 │
│ Prepared: 3:20PM              Date: 11/02/99     │
│                                                 │
│               Rate: 25  ML/HR                   │
│ DEXTROSE 5%  500  ML                            │
│ HEPARIN SODIUM  1000  UNITS                      │
│                                                 │
│                                                 │
│ AS:                                             │
│ FREQ:                                           │
│                                                 │
│ Expiration: 11/03/99  3:20PM          By:       │
└────────────────────────────────────────────────┘
```

Name _____ Date _____

IV Preparation

   a. Gather the materials needed to make this medication.

   b. Wash hands properly.

   c. Clean the hood properly.

   d. Prepare the medication.

(✓)	START HERE	DATE 1/29	TIME 3:00 (A.M.) P.M.	PROFILED BY:	FILLED BY:	CHECKED BY:	PATIENT NAME AND I.D.
	Start Cefobid 1g Q12 hrs						C. Jones 982736 Rm 371
		M.J. Smith. M.D.					

   e. Write a label.

Mt. Hope Pharmacy Services

Patient: _____ ID. No. _____ Rm. No. _____

Prepared: _____ Date: _____

Expiration: _____   By:

Chapter 11, continued

RECONSTITUTION AND PROTOCOL CHARTS

This exercise will demonstrate accurate reading and information utilization of Reconstitutions and Minibag Administration Protocol charts (use the charts included under the exercise for Small Fluid Volumes, pp. A-34–A-38). Answer questions 1–5 related to utilizing chart information.

Question 6 will provide an opportunity to utilize medication charts, do appropriate calculation, if necessary, gather materials, and prepare the admixture. (Preparing a label will be at the instructor's discretion.) Your instructor may wish to vary the drug strength, thus requiring a calculation and a variance in dose.

Questions 7 and 8 offer additional opportunities to acquire information from orders, prepare labels, and compound the admixture.

1. How many mLs are used to reconstitute:

   Mandol 1 g _____

   Ticar 3 g _____

   Zinacef 1.5 g _____

2. What are the resulting concentrations?

   Mandol 1 g _____

   Ticar 3 g _____

   Zinacef 1.5 g _____

3. What type of fluid would be used to administer the medication, and how many mLs?

   Mandol 1 g _____

   Ticar 3 g _____

   Zinacef 1.5 g _____

4. What infuse over time would be printed on the label?

   Mandol 1 g _____

   Ticar 3 g _____

   Zinacef 1.5 g _____

5. What special label information should the following medications contain:

   Septra _____

   Furosemide _____

   Flagyl _____

Name _____ Date _____

6. Please gather the materials to make the following:

   Unasyn 3 g q6h to start at 1200 today.

   Reconstitute the vial and give the resulting concentration. _____

   What fluid volume will be used to reconstitute? _____

   What fluid will the drug be placed in and what volume? _____

7. Read the order closely and answer the questions.

(✓)	START HERE →	DATE 2/4	TIME 11:00	A.M. P.M.	PROFILED BY:	FILLED BY:	CHECKED BY:	PATIENT NAME AND I.D.
								Adams, Luke 38920 Rm 411

Hang Aminophylline 250 mg in D₅W 500 mL to start now. Infuse at 35 mL/hr

a. Is this a large volume or minibag?

b. What size bag is needed?

c. How long will one bag last?

d. How many bags (approximately) will be needed every 24 hours?

Prepare a label.

Mt. Hope Pharmacy Services

Patient: _____ ID. No. _____ Rm. No. _____

Prepared: _____ Date: _____

Expiration: _____ By: _____

Prepare this order.

8. Read the order closely and answer the questions.

(✓)	START HERE →	DATE 2/4	TIME 9:00	A.M. P.M.	PROFILED BY:	FILLED BY:	CHECKED BY:	PATIENT NAME AND I.D.

Start 1 LLR with 20 mEq KCl at 125 mL/hr

Jones, Mary
369752 Rm 110-1

a. Is this a large volume or minibag?

b. What size bag is needed?

c. How long will one bag last?

d. How many bags (approximately) will be needed every 24 hours?

Prepare a label.

Mt. Hope Pharmacy Services

Patient: _____ ID. No._____ Rm. No. _____

Prepared: _____ Date:_____

Expiration: _____ By:

Prepare this order.

Name _____ Date _____

Chapter 11, continued

PEDIATRIC DOSING

Calculate dosage strengths for the following pediatric patients. Calculations will be reviewed by the instructor.

1. J.B. is a three-year-old weighing 37 lbs. What is his weight in kg?

2. How many grams are in 1 lb?

3. A.K. is a 21-day-old neonate weighing 2.6 lbs.

    a. Physician order reads ampicillin 100 mg/kg/dose IV q6h. How much ampicillin should be sent up per dose for this baby?

    b. Physician orders gentamicin 5 mg/kg/day IV q12h. How much gentamicin should be sent up per dose?

4. T.N. is a 14-month-old girl weighing 25 lbs. A normal dose for ceftriaxone is 50 mg/kg/day IV given once a day. What would her dose be?

5. S.R. is a three-year-old weighing 35 lbs. Physician writes for amoxicillin PO 50 mg/kg/day t.i.d. Amoxicillin comes as 125 mg/5mL suspension. How much amoxicillin would be dispensed in an oral syringe for one dose? What is this in mg and mL?

6. B.B. is a 53-day-old neonate weighing 2.5 kg.

    a. Physician orders aminophylline 6 mg/kg IV loading dose, then 2 mg/kg dose IV q8h. How many mg for each dose would you give?

    b. Physician then writes for morphine 0.37 mg IV 12-24hrs PRN pain. How many mg/kg/dose is this?

7. T.B. is a 15-year-old boy brought in for seizures. He weighs 120 lbs. The physicians want to load him with phenobarbital at 15 mg/kg and then 12 hours later start 3 mg/kg/day on a bid schedule. What is his loading and daily maintenance dose?

8. D.A. is a one-day-old neonate weighing 800 grams. Physician orders cefotaxime 150 mg/kg/day IV q8h. How many mg/kg/dose is this?

9. Q.P is a ten-year-old girl admitted for asthma. She weighs 90 lbs. Physician orders methylprednisolone (Solu-Medrol) 2 mg/kg/day IV q6h.

   a. What is her total daily dose?

   b. How many mg are in one dose for her?

10. E.M. is an eight-year-old girl weighing 63 lbs. Physician orders amoxicillin 40 mg/kg/day PO t.i.d. The amoxicillin you will use is 250 mg/5mL suspension.

   a. How many mg will one dose be?

   b. How many mLs will one dose be?

Name _____ Date _____

Chapter 11, continued

NEONATAL NUTRITIONAL CALCULATIONS AND PREPARATIONS

In this exercise you will calculate ingredient levels for neonatal parenteral feeding. Your instructor will review your calculations. The instructor may assign a pediatric TPN (Total Parenteral Nutrition) to be compounded, or design one for student preparation. Use the Pharmacy Supply Sheet as a reference to make calculations for materials in the laboratory actually used in preparing a TPN.

   If the order was received for baby Brown weighing 1264 grams and you were to prepare the lipids at 2 g/kg for 20 hours, what volume of lipids would be drawn up in a syringe if 20% lipids are used? (See the Pediatric Fluid Calculations Example below.)

PEDIATRIC FLUID CALCULATIONS EXAMPLE

*** CALCULATE TO THREE SIGNIFICANT FIGURES (THREE DIGITS)
   (i.e., 101, 10.1, 1.01, 0.101)

CALCULATE MLS OF EACH

GIVEN: TROPHAMINE 6% AMINO ACIDS	1.6 GRAMS	_____
DEXTROSE	10%	_____
SODIUM CHLORIDE	8 MEQ	_____
POTASSIUM PHOSPHATE	4.4 MEQ	_____
POTASSIUM CHLORIDE	2 MEQ	_____
MAGNESIUM SULFATE	1 MEQ	_____
CALCIUM GLUCONATE	2 MEQ	_____
PEDIATRIC MULTIVITAMINS	6.5 MLS	_____
PEDIATRIC TRACE ELEMENTS	0.1 MLS	_____
OTHER: HEPARIN 1/2 U/CC		_____
STERILE WATER TO BE ADDED		_____

TAV = 200 MLS

RATE = 6.5 ML/HR

1)   CALCULATE VOLUME OF COMPONENTS
2)   ADD ALL VOLUMES TOGETHER
3)   SUBTRACT VOLUME OF COMPONENTS FROM TAV

   TAV – VOLUME OF COMPONENTS = VOLUME OF STERILE WATER TO ADD TO ORDER

4)   ADD VOLUME OF STERILE WATER

Name _____ Date _____

Pediatric Fluid Practice

1. How many grams of amino acids are there if you have a 6% amino acid solution, 250 mL volume?

2. How many grams of dextrose are there in a 500 mL 10% solution?

3. Calculate the following:

    a) NaCl 154 mEq

    b) Potassium phosphate 20 mEq

    c) Mag Sulfate 10 mEq

4. A bag of TPN has 500 mL left in it at 11:00 a.m. today; the rate is 75 mL/hr. When is the next bag due?

    Day _____   Time _____

5. How long will a 250 mL bag last if the rate is 15 mL/hr?

6. How many grams of dextrose are there if you have 500 mL of a 70% dextrose solution?

7. Calculate this neonatal TPN.

    Amino acids 10% 9 grams   _____

    Dextrose 12.5% 20%   _____

    Sodium chloride 23 mEq   _____

    Potassium phosphate 4.4 mEq   _____

    Potassium chloride 2 mEq   _____

    Magnesium sulfate 2 mEq   _____

    Calcium gluconate 0.5 mEq   _____

    Pediatric multivitamins 5mL   _____

    Pediatric trace elements 0.15 mL   _____

    Other: Heparin 1 unit/mL

    TAV = 480 mL

    Rate = 18 mL/hr

Sterile water to be added: _____

Neonatal Nutrition

1. How many grams of Dextrose are there in 250 mL of 10% solution?

2. How many grams of protein are there in 500 mL of a 6% Trophamine solution?

3. If a TPN order calls for 12.5% Dextrose, how many mL of the stock 50% Dextrose will you need to fill this order TAV 275 mL?

4. How many grams of fats are in 200 mL of a 20% solution?

5. Baby boy Green is a 26-week gestation neonate weighing 700 grams and is three days old. He is being treated for prematurity, respiratory distress syndrome, and can rule sepsis. He is in critical condition and on a ventilator. A neonatologist has ordered hyperalimentation for him beginning today. Review the order. Calculate the caloric content ordered.

Caloric Content Calculation			
1) Dextrose	3.4 kcal/gm	= _____	kcal/day
2) Lipid	9 kcal/gm	= _____	kcal/day
3) Protein	4 kcal/gm	= _____	kcal/day
4) Total		= _____	**kcal/day**

6. Review the neonatal hyperalimentation order for baby Green. Using the Pharmacy Supply Sheet, calculate the amount in milliliters (mL) of each ingredient to add. The lipids will be infused separately, but calculate the volume to be infused.

INGREDIENTS	AMOUNT IN (ML)
Tropamine 6%	
Dextrose 10%	
Sodium Chloride	
Potassium Phosphate	
Potassium Chloride	
Potassium Acetate	
Magnesium Sulfate	
Calcium Gluconate	
Pediatric Multivitamin Injection	
Neotatal Trace Elements	
Heparin Beef	
Sterile Water	
Lipids 20%	

7. Baby girl Taylor is a 30-week gestational neonate weighing 1500 grams. She is seven days old and being treated for prematurity and pneumonia. She is on a ventilator and has a central percutaneous catheter (i.e., central line). Review the ordered TPN.

   a. Calculate the calorie content.

Caloric Content Calculation		
1) Dextrose	3.4 kcal/gm	= _____ kcal/day
2) Lipid	9 kcal/gm	= _____ kcal/day
3) Protein	4 kcal/gm	= _____ kcal/day
4) Total		= _____ **kcal/day**

Name _____ Date _____

b   Calculate the amount in mL of ingredients ordered.

INGREDIENTS	AMOUNT IN (ML)
Tropamine 6%	
Dextrose 17%	
Sodium Chloride	
Potassium Phosphate	
Potassium Chloride	
Potassium Acetate	
Magnesium Sulfate	
Calcium Gluconate	
Pediatric Multivitamin Injection	
Neotatal Trace Elements	
Heparin Beef	
Sterile Water	
Lipids 20%	

8.   Your instructor will divide the class into groups. In a laminar flow hood and using aseptic technique, add the electrolytes to the hyperalimentation provided. Let the instructor watch your technique.

9.   Review the TPN order for Baby X. Calculate the amount in mLs of ingredients ordered.

PHARMACY SUPPLY SHEET

Trophamine 6%

Dextrose 50%

Lipids 20%

Sterile Water

Sodium Chloride   4 mEq/mL

Sodium acetate   2 mEq/mL

Sodium Phosphate   4 mEq/mL

Potassium Phosphate   4.4 mEq/mL

Potassium Chloride   2 mEq/mL

Potassium Acetate   2 mEq/mL

Magnesium Sulfate   4.06 mEq/mL

Calcium Gluconate   0.47 mEq/mL

Pediatric MVI

Neonatal Trace Elements

Heparin Beef   1000 units/mL

Sterile empty IV bags

Name _____ Date _____

MT. HOPE HOSPITAL
SPECIAL FLUID ORDER SHEET

DATE: *Nov. 10*   **NICU**   **TIME:**

PATIENT NO: **WEIGHT (KILOGRAMS)** *0.7*

PATIENT NAME *Baby Green*   **AGE (DAYS)**

COMPONENT	AMOUNT/ KG/24HR	LABEL	TOTAL
ML			
AMINO ACIDS *Trophamine*	0.5	*0.35gm*	
DEXTROSE (%) *50%*		*10%*	
SODIUM CHLORIDE	*1mEq*	*0.7mEq*	
POTASSIUM PHOSPHATE	*1.4mEq*	*0.98mEq*	
POTASSIUM CHLORIDE	*0.5mEq*	*0.35mEq*	
MAGNESIUM SULFATE	*0.25mEq*	*0.175mEq*	
CALCIUM GLUCONATE	*1mEq*	*0.7mEq*	
PEDIATRIC MULTIVITAMINS			*6.5*
TRACE ELEMENTS			*0.07*
HEPARIN (BEEF)	*1U/mL*	*75U*	
		TAV (TOTAL ACTUAL VOLUME)	
		TOTAL COMPONENTS	
STERILE WATER			

Fluid Infusion rate (mL/hr):	*3*	**IV LIPIDS**
Volume of Fluids (TAV in mL):	*75*	**Lipids (gm/Kg/24hr):** *0.5*
Osmolarity:		**Percent Lipid:** *20%*
Location of Line: (Peripheral) (Central)		**Volume Lipid:**
Infusion (hrs.):	*20*	

Dr. *Smith*

MT. HOPE HOSPITAL
SPECIAL FLUID ORDER SHEET

DATE: _June 11_   NICU   TIME: _____

PATIENT NO: _____   WEIGHT (KILOGRAMS) __1.5__

PATIENT NAME ___Taylor Girl___   AGE (DAYS) _____

COMPONENT	AMOUNT/ KG/24HR	LABEL	TOTAL
ML			
AMINO ACIDS _Trophamine_	2	3gm	
DEXTROSE (%) 50%		17%	
SODIUM CHLORIDE	4mEq	6mEq	
POTASSIUM PHOSPHATE	2mEq	3mEq	
POTASSIUM CHLORIDE	2mEq	3mEq	
MAGNESIUM SULFATE	1mEq	1.5mEq	
CALCIUM GLUCONATE	1.75mEq	2.63mEq	
PEDIATRIC MULTIVITAMINS			6.5
TRACE ELEMENTS			0.15
HEPARIN (BEEF)			
		TAV (TOTAL ACTUAL VOLUME)	
		TOTAL COMPONENTS	
STERILE WATER			

Fluid Infusion rate (mL/hr): __8.9__   **IV LIPIDS**

Volume of Fluids (TAV in mL): __214__   Lipids (gm/Kg/24hr): __1.5__

Osmolarity: _____   Percent Lipid: __20%__ _____

Location of Line: (Peripheral) (Central)   Volume Lipid: _____

Infusion (hrs.): __20__

Dr. ___Smith___

Name _____ Date _____

MT. HOPE HOSPITAL
SPECIAL FLUID ORDER SHEET

DATE: NICU   TIME:

PATIENT NO: WEIGHT (KILOGRAMS) _____1_____

PATIENT NAME _____*Baby X*_____   AGE (DAYS) _____

COMPONENT	AMOUNT/ KG/24HR	LABEL	TOTAL
MLS			
AMINO ACIDS *Trophamine*	2.5	2.5gm	_____
DEXTROSE (%) 50%		12.5%	_____
SODIUM CHLORIDE	6mEq	6mEq	_____
POTASSIUM PHOSPHATE	2.8mEq	2.8mEq	_____
POTASSIUM CHLORIDE	2mEq	2mEq	_____
MAGNESIUM SULFATE	3mEq	3mEq	_____
CALCIUM GLUCONATE	3.2mEq	3.2mEq	_____
PEDIATRIC MULTIVITAMINS	_____	_____	6.5
TRACE ELEMENTS	_____	_____	0.1
HEPARIN (BEEF)	_____	_____	_____
		TAV (TOTAL ACTUAL VOLUME)	_____
		TOTAL COMPONENTS	_____
STERILE WATER			_____

		IV LIPIDS	
Fluid Infusion rate (mL/hr):	3.3		
Volume of Fluids (TAV in mL):	80	Lipids (gm/Kg/24hr):	Ø
Osmolarity:	_____	Percent Lipid:	_____ _____
Location of Line: (Peripheral) (Central)		Volume Lipid:	_____
Infusion (hrs.):	24		

Dr. _____*Smith*_____

MT. HOPE HOSPITAL
SPECIAL FLUID ORDER SHEET

DATE: NICU   **TIME:**

PATIENT NO: **WEIGHT (KILOGRAMS)** _____

PATIENT NAME _____   **AGE (DAYS)** _____

COMPONENT	AMOUNT/ KG/24HR	LABEL	TOTAL
MLS			
AMINO ACIDS _____	_____	_____	_____
DEXTROSE (%)	_____	_____	_____
SODIUM CHLORIDE	_____	_____	_____
POTASSIUM PHOSPHATE	_____	_____	_____
POTASSIUM CHLORIDE	_____	_____	_____
MAGNESIUM SULFATE	_____	_____	_____
CALCIUM GLUCONATE	_____	_____	_____
PEDIATRIC MULTIVITAMINS	_____	_____	_____
TRACE ELEMENTS	_____	_____	_____
HEPARIN (BEEF)	_____	_____	_____

TAV (TOTAL ACTUAL VOLUME) _____

TOTAL COMPONENTS _____

STERILE WATER   _____

Fluid Infusion rate (mL/hr):   _____   **IV LIPIDS**

Volume of Fluids (TAV in mL):   _____   **Lipids (gm/Kg/24hr):** _____

Osmolarity: _____   **Percent Lipid:**   _____ _____

Location of Line: (Peripheral) (Central)   **Volume Lipid:**   _____

Infusion (hrs.):   _____

Dr. _____

Name _____ Date _____

Chapter 11, continued

ADULT TOTAL PARENTERAL NUTRITION

Calculate volumes of each component that will constitute the adult TPN. Queen TPN will be formulated using peripheral formulation for peripheral administration. Dextrose 40% will be used to formulate a 6% solution with a total volume of 1100 mL. Use 50mL of 10% Lipids. Calculations will be checked by your instructor and technique observed during compounding.

Itchy TPN will be a special formulation using 8.5% Amino Acids, Dextrose prepared to 20%, and 20% Lipids. The Lipids will not be mixed as was the case in the 3-in-1 fluids, but in this instance sent to the floor in the original bottle. Total volume will be 1000 mL. Calculations will be checked by the instructor and technique observed during compounding.

It is suggested that students work independently on calculations, but be assigned to groups for preparation of the product. Each student in a group should have a part in measuring components and introduction into the fluid admixture.

PHARMACY SUPPLY SHEET

Trophamine 6%

Dextrose 50%

Lipids 20%

Sterile Water

Sodium Chloride	4 mEq/mL
Sodium acetate	2 mEq/mL
Sodium Phosphate	4 mEq/mL
Potassium Phosphate	4.4 mEq/mL
Potassium Chloride	2 mEq/mL
Potassium Acetate	2 mEq/mL
Magnesium Sulfate	4.06 mEq/mL
Calcium Gluconate	0.47 mEq/mL

Pediatric MVI

Neonatal Trace Elements

Heparin Beef	1000 units/mL

Sterile empty IV bags

Mt. Hope Hospital
My Town, SC
Adult Parenteral Nutrition Order Form

QUEEN, DIXIE

RM 306-B

Date: _____ Time: __3.30__ (PM) (AM)

☐ **Consult Nutritional Support Service (Beeper 0349)**
☐ **Conduct Indirect Calorimetry Test**

Central Formula (per liter)	Peripheral Formula (per liter)
Amino Acids 40gm	Amino Acids 25gm
Dextrose 17.5% (600 Kcals)	*40%* Dextrose 6% (200 Kcals)
Fat 20% 125mL (250 Kcals)	~~Fat 20%~~ *10%* ~~200mL (400 Kcals)~~ *50mL*
Standard Electrolytes*	~~Standard Electrolytes*~~ *See below*
Trace Elements - 4 1mL/Day	Trace Elements - 4 1mL/Day
Multivitamins - 12 10mL/Day	Multivitamins - 12 10mL/Day Osmolarity: 740 mOsm/L

Total Volume _____ mL/Day   Total Volume __1100__ mL/Day

*Standard Electrolytes (per liter) Na - 50mEq, Ca - 7.5mEq, Cl - 45mEq, Acetate - 45 mEq, Phos - 9mM

(Indicate Total Daily Requirements)   Guidelines   General Rule

1. **Amino Acids** _____ gm/Day   0.5 - 2.5 gm/Kg/Day   1 gm/Kg/Day

    Type _____

2. **Total Nonprotein**

    Calories _____ Kcals/Day*   10-40 Kcals/Kg/Day   25 Kcals/Kg/Day

    Dextrose _____ %   0-100%   65%

    Fat _____ %   0-65%   35%

    100%

3. **Total Volume** _____ mL/Day   Minimum Volume: 1Kcal/1.0mL

*Substrate must equal 100%

Special Formulation - Electrolytes (check one)

☐ **Standard Electrolytes/Liter**   ☐ **Standard Electrolytes plus Additional Electrolytes**

☐ **Standard Electrolytes/Liter - No Potassium**   ☑ **Custom Electrolytes**

Sodium Acetate	_____ mEq/Day		Potassium Acetate	_____ mEq/Day
Sodium Chloride	_10_ mEq/Day		Potassium Chloride	_20_ mEq/Day
Sodium Phosphate	_____ mEq/Day		Potassium Phosphate	_____ mEq/Day
Magnesium Sulfate	_8_ mEq/Day		Calcium Gluconate	_____ mEq/Day

Multivitamins - 12 (10mL) per _____   Other _____

Trace Elements - 4 (1mL) per _____   Other _____

HUMAN REGULAR INSULIN __30__ units/Day

Phytonadione (Vit. K) 10 mg IM per __week__

OTHER _____

Special Instructions _____ .

Dr. Smith Jones

M.D.

76016153

Pharmacy Must Receive TPN Orders by 12 Noon

Name _____ Date _____

Mt. Hope Hospital
My Town, SC
Adult Parenteral Nutrition Order Form

ITCHY, JOHNNY

RM 457-A

Date: _____ Time: _10:45_ (PM) ((AM))

☐ **Consult Nutritional Support Service (Beeper 0349)**
☐ **Conduct Indirect Calorimetry Test**

Central Formula (per liter)
Amino Acids 40gm
Dextrose 17.5% (600 Kcals)
Fat 20% 125mL (250 Kcals)
Standard Electrolytes*
Trace Elements - 4 1mL/Day
Multivitamins - 12 10mL/Day

Peripheral Formula (per liter)
Amino Acids 25gm
Dextrose 6% (200 Kcals)
Fat 20% 200mL (400 Kcals)
Standard Electrolytes*
Trace Elements - 4 1mL/Day
Multivitamins - 12 10mL/Day Osmolarity: 740 mOsm/L

Total Volume _____ mL/Day Total Volume _____ mL/Day
*Standard Electrolytes (per liter) Na - 50mEq, Ca - 7.5mEq, Cl - 45mEq, Acetate - 45 mEq, Phos - 9mM

(Indicate Total Daily Requirements) Guidelines General Rule

1. Amino Acids _30_ gm/Day 0.5 - 2.5 gm/Kg/Day 1 gm/Kg/Day
   Type _8.5 Travasol_

2. Total Nonprotein
   Calories _920_ Kcals/Day* 10-40 Kcals/Kg/Day 25 Kcals/Kg/Day
   Dextrose _70_ % 0-100% 65%
   Fat _30_ % 0-65% 35%
   100%

3. Total Volume _1000_ mL/Day Minimum Volume: 1Kcal/1.0mL
*Substrate must equal 100%

Special Formulation - Electrolytes (check one)

☐ **Standard Electrolytes/Liter**   ☐ **Standard Electrolytes plus Additional Electrolytes**

☐ **Standard Electrolytes/Liter - No Potassium**   ☑ **Custom Electrolytes**

Sodium Acetate	_____ mEq/Day		Potassium Acetate	_____ mEq/Day
Sodium Chloride	_20_ mEq/Day		Potassium Chloride	_40_ mEq/Day
Sodium Phosphate	_____ mEq/Day		Potassium Phosphate	_____ mEq/Day
Magnesium Sulfate	_4_ mEq/Day		Calcium Gluconate	_10_ mEq/Day

Multivitamins - 12 (10mL) per _____   Other _____
Trace Elements - 4 (1mL) per _Day_   Other _____

HUMAN REGULAR INSULIN _____ units/Day

Phytonadione (Vit. K) 10 mg IM per _____

OTHER _____

Special Instructions _____ .
Dr. Smith Jones
M.D.
76016153

Pharmacy Must Receive TPN Orders by 12 Noon

Mt. Hope Hospital
My Town, SC
Adult Parenteral Nutrition Order Form

Date: _____ Time: _____ (PM) (AM)

☐ **Consult Nutritional Support Service (Beeper 0349)**
☐ **Conduct Indirect Calorimetry Test**

Central Formula (per liter)
  Amino Acids 40gm
  Dextrose   17.5% (600 Kcals)
  Fat 20%   125mL (250 Kcals)
  Standard Electrolytes*
  Trace Elements - 4 1mL/Day
  Multivitamins - 12 10mL/Day

Peripheral Formula (per liter)
  Amino Acids 25gm
  Dextrose   6% (200 Kcals)
  Fat 20%   200mL (400 Kcals)
  Standard Electrolytes*
  Trace Elements - 4 1mL/Day
  Multivitamins - 12 10mL/Day   **Osmolarity: 740 mOsm/L**

    Total Volume _____ mL/Day **Total Volume** _____ mL/Day
*Standard Electrolytes (per liter) Na - 50mEq, Ca - 7.5mEq, Cl - 45mEq, Acetate - 45 mEq, Phos - 9mM

(Indicate Total Daily Requirements)   Guidelines   General Rule

1.   **Amino Acids** _____ **gm/Day**   **0.5 - 2.5 gm/Kg/Day**   **1 gm/Kg/Day**
    Type _____

2.   **Total Nonprotein**
    Calories _____ **Kcals/Day***   **10-40 Kcals/Kg/Day**   **25 Kcals/Kg/Day**
        Dextrose _____ **%**   **0-100%**   **65%**
        Fat _____ **%**   **0-65%**   **35%**
            100%

3.   **Total Volume** _____ **mL/Day**   **Minimum Volume: 1Kcal/1.0mL**
*Substrate must equal 100%

Special Formulation - Electrolytes (check one)

☐ **Standard Electrolytes/Liter**   ☐ **Standard Electrolytes plus Additional Electrolytes**

☐ **Standard Electrolytes/Liter - No Potassium**   ☐ **Custom Electrolytes**

    Sodium Acetate _____ **mEq/Day**   **Potassium Acetate** _____ **mEq/Day**
    Sodium Chloride _____ **mEq/Day**   **Potassium Chloride** _____ **mEq/Day**
    Sodium Phosphate _____ **mEq/Day**   **Potassium Phosphate** _____ **mEq/Day**
    Magnesium Sulfate _____ **mEq/Day**   **Calcium Gluconate** _____ **mEq/Day**

    Multivitamins - 12 (10mL) per _____   **Other** _____
    Trace Elements - 4 (1mL) per _____   **Other** _____

HUMAN REGULAR INSULIN _____ **units/Day**

Phytonadione (Vit. K) 10 mg IM per _____

OTHER _____

Special Instructions _____ .

_____

M.D.
76016153

                Pharmacy Must Receive TPN Orders by 12 Noon

Name _____ Date _____

Chapter 11, continued

CHEMOTHERAPY

Chemotherapy has its own special procedures and techniques. This exercise includes chemo orders in which you will utilize the Chemotherapy Preparation and Dispensing Guidelines to answer questions concerning the order. A label is then to be written for the order. A drug not listed on the chart will require a reference search.

It is suggested that a simulated chemo drug, Taxol 30 mg/5mL, be prepared for practice. Practice should occur under a vertical flow hood if available. Otherwise, simulate the conditions as nearly as possible. Caps, gowns, gloves, and masks should be available for use during this exercise.

Answer the questions about each chemo agent preparation; then make a label for each.

Chemo Order #1

(✓)	START HERE	DATE 2.25	TIME 8:00	A.M. P.M.	PROFILED BY:	FILLED BY:	CHECKED BY:	PATIENT NAME AND I.D.
								Knightly, Lisa 743125 Rm. 681

Please give Thiotepa 15mg at 11:00 A.M. today

Dr. G. Jones

a. Reconstitute with _____.

b. Vial concentration _____.

c. Dilute to dispense in _____.

d. Infuse over _____

_____.

e. Expires in _____.

f. Special labeling _____

_____.

Mt. Hope Pharmacy Services

Patient: _____ ID. No. _____ Rm. No. _____

Prepared: _____ Date: _____

Expiration: _____ By: _____

Chemo Order #2

(✓)	START HERE →	DATE 2/25	TIME 10:00	A.M. P.M.	PROFILED BY:	FILLED BY:	CHECKED BY:	PATIENT NAME AND I.D.

Cisplatin 45 mg
dose to start today

Dr. Smith

Boyd, Franklin
387216   Rm. 672

a. Reconstitute with _____.

b. Vial concentration _____.

c. Dilute to dispense in _____.

d. Infuse over _____.

e. Expiration _____.

f. Special labeling _____.

Mt. Hope Pharmacy Services

Patient: _____ ID. No._____ Rm. No. _____

Prepared: _____ Date:_____

Expiration: _____   By: _____

Chemo Order #3

Patient Woody Lee, Room #1162, Acct #36521
Prepare Taxol 15 mg dose in D5W to make a final concentration of 0.3 mg/mL. Use correct vertical flow hood technique and gather all materials needed to prepare before entering the hood. Show calculations.

Name _____ Date _____

CHEMOTHERAPY PREPARATION AND DISPENSING GUIDELINES

AGENT	RECONSTITUTION	DILUTION FOR DISPENSING	AUXILIARY INFORMATION
Asparaginase (Elspar)	10,000 unit vial IM: Add 1mL NS (10,000u/mL) IV: Add 5mL NS (2000u/mL)	*IM: Final Conc 10,000u/mL in Syr. IV Push: Final Conc 2000u/mL in Syr. IV Infusion: Place dose in 50mL (NS only) Infuse over 30 min or more	Exp. 8 hr R.T. Do not shake vial Not stable in D5W
Bleomycin (Blenoxane) Bleomycin	15 unit vial Add 1.5mL SWFI (100/mL)	S.C., IM: Final Conc. 100/mL in Syr. IV Push: Final Conc 100/mL in Syr. *IV Infusion: Place dose in 50mL (D5W, NS); Infuse over 15 min or more	Exp. 24 Hr R.T. Dispense in Glass 1 Hr Exp Date if dispensed in PVC Container
Carboplatin (Paraplatin) Carboplatin	50mg, 150mg, 450mg vial Add 5mLs, 15mL, 45mL, SWFI Respectively (10mg/mL)	*IV Infusion: Prepare as follows Place dose in 100mL (D5W) Infuse over 30 min or more	Exp. 24 hr R.T. in D5W Exp. 8 hr R.T. in NS
Carmustine (BICNU) Carmustine (BICNU)	100mg vial See vial to reconstitute*	*IV Infusion: Prepare as follows Dose < 20mg: 100mL (D5W, NS); Dose 20mg-100mg:250mL (D5W, NS) Dose >100mg: 500mL (D5W, NS)	Exp. 8 hr R.T. Dispense in glass Protect from light Must be diluted, IV Push Not recommended
Cisplatin (Platinol) Cisplatin	10mg, 50mg vials Add 10mL and 50mL SWFI Respectively (1mg/mL). This also forms a NS concentration due to NaCl present in the vials	*IV Infusion: Prepare as follows Dose < 50mg: 250mL (NS) Dose > 50mg: 500mL NS Infuse over 2 hrs or more	Exp. 24 hr R.T At least 1/4 NS must be present for stability Do not refrigerate Avoid aluminum needles
Cyclophosphamide (Cytoxan)	100mg, 200mg, 500mg vials Add 5mL, 10mL, 25mL SWFI Respectively (20mg/mL)	IV Push: Conc. to be 20mg/mL in syr *IV infusion: Prepare as follows Dose < 500mg: 50mL (D5W, NS) Dose 500mg - 1gm: 100mL Dose > 1gm: 250mL (D5W, NS) Infuse at 200mg/min or less	Exp. 24 hr R.T.

CHEMOTHERAPY PREPARATION AND DISPENSING GUIDELINES

AGENT	RECONSTITUTION	DILUTION FOR DISPENSING	AUXILIARY INFORMATION
Cytarabine (Cytosar V) (ARA-C)	For IV use reconstitute as follows: 100mg vial: Add 5mL SWFI (20mL/mL)1; 500mg vial add 10mL SWFI (50mg/mL); for SC, IM use reconstitute as follows: 100mg vial - Add 1mL SWFI (100mg/mL)	SC, IM: Conc to be 100mg/mL in syr IV Push: As follows - Conc can be 20mg/mL in syr. or 50 mg/mL in syringe as per vial used	Exp. 24 hr R.T. Do not refrigerate Call for pediatric dispensing guidelines per patient if not given
Dacarbazine (DTIC)	200mg vial See vial for reconstitution*	*IV Infusion: Prepare as follows Dose < 100mg; Place in 100mL (D5W, NS) Dose 100mg-200mg; 250mL (D5W, NS) Dose > 200mg: 500mL Infuse over 30 min or more	Exp. 8 hr R.T. Protect from light Avoid Extravasation
Dactinomycin (Cosmegen) (Actinomycin-D)	0.5mg vial See vial for reconstitution*	*IV Push: Reconstitute to be 0.5mg/mL in syringe: IV Infusion: Place dose in 50mL (D5W, NS); Infuse over 15 min more.	Exp. 24 hr R.T. Avoid Extravasation
Daunorubicin (Cerubidine)	20mg vial Add 4mL SWFI (5mg/mL)	*IV Push: Conc. to be 5mg/mL in Syr IV Infusion: Place dose in 50mL (D5W, NBS)	Exp. 24 hr R.T Avoid Extravasation
Doxorubicin (Adriamycin)	See vial*	*IV Push: Conc. to be 2mg/mL in Syr IV Infusion: Prepare as follows: Dose < 50mg; Place in 50mL (D5W, NS) Dose > 50mg; Place in 100mL (D5W, NS) Infuse over 15 min or more	Exp. 24 hr. R.T. Protect from light Avoid Extravasation Call for pediatric dispensing guidelines if not given.

Name _____ Date _____

CHEMOTHERAPY PREPARATION AND DISPENSING GUIDELINES

AGENT	RECONSTITUTION	DILUTION FOR DISPENSING	AUXILIARY INFORMATION
Etoposide (Vepesid) (VP-16)	See vial*	*IV Infusion only 1: Prepare as follows: Dose, 100mg: Place in 250mL (D5W, NS; 100mg < Dose < 200mg Place in 500mL (D5W, NS) Conc. < 0.4mg/mL Infuse over at least 60 minutes.	Exp. dates vary as follows: Conc. < 0.4mg/mL Exp. 24 hr. R.T. 0.4mg/mL <Conc. < 0.6mg/mL Exp. 8 hrs R.T. Conc. > 0.6mg/mL Exp. 2 hrs. R.T
Flouridine (FUOR)	500mg vial Add 5mL SWFI (100mg/mL)	*IV Infusion: Place dose in 250mL (D5W, NS) Infuse at least over 60 min.	Exp. 24 hrs. R.T. Do not refrigerate
Fluorouracil (5-FU)	See vial*	*IV Push: Conc. to be 50mg/mL in syr. (See Note *); IV Infusion: prepare as follows: Dose< 1200mg: place in 50mL (D5W, NS): 1200mg < Dose < 2500mg: Place in 100mL (D5W, NS); Dose > 2500mg: Place in 250mL (D5W, NS); Infuse at least over 15 min.	Exp. 24 hrs R.T. Do not refrigerate *NOTE: Most 5FU is given by continuous infusion in LVPs. Please clarify first.
Ifosfamide (Ifex)	1 gram vial Add 20mL SWFI (50mg/mL)	IV Push: Conc. to be 50mg/mL in syr. *IV Infusion: Prepare as follows: Dose < 1 gm: Place in 100mL (D5W, NS); 1 gm < dose < 3gm: Place in 250mL (D5W, NS); Dose > 3 gm: Place in 500mL (D5W, NS); Infuse over at least 30 min.	Exp. 24 hrs. R.T.
Mechlorethamine (Mustargen) (Nitrogen Mustard)	See vial*	To be mixed on floor prior to use Dispense vial with Non-Bacteriostatic Normal Saline and instruct RN to mix only prior to administration	Exp. 30 min R.T. Avoid Extravasation

CHEMOTHERAPY PREPARATION AND DISPENSING GUIDELINES

AGENT	RECONSTITUTION	DILUTION FOR DISPENSING	AUXILIARY
Methotrexate (MTX)	See vial*	IV Push: Conc. to be 25mg/mL in syringe *IV Infusion: Prepare as follows: Dose < 500mg; Place in 50mL (D5W, NS); 500mg < Dose , 1000mg; Place in 250mL (D5W, NS); Dose > 1000mg: Place in 250mL (D5W, NS); Infuse over at least 30 min.	Exp. 24 hrs R.T.
Mitomycin (Mutamycin) (Mitomycin C)	See vial*	*IV Push: Conc. to be 0.5mg/mL in Syringe IV Infusion: Place dose in 50mL (NS **) Infuse at least over 15 minutes	Exp. 12 hrs R.T. Avoid Extravasation Do not dilute in D5W Protect from light
Mitoxantrone (Novantrone)	See vial*	*IV Infusion: Place dose in 50mL (D5W, NS) Infuse at least over 15 minutes	Exp. 24 hrs R.T. IV Push not recommended
Plicamycin Mithracin (Mithramycin)	See vial*	*IV Infusion: Prepare as follows: Dose < 2.5mg: Place in 500mL (D5W, NS) Dose > 2.5mg: Place in 1000mL (D5W, NS) Infuse over 4 to 6 hours	Exp. 24 hrs R.T. Avoid Extravasation
Thiotepa	15mg vial Add 1.5mL SWFI (10mg/mL)	*IV Push: Conc. to be 10mg/mL in syr. IV Infusion: Place dose in 50mL (D5W, NS); Infuse over at least 15 min.	Exp. 24 hrs R.T.
Vinblastine (Velban)	10mg vial Add 10mL NS (1mg/mL)	*IV Push: Conc. to be 1mg/mL in syr. IV Infusion: Place dose in 50mL (D5W, NS); Infuse at least over 15 min.	Exp. 24 hrs R.T. Protect from light Avoid extravasation
Vincristine (Oncovin)	See vial*	*IV Push: Conc. to be 1mL/mL syr. IV Infusion: Place dose in 50mL (D5W, NS); Infuse over at least 15 min.	Exp. 24 hrs R.T. Protect from light Avoid Extravasation

*Dispensing format unless otherwise stated per doctor's order or written request for nursing staff.

Name _____ Date _____

Chapter 11, continued

This is an exercise in repackaging drug products for oral dosing. References for repackaging guidelines are found in the USP and ASHP Technical Assistance bulletin on Single Unit and Unit Dose Packages of Drugs.

This exercise includes completing the unit dose Repackaging Control Log for the 10 drugs listed for preparation. An example sheet is included that demonstrates correct label construction and information as well as ancillary labels. Additional materials that may be required include labels, oral syringes, and/or oral unit dose bottles. Bottle liquid dispensing devices may also be used.

You will record all 10 drugs on the log, as if a three-day supply were to be prepared. Two tablets and two liquids, only, are to be selected by each student to prepare as unit dose forms with labels. Scored tablets are to be broken.

Expirations:

- **ALL LIQUIDS UNLESS OTHERWISE STATED GET 30-DAY EXPIRATION.**

- **ALL TABLETS UNLESS OTHERWISE STATED GET 90-DAY EXPIRATION.**

- Syringes kept at room temperature get 30-day expiration (anything up to and including 10 mL).

- Reconstituted antibiotics get 5 days expiration in syringes and go into the refrigerator.

- Reconstituted bottles of antibiotics usually get 14 days expiration. Read the label.

- Oral specials over 10 mL go into bottles and are good for 90 days at room temperature.

Include all auxiliary labels that apply. Prepare the doses and labels. Have the work checked by the instructor.

*Note the example sheet with log and labels for Reglan 0.25 mg liq q6h (note the brand name is not available, so the generic metoclopramide is used) and Capoten 6.25 mg po t.i.d.

Drug Orders to Prepare

1. Nystatin 500,000 units per NG t.i.d.
2. Isoptin 60 mg q8h m (from 120 mg tab)
3. Corgard 80 mg 1/2 tab bid
4. Isoptin 40 mg q8h (from 80 mg tab)
5. Diphenhydramine Elixir 12.5 mg per NG qid
6. Potassium Chloride solution 40 mEq bid
7. Lanoxin elixir 25 mcg qd
8. Septra DS liquid 160 mg q6h
9. Cisapride Suspension 1 mg q6h
10. Diabeta 2.5 mg bid (from 5 mg tab)

REPACKAGING CONTROL LOG
DEPARTMENT OF PHARMACEUTICAL SERVICES

PHARMACY LOT NUMBER	DRUG-STRENGTH DOSAGE FORM	MANUFACTURER AND LOT NUMBER	EXP. DATE MANUF. MTC	RESULTING CONC.	QUANTITY	PREP. BY CK'D
MTC 7030501	Metoclopramide Oral soln	Roxane 194AB1	3-98 / 4-4-97	0.25mg (5mg) / 0.25mL (5mL)	12	AVT
MTC 7030502	Captopril 12.5mg tabs	Squibb 12RAV8	7-99 / 6-5-97	6.25mg (12.5mg) / 1/2 tab (1 tab)	9	AVT

```
METOCLOPRAMIDE
  (USE FOR REGLAN SYRI)
0.25MG/0.25ML
  (5MG/5ML)
MTC7030501
EXP: 4-5-97

        ORAL
```

```
CAPOTEN
  (CAPTOPRIL)
6.25MG/   1/2 TABLET
  (12.5MG/  1 TABLET)
MTC7030502
EXP:  6/05/97

        ORAL
```

Name _____ Date _____

REPACKAGING CONTROL LOG
DEPARTMENT OF PHARMACEUTICAL SERVICES

PHARMACY LOT NUMBER	DRUG-STRENGTH DOSAGE FORM	MANUFACTURER AND LOT NUMBER	EXP. DATE <u>MANUF.</u> MTC	RESULTING CONC.	QUANTITY	PREP. BY CK'D

Name _____ Date _____

Chapter 11, continued

IV SPECIALS

The IV special is a single dose in a syringe prepared aseptically and labeled. The product is therefore prepared under sterile conditions, that is, under air from hood conditions. The syringe is given an overfill volume of 0.1 mL to account for drug volume lost in the needle and syringe hub when the needle is attached and the drug administered. The overfill **is not** indicated on the log.

Expiration dates will depend on the agent being prepared. Information concerning Reconstitutions can be found in the chart on pages A-34–A-35. Expiration dates will be obtained from the Minibag Administration Protocol chart (pages A-36–A-38). Read the extreme right column, headed IVS, to determine if the drug can be prepared as an IV special. The determined expiration date is reduced by one day (24 hours). The prepared syringe is generally maintained in the patient tray and not refrigerated. If the drug is unused, returned to the pharmacy, and still is within date, it is not recycled to another patient; instead, it is destroyed.

Generally, a three-day supply is prepared. However, the procedure may vary from institution to institution.

Some drugs cannot be refrigerated and therefore will not be made as an IVS for storage under refrigeration.

The log number will list I (for IV), the last number in the year, the month, the day, and the number of the drug prepared (01 for the first of the day, 02 for the second, 03 for the third, etc.). Example for March 3, 2002, and the fifth drug prepared: **I2030305**.

The IVS label will contain the following information:

- stock bottle name

- generic or trade name as ordered

- amount ordered

- concentration of stock bottle

- log number (start with I)

- expiration date and time

- auxiliary labels/notes (e.g., must dilute further)

When preparing the drug use the smallest syringe possible. **Remember, each IVS will contain 0.1 mL overfill.**

- If the total volume including overfill is less than or equal to 1 mL, use a TB (1 mL) syringe.

- If the total volume including overfill is greater than 1 mL but less than or equal to 3 mL, then use a 3 mL syringe.

- If the total volume including overfill is greater than 3 mL but less than or equal to 5 mL, then use a 5 mL syringe.

- If the total volume including overfill is greater than 5 mL but less than or equal to 10 mL, then use a 10 mL syringe.

Name _____ Date _____

Standardization dosing will decrease errors and decrease the number of dosages to be made. Example:

Standard Dosage for Pediatric Patients Dexamethasone Injection (0.5 mg/mL)			
Dosage Range	**Standard Dose**	**Volume**	**Weight**
0.45-0.55 mg	0.50 mg	0.1 mL	(Weight range of patient)
Approved by institutions and physicians.			

Log all eight of the listed medications, in the order listed below. You will need to calculate some of the medications to arrive at a final concentration. Log each med for a three-day supply. Use the log sheet with Lanoxin as the first medication.

Your instructor will select three of the medications to be prepared as IVS syringes. Prepare only one unit of each of the selected medications and cap with a syringe cap. Write a label for each and atttach it to the prepared syringe. Make an additional copy of the labels to use as a study copy.

MEDICATIONS TO BE PREPARED AS INTRAVENOUS SPECIALS (IVS)	
	Concentration to use:
1. Gentamicin 5 mg IV q12h (Dilute for IV use)	20 mg/2 mL
2. Vancomycin 20 mg IV q24h	50 mg/mL
3. Tobramycin 48 mg IV q8h	40 mg/mL
4. Heparin 3000 units SQ q12h	5000 units/mL
5. Dexamethasone 0.8 mg IV q12h	4 mg/mL
6. Penicillin 50,000 units IV q12h	250,000 units/mL
7. Claforan 200 mg IV q8h	200 mg/mL
8. Phenobarbital 9 mg IV q24h	65 mg/mL

REPACKAGING CONTROL LOG
DEPARTMENT OF PHARMACEUTICAL SERVICES

PHARMACY LOT NUMBER	DRUG-STRENGTH DOSAGE FORM	MANUFACTURER AND LOT NUMBER	EXP. DATE MANUF. MTC	RESULTING CONC.		QUANTITY	PREP. BY CK'D
I8031601	(Digoxin) Lanoxin 250mcg/mL	BW A49381	9-99 / 4-16-98	0.25mg/mL	0.125mg/0.5mL	3	D AB

```
LANOXIN INJECTION
 (DIGOXIN)
0.125MG/0.5ML
 (0.25MG/ML)
I8031601
EXP 4/16/98    4P

        ORAL
```

Name _____ Date _____

IV Special Label

Write labels with the following information for gentamycin, heparin, and phenobarbital:

Drug injection

Concentration of dose ordered

(Orginal concentration used)

Lot: Number from log

Exp: Date and time

Mt. Hope Pharmacy Services

Patient: _____ ID. No. _____ Rm. No. _____

Prepared: _____ Date: _____

Expiration: _____ By: _____

Mt. Hope Pharmacy Services

Patient: _____ ID. No. _____ Rm. No. _____

Prepared: _____ Date: _____

Expiration: _____ By: _____

Mt. Hope Pharmacy Services

Patient: _____ ID. No. _____ Rm. No. _____

Prepared: _____ Date: _____

Expiration: _____ By: _____

Name _____ Date _____

GUIDELINES FOR PREPARING INTRAVENOUS SPECIALS (IVS)

EXPIRATION DATES:

The table outlines specific expiration dates. The time used for preparing IVS is **4PM**. This corresponds to the present cart exchange time. Therefore, all IVS will have the appropriate expiration date and the time of expiration of 4PM. This only affects IVS, not dilutions made by the pharmacy.

MEDICATION	CONCENTRATION	EXPIRATION DATE
Aminophylline Dilution	10mg/mL 3mL TAV	1 day
Cefazolin (Ancef, Kefzol)	200mg/mL	4 days (-) 1 day
Cefotaxime (Claforan)	200mg/mL	5 days (-) 1 day
Cephalothin (Keflin)	166.66 mg/mL	4 days (-) 1day
Cimetidine (Tagamet) minibag	6mg/mL minibag	7 days
Chloramphenicol inj	100mg/mL	1 month (-) 1 day
Dexamethasone (Decadron)	4mg/mL	1 month (-) 1 day
Dexamethasone Dilution	0.5mg/mL Dilution	7 days
Digoxin	250mcg/mL (Adult) 100mcg/mL (Pediatric)	1 month (-) 1 day
Digoxin Dilution	20mcg/mL Dilution	7 days
Gentamicin	10mg/mL (Pediatric) 40mg/mL (Adult)	20 days (-) 1 day
Heparin	10,000 units/mL	1 month (-) 1 day
Penicillin G Potassium (Aqueous)	250,000 units/mL	7 days (-) 1 day
Phenobarbital	65mg/mL	1 month (-) 1 day
Phenobarbital Dilution	10mg/mL Dilution	7 days
Tobramycin	10mg/mL (Pediatric) 40mg/mL (Adult)	4 days (-) 1 day
Vancomycin	50mg/mL	4 days (-) 1 day
Aminophylline Dilution	10mg/mL 3mL TAV	1 day
Candida Albicans Antigen Skin Test	0.1mL	1 month
Mumps Antigen Skin Test	0.1mL	1 month
Diptheria-Tetanus-Pretussis Vaccine	0.5mL	1 month
Glycerin USP 99% (must be Autoclaved)	2mL	3 months

Name _____ Date _____

Chapter 11, continued

MEDICATION DISTRIBUTION SYSTEM

A unit of dose is an ordered amount of medication in a dosage that is in as ready-to-administer form as possible. Usually a 24-hour supply is delivered to or made available at patient care units.

This exercise will give you an opportunity to review orders to determine important pharmacy-related information; evaluate patient drawers for needs in filling a 24-hour supply; and practice filling patient drawers.

Unit Dose Orders

Identify and list, from each of the following inpatient physician orders, the items of importance to pharmacy. Record the number(s) of units needed for a 24-hour supply.

(✓)	START HERE	DATE 10/16/99	TIME 1500	A.M. P.M.	PROFILED BY:	FILLED BY:	CHECKED BY:	PATIENT NAME AND I.D.
		Continue home meds:						Erwin, Tammy 00293-45 Rm. 300
		(1) Capoten 12.5mg PO q12						
		(2) Nystatin cream to affected area tid						
		(3) Digoxin 0.125mg PO qd						
		(4) Nafcillin 1gm IV q6h						
		(5) Enteric coated aspirin X gr PO qd						
				Smith, MD				

Items for pharmacy:

No. of medication units:

(✓)	START HERE ➡	DATE 10/16/99	TIME 1300	A.M. P.M.	PROFILED BY:	FILLED BY:	CHECKED BY:	PATIENT NAME AND I.D.

Start following meds ASAP:

1. Hydralazine 10mg IV q6h
2. Emetecon IM q2-3h prn Nausea
3. D5 1/2 NS c̄ 20mEq KCl at 50mL/hr
4. Vital signs q shift
5. NPO after 12M

Blood, MD

Patient Name: Brooks, Thomas 00261-13 Rm 502-2

Items for pharmacy:

No. of medication units:

(✓)	START HERE ➡	DATE 10/16/99	TIME 1000	A.M. P.M.	PROFILED BY:	FILLED BY:	CHECKED BY:	PATIENT NAME AND I.D.

1. X-Ray 2 kidney
2. Fluids ad lib
3. Pyridium 200mg PO tid
4. Urinalysis AM
5. TMP-SMZ 160/800 PO bid
6. Movement ad lid

Jones, MD

Patient Name: Wise, Kerry 00338-89 Rm 504

Items for pharmacy:

No. of medication units:

Name _____ Date _____

(✓)	START HERE →	DATE 10/16/99	TIME 1400	A.M. P.M.	PROFILED BY:	FILLED BY:	CHECKED BY:	PATIENT NAME AND I.D.
	① Hydromorphone 2mg q6h prn Pain							
								Morris, Ronald
	② Lasix 20mg AM							00334-83
	③ Keep L foot elevated							
	④ P÷ AM							Rm 128-2
	⑤ Zovirax Ointment 5% apply to lesions q3h							
	Smith, MD							

Items for pharmacy:

No. of medication units:

(✓)	START HERE →	DATE 10/16/99	TIME	A.M. P.M.	PROFILED BY:	FILLED BY:	CHECKED BY:	PATIENT NAME AND I.D.
	① Respiratory Therpy Treatments bid							Johnson, Tony
								00325-77
	② Ventolin 4mg q12h							
								Rm 404-1
	③ Acetaminophen 650mg q4-6h prn							
	④ Fluids ad lid							
	⑤ Demonstrate use of ventolin inhaler Hart, MD							

Items for pharmacy:

No. of medication units:

CART-FILLING EXERCISE:
WHAT IS NEEDED IN THE PATIENT DRAWER

Directions: Complete total Daily Quantity ordered and amount to (Post) Add

	Daily Quantity	(Post) Add
1. Ibuprofen 600 mg PO Q8h Two were left in the drawer	( )	( )
2. Colace 100 mg Liq PO bid POS* One was left in the drawer	( )	( )
3. Ferrous sulfate 325 mg PO tid None were left in the drawer	( )	( )
4. Doxycycline 100 mg PO q12h One was left in the drawer	( )	( )
5. Prednisone 7.5 mg PO qAM None were left in the drawer	( )	( )
6. Benadryl 25 mg PO qhs One was left in the drawer	( )	( )
7. Amoxil 250 mg PO tid None were left in the drawer	( )	( )
8. Lasix 40 mg PO qAM One was left in the drawer	( )	( )
9. Zantac 150 mg PO bid Two were left in the drawer	( )	( )
10. Dexamethasone 2 mg IV q6h IVS One was left in the drawer	( )	( )
11. Heparin flush IV q8h PRN None were left in the drawer	( )	( )
12. Reglan 10 mg PO ac&hs Two were left in the drawer	( )	( )
13. Aldomet 25 mg PO q8h One was left in the drawer	( )	( )
14. Hydralazine 75 mg PO q12h None were left in the drawer	( )	( )
15. Clinoril 200 mg PO q12h Two were left in the drawer	( )	( )
16. Allopurinol 300 mg PO qAM None were left in the drawer	( )	( )

* POS = Oral special.

Name _____ Date _____

	Daily Quantity	(Post) Add
17. Captopril 6.25 mg PO 18h PRN None were left in the drawer	( )	( )
18. Heparin flush IV q4h Three were left in the drawer	( )	( )
19. Zantac 150 mg PO bid None were left in the drawer	( )	( )
20. Reglan 10 mg PO ac&hs Two were left in the drawer	( )	( )
21. Theo-Dur 200 mg PO bid One was left in the drawer	( )	( )
22. Vistaril 25 mg PO Q4h PRN Three were left in the drawer	( )	( )
23. Lopressor 25 mg PO q8h POS* None were left in the drawer	( )	( )
24. DiaBeta 5 mg PO qAM None were left in the drawer	( )	( )
25. Clinoril 200 mg PO tid One was left in the drawer	( )	( )
26. Procardia 10 mg Bite and swallow q4h PRN Two were left in the drawer	( )	( )
27. Propranolol 10 mg PO q8h None were left in the drawer	( )	( )
28. Keflex 500 mg PO q6h Two were left in the drawer	( )	( )
29. Heparin 3000 units sq q12h POS* None were left in the drawer	( )	( )
30. Lopressor 25 mg PO q12h POS* None were left in the drawer	( )	( )
31. Aldomet 125 mg liq PO q8h One was left in the drawer	( )	( )
32. Pen-Vee K 500 mg PO q6h Two were left in the drawer	( )	( )

* POS = Oral special.

Name _____ Date _____

UNIT DOSE FILLING:
PATIENT FILL LIST

Your instructor will partially fill some or all of these patient drawers. Fill drawers with appropriate quantities of medications and record on the fill list the units added to each drawer. Some drawers may be left empty to indicate a new patient.

1. (Name) **Commons, Beth**   00276-28   (Rm) **420-1**
   Benylin Cough Syrup Q6H   (4)   (   )
   Cipro 750 mg Q12 H   (2)   (   )
   Dalmane 15 mg QD HS   (1)   (   )
   Norgesic Forte QD AM   (1)   (   )

   Filled by:_____

2. (Name) **Reese, Michael**   00335-79   (Rm) **211-2**

   Reglan Syrup 7 mg TID AC   (3)   (   )
   Motrin 800 mg Q6H   (4)   (   )
   Dalmane 30 mg QD HS   (1)   (   )
   MOM PRN   (1)   (   )
   Allopurinol 200 mg QD AM   (1)   (   )

   Filled by:_____

3. (Name) **Love, Tanya**   00333-90   (Rm) **361-1**

   Lasix 40 mg QD AM   (1)   (   )
   Procardia 10 mg TID   (3)   (   )
   Valium 2 mg QD HS   (1)   (   )
   Keflex 500 mg Q6H   (4)   (   )

   Filled by:_____

4. (Name) **Stallone, Stacy**   00336-88   (Rm) **117**

   Tenormin 100 mg Q12H   (2)   (   )
   Acetaminophen 325 mg Q6H   (4)   (   )
   Dimatapp Tab PO Q12H   (1)   (   )
   Diuril 500 mg PO BID   (2)   (   )

   Filled by:_____

5. (Name) **Roof, William**   00335-88   (Rm) **112-1**

   Aventyl 10 mg QD AM   (1)   (   )
   Ascorbic Acid 250 mg QD   (1)   (   )
   Mycelex-7 Trouch QID   (1)   (   )
   Guaifenesin 200 mg Syrup Q4H   (6)   (   )

   Filled by:_____

6. (Name) **Cutt, Carrie**   00283-35   (Rm) **272**

   Sucralfate 1000 mg QD AM   (4)   (   )
   Motrin 400 mg Q6H   (4)   (   )
   Zyloprim 100 mg BID   (2)   (   )
   Multivitamin QD   (1)   (   )

   Filled by:_____

Name _____ Date _____

Complete units required. Your instructor will partially fill some or all of these patient drawers.

Complete the filling by recording the correct number of units to dispense, then place the appropriate drug and strength in each drawer. Make drawer name tabs for these patients. Some drawers may be left empty to indicate a new patient.

7.   (Name) **Cato, Inez**   00270-22   (Rm) **206-1**

    Doxycycline Caps 100 mg Q12H   ( )   ( )
    Multivitamins QD   ( )   ( )
    Ibuprofen 400 mg Q8H   ( )   ( )
    Dulcolax 5 mg Suppository QD HS ( )   ( )
    Diabeta 1.25 mg QD AM   ( )   ( )

                                                Filled by:_____

8.   (Name) **Jeffery, George**   00320-72   (Rm) **501-2**

    Procardia 30 mg XL QD   ( )   ( )
    Dyazide BID   ( )   ( )
    Naldecon Tabs Q12H 1 now   ( )   ( )
    Dalmane 15 mg QD HS   ( )   ( )

                                                Filled by:_____

9.   (Name) **Rish, Randy**   00335-82   (Rm) **550**

    Cipro 250 mg TID   ( )   ( )
    Voltaren 50 mg TID   ( )   ( )
    Mylanta 60 ml AC&HS   ( )   ( )
    Reglan 10 mg Q6H 30 min AC   ( )   ( )

                                                Filled by:_____

10.   (Name) **Erwin, Tammy**   00293-45   (Rm) **300**

    Coumadin 2 mg QD AM   ( )   ( )
    MS Contin 30 mg Q4H   ( )   ( )
    Diltiazem 180 mg TID   ( )   ( )
    Glycerin Suppository PRN   ( )   ( )

                                                Filled by:_____

11.   (Name) **Murphy, Peggy**   00334-84   (Rm) **321-2**

    Zantac 300 mg BID   ( )   ( )
    Cytotec 100 mg Q6H   ( )   ( )
    Feldene 40 mg Q12H   ( )   ( )
    Dalmane 15 mg HS PRN   ( )   ( )

                                                Filled by:_____

12.   (Name) **Hine, Herman**   00311-63   (Rm) **380**

    Benadryl 25 mg QHS   ( )   ( )
    Allopurinol 300 mg QAM   ( )   ( )
    Vistaril 25 mg Q4H   ( )   ( )
    Propranolol 10 mg Q8H   ( )   ( )
    Lotrimin 1% Cream TID   ( )   ( )

                                                Filled by:_____

Chapter 11, continued

MEDICATION PROFILING

This exercise provides you with an opportunity to practice entering medications into a patient medication profile. If a computer is available, the instructor may want each student to enter the following orders into a computerized profiling system. However, with or without a computer system, write in the required information on each of these profile forms. This provides practice in extracting and entering appropriate information while building a profile. (Refer to the Minibag Administration Profile chart on pages A-36–A-38.)

(✓)	START → HERE	DATE	TIME	A.M. P.M.	PROFILED BY:	FILLED BY:	CHECKED BY:	PATIENT NAME AND I.D.
	D₅W - 1/2 NS w/ 20mEq KCl/L at 125cc/hr							James, Art Rm. 1049-1
	Septra DS ÷ BID X 7 days							
	HCTZ 50mg QAM							
	Dilantin 100mg IV tid							
	MOM 30mL prn constipation							
					Dr. Blood			

Name _____ Date _____

(✓)	START HERE →	DATE	TIME	A.M. P.M.	PROFILED BY:	FILLED BY:	CHECKED BY:	PATIENT NAME AND I.D.

Morphine 8mg IV Q6-8h prn pain
Ancef 1gm IV Q8h X 48hrs
D₅LR + 10mEq KCl/L at 75cc/hr

Vasotec 2.5mg IV Q8h prn   Systolic BP >150
                            Diastolic BP >110
Tylenol ES ÷ Q4h prn temp >101°
Procardia 10mg SL prn

                                    Dr. Shoe

PATIENT NAME AND I.D.: Taylor, Matt Rm 609-1

(✓)	START HERE →	DATE	TIME	A.M. P.M.	PROFILED BY:	FILLED BY:	CHECKED BY:	PATIENT NAME AND I.D.

D₅NS + 40grams Mag Sulfate at 50cc/hr
Ampicillin 2 grams IV Q6h

Brethine 2.5mg PO Q4h
Pericolace ÷ bid prn Constipation
PNV ÷ Q day
Vistaril 50mg Q6h prn

Phenergan 25mg PR Q6h prn N&V

PATIENT NAME AND I.D.: Adams, Ashley Rm 403-1

Name _____ Date _____

Complete the following profiles for each attached physician order.

Patient Name:
Room Number:
ID:
Allergy:

Medication Ordered	Med/ Soln	Type Soln	Fluid	Route	Frequency/ Rate	Expiration of Soln	Duration	Comments	

Name _____ Date _____

Patient Name:
Room Number:
ID:
Allergy:

Medication Ordered	Med/ Soln	Type Soln	Fluid	Route	Frequency/ Rate	Expiration of Soln	Duration	Comments	

Name _____ Date _____

Patient Name:
Room Number:
ID:
Allergy:

Medication Ordered	Med/ Soln	Type Soln	Fluid	Route	Frequency/ Rate	Expiration of Soln	Duration	Comments	

Name _____ Date _____

Chapter 11, continued

MEDICATION ADMINISTRATION RECORD (MAR)

The Medication Administration Record (MAR) documents the medication administered to patients. This document will list items such as the route of administration, time to start each med, and time to stop (if included in the order), and is a duplicate copy of the medication order. This is part of the patient chart and is a legal document. These records are usually printed on a 24-hour basis and list the meds and times for 24 hours. Q generally means around the clock (q8h), while tid (times per day) will mean during waking hours. Scheduled drugs have listed times of administration, but PRN drugs do not have listed times.

This exercise will give you an opportunity to build a patient MAR by reading the included orders and placing the appropriate information in the columns provided. If computers with pharmacy software are available, the instructor may want the student to enter these orders into a computerized MAR. An example of a computerized MAR is included.

(✓)	START HERE →	DATE 3/6/99	TIME 0540	A.M. P.M.	PROFILED BY:	FILLED BY:	CHECKED BY:	PATIENT NAME AND I.D.
	Admit to 7E or 7W							Ruff, Mary 7942153 Rm: 748-1
	Dx 2° burns to hands, arms, face							
	All - NKA							
	Whirlpool in AM							
	Silvadene cream BID to wounds							
	D₅ 1/2 NS w/ 20 KCl/L at 125cc/hr							
	Zantac 50mg IV Q8°							
	MSO4 2-4mg IV Q2° prn pain							
	Ampicillin 1gm IV Q6°							
	Gentamicin 85mg IV Q8°							
							Dr. P. Brown	

(✓)	START HERE →	DATE	TIME	A.M. P.M.	PROFILED BY:	FILLED BY:	CHECKED BY:	PATIENT NAME AND I.D.
	Procardia 10mg Bite and swallow prn					Sys >150		
						Dias >110		
	MVI ÷ PO QD							
	Zinc 200mg PO QD							
	Reg diet							
	When taking po Percocet Q4-6 prn							

Name _____ **Date** _____

(✓)	START → HERE	DATE 4/6/99	TIME 0730	A.M. P.M.	PROFILED BY:	FILLED BY:	CHECKED BY:	PATIENT NAME AND I.D.
		Admit Dr. Cook						Johnson, Steve
		Dx MI						2687013
		Allergy Codeine						Rm 328
		Nitrol 2% 1/2" Q6° Off 12M-6A						
		Nitro 0.4mg SL SBP >170 DBP >100						
		Tylenol gr X po Q6° prn						
		MDM 30mL prn						
		1/2 NS w/20mEq KCl /L at 50mL/Hr						
							Dr. Cook	

(✓)	START → HERE	DATE 4-5-99	TIME 1000	A.M. P.M.	PROFILED BY:	FILLED BY:	CHECKED BY:	PATIENT NAME AND I.D.
		Admit						Shoker, Tom
		Dx Pneumonia						1049324
								Rm: 232
		Claforan 1gm IV Q8°						
		Erythromycin 500mg IV Q6°						
		D5 1/2 NS at 125cc/hr						
		Tylenol 650mg Q4° prn pain or temp >101						
							G. Roger, MD	

(✓)	START → HERE	DATE	TIME	A.M. P.M.	PROFILED BY:	FILLED BY:	CHECKED BY:	PATIENT NAME AND I.D.
		Continue home meds						
		Digoxin 0.125mg Q day						
		Hydralazine 75mg po tid						
		Zantac 150mg BID						
		ASA EC Q day						
		Maalox 30cc Q4° prn indigestion						

Name _____ Date _____

(✓)	START HERE →	DATE	TIME	A.M. P.M.	PROFILED BY:	FILLED BY:	CHECKED BY:	PATIENT NAME AND I.D.
	Admit to Dr. Cook							
	Solu-Medrol 125mg IV PB Q8° X 4 doses							
	Albumin 25gm IV PB follow w/40mg Lasix							
	Biaxin 500mg po Q12h							
	Rocephin 1gm IV PB Q day							
	Albuterol Aerosol Q4° WA							
	D₅ 1/2 NS at 100cc/hr X 4 then 60cc/hr							
	Tylenol gr X PO Q4° T° >101 or mild pain							
	Restoril 15mg Q HS							
	Zantac 150mg Bid 30min Ac & HS							

Patient I.D.: Taylor, Mark 7642197 Rm: 649-1

(✓)	START HERE →	DATE	TIME	A.M. P.M.	PROFILED BY:	FILLED BY:	CHECKED BY:	PATIENT NAME AND I.D.
	KCl 10mEq ii po QAM							
				J. Cook, MD				

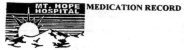

MEDICATION RECORD

IM		SQ	
A-Left Deltoid	E-Left Gluteus	J-Abdomen	M-LT Arm
B-Right Deltoid	F-Right Gluteus	K-RT Arm	N-LT Leg
C. Left Thigh	G-RT Ventrogluteal	L- RT Leg	
D- Right Thigh	I-LT Ventrogluteal		

03/15/   0800 to 03/16/   0759

NURSE VERIFICATION SIGNATURE:

START DATE & TIME TO STOP DATE & TIME	GENERIC NAME, STRENGTH, DOSAGE FORM DOSE DIRECTIONS TRADE NAME(S), COMMENTS		TBG ≐/ INITIAL	ROUTE FREQ.	1ST 0730-1530	2ND 1530-2330	3RD 2330-0730

03/03 0000
03/22 2359
#47
	NS
	AMPICILLIN/SULBACTAM
	   INFUSE OVER: 60MIN
	      USE FOR UNASYN
		50 ML
		1.5 GM
			/	IV
				
				Q6H
				PGY
					12	18	00
							
							06

03/08 0600
 	
#62
	DEXTROSE 5%
	METHYLDOPATE
	   INFUSE OVER: 60MIN
	
	   ALDOMET
		100 ML
		500 MG
			/	IV
				
				Q6H
				PGY
					12	18	00
							
							06

			/				
03/03 0900 #49	FAMOTIDINE 40MG/5ML GIVE: 20 MG=2.5 ML PEPCID		/	NG Q12H	09	21	
03/03 1400 #50	PHENYTOIN 100MG/4ML GIVE: 100 MG=4 ML DILANTIN SUSP		/	NG Q8H		14	22	06
03/05 0800 #57	METOCLOPRAMIDE HCL 5MG/ML GIVE: 10 MG=2 ML REGLAN		/	IV Q6H	08 14	20	02

03/05 1400
 	
#59
	NIFEDIPINE 10MG
	   GIVE: 10 MG=1 CAPSULE
	ADALAT/PROCARDIA
	   USE FOR PROCARDIA
			/	ORAL
				Q8H
						14	22	06

03/10 2100 #71	DOCUSATE SODIUM 100MG/30ML GIVE: 100 MG=30 ML DSS/COLACE		/	ORAL BID	09	21	

02/25 0400
 	
#5
	ACETAMINOPHEN 325MG
	   GIVE: 650 MG=2 TABLET
	TYLENOL
	   PRN T ＞ 101
			/	ORAL
				Q4H
				PRN			

02/27 1900
 	
#13
	MAGNESIUM HYDROXIDE SUSP 30ML U/D
	   GIVE: 30 ML
	LOC/MOM
	   FOR CONSTIPATION
	   MOM
			/	ORAL
				DAILY
				PRN			

02/27 1900 #14	AL-MG OH &SIMETHICONE SUSP 30ML U/D GIVE: 30 ML MAALOX PLUS/MYLANTA		/	ORAL DAILY PRN			

02/28 1000
 	
#23
	ENALAPRILAT 1.25MG/ML
	   GIVE: 1.25 MG=1 ML
	VASOTEC
	   SBP ＞ 150
			/	IV
				Q6H
				PRN			

ALLERGIES: NKA
PT: HUDSON, LANDER
   ACCOUNT # 32547698   RM: 275-2
   MD: BLADDER, GALLE
   NSI

DX: INT. RA CEREBRAL BLEEDING
PAGE 1   *CONTINUED*

Name _____ Date _____

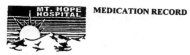

MEDICATION RECORD

IM
A-Left Deltoid
B-Right Deltoid
C. Left Thigh
D- Right Thigh

E-Left Gluteus
F-Right Gluteus
G-RT Ventrogluteal
I-LT Ventrogluteal

SQ
J-Abdomen
K-RT Arm
L- RT Leg

M-LT Arm
N-LT Leg

NURSE VERIFICATION SIGNATURE:

03/15/ 0800 to 03/16/ 0759

START DATE & TIME TO STOP DATE & TIME	GENERIC NAME, STRENGTH, DOSAGE FORM DOSE DIRECTIONS TRADE NAME(S) COMMENTS	TBG Δ/ INITIAL	ROUTE FREQ.	1ST 0730-1530	2ND 1530-2330	3RD 2330-0730
03/02 2100 #48	ARTIFICIAL TEARS OPTH SOL 15ML 8TL GIVE: *AS DIRECTED TEARS/LIQUIFILM		OPH DAILY PRN	Y		
03/04 1000 #52	BISACODYL 10MG GIVE: 10 MG=1 SUPPOSITORY DULCOLAX		RTL PRN			
03/05 1100 #60	NIFEDIPINE 10MG GIVE: 10 MG=1 CAPSULE ADALAT/PROCARDIA PRN SBP) 150 *SL/NG**		ORAL Q2H PRN			
03/07 2334 #63	PROMETHAZINE HCL 25MG/ML GIVE: 12.5 MG=0.5 ML PHENERGAN MAY CAUSE DROWSINESS		IV Q2H PRN			
03/08 1600 #63	PROMETHAZINE HCL 25MG/ML GIVE: 25 MG=1 ML PHENERGAN MAY CAUSE DROWSINESS **MAY GIVE IV OR IM **		IM Q4H PRN			
03/09 1800 #67	LORAZEPAM 2MG/ML GIVE: 1-2 MG=0.5-1 ML ATIVAN PRN AGITATION, VENT DYSYNCHONY		IV Q4H PRN			

**ALLERGIES: NKA **
PT: HUDSON, LANDER
ACCOUNT # 32547698   RM: 275-2
MD: BLADDER, GALLE
NSI

DX: INT. RA CEREBRAL BLEEDING
PAGE 2

CONTINUED

Name _____ Date _____

MOST FREQUENT MAR ADMINISTRATION TIMES

FREQUENCY CODE	ADMINISTRATION TIME*	
QD, QAM	9 AM (0900)	
QOD, Q48	9 AM (0900) on day to be given	
Q3D, Q4D, Q5D, Q6D	Every 3rd, 4th, 5th, or 6th day	
QW	Every week	
Q4W	Every 4 weeks (or once a month)	
MXW	Multiple days of the week	
COUMADIN DOSED QD (QD6P)	6 PM (1800)	
QPM	7 PM (1900)	
QHS	9 PM (2100)	
BID	9A-9P	(0900,2100)
TID	9A-1P-5P	(0900,1300,1700)
QID	9A-1P-5P-9P	(0900,1300,1700,2100)
Q4	1A-5A-9A-1P-5P-9P (0600,1000,1400,1800,2200)	
5XD	6A-10A-2P-6P-10P (0600,1000,1400,1800,2200)	
Q6A	6A-12N-6P-12M	(0600,1200,1800,0000)
Q6B	5A-11A-5P-11P	(0500,1100,1700,2300)
Q6C	2A-8A-2P-8P	(0200,0800,1400,2000)
Q8A	6A-2P-10P	(0600,1400,2200)
Q8B	1A-9A-5P	(0100,0900,1700)
Q12A	9A-9P	(0900,2100)
Q12B	6A-6P	(0600,1800)
Q12C	5A-5P	(0500,1700)
Q12D	11A-11P	(1100,2300)
Q12E	2A-2P	(0200,1400)

Q2O - O = ODD HOURS
Q2E - E = EVEN HOURS

DESIGNATED TIMES BY UNIT, DEPENDING ON DELIVERY OF MEAL TRAYS

For Insulin dosing QAMI – 30 minutes before unit gets breakfast
QPMI – 30 minutes before unit gets supper

WM1 - WITH MEALS ONCE A DAY - Use for daily with a meal
WM2 - WITH MEALS TWICE A DAY - Use for bid with meals
WM3 - WITH MEALS THREE TIMES A DAY - Use for tid with meals

*Standard times unless physician order states otherwise.

Name _____ Date _____

Medication AdministrationRecord

Allergy:

Start date & time to stop date & time	Generic Name, Strength, Dosage Form Dose Directions, Trade Names, Comments	Route Freq.	First 0730-1530	Second 1530-2330	Third 2300-0730

Name _____ Date _____

on AdministrationRecord

& time & time	Generic Name, Strength, Dosage Form Dose Directions, Trade Names, Comments	Route Freq.	First 0730-1530	Second 1530-2330	Third 2300-0730

Name _____ Date _____

Medication AdministrationRecord

Start date & time to stop date & time	Generic Name, Strength, Dosage Form Dose Directions, Trade Names, Comments	Route Freq.	First 0730-1530	Second 1530-2330	Third 2300-0730

Name _____ Date _____

on AdministrationRecord

Allergy:

time & time	Generic Name, Strength, Dosage Form Dose Directions, Trade Names, Comments	Route Freq.	First 0730-1530	Second 1530-2330	Third 2300-0730

Name _____ Date _____

appendix B

COMMON CATEGORIES OF DRUGS

Note: Examples include generic drug names followed in parentheses by a brand-name drug.

Absorbent. Drug given to absorb, or take up, other chemicals of a toxic nature. Example: polycarbophil, a gastrointestinal absorbent. Absorbents are often added to tablets and capsules.

Adrenergic. Drug that activates organs affected by the sympathetic nervous system. Example: epinephrine (Adrenalin)

Adsorbent. Drug that binds other chemicals to its surface; used to reduce amount of toxic chemical in the body. Example: kaolin and pectin (Kaodene)

Alcohol Abuse Inhibitor. Drug that causes an adverse reaction to the ingestion of alcohol. Example: disulfiram (Antabuse)

Alkalinizer. Drug that raises internal pH, making the blood and tissues more alkaline. Example: sodium bicarbonate (Neut Injection)

Anabolic Steroid. Drug used to treat catabolic disorders, in which living tissue is turned into energy and waste products. Example: methandrostenolone

Analeptic. Drug used to stimulate central nervous system. Example: doxapram hydrochloride (Dopram Injection)

Analgesic. Drug used to suppress pain without rendering the patient unconscious. Examples: morphine sulfate, aspirin

Androgen. Hormone affecting male reproductive functions and sexual characteristics. Example: testosterone (Duratest Injection)

Anesthetic. Drug given to reduce or eliminate pain. A **general anesthetic** renders the patient unconscious. Example: ether. A **local anesthetic** affects pain in a particular location. Example: procaine. A **topical anesthetic** is a local anesthetic that affects the mucous membranes. Example: tetracaine

Anorexic. Drug that elevates mood to suppress appetite. Example: phendimetrazine

Antacid. Drug that neutralizes excess gastric acid. Example: aluminum hydroxide (Amphojel)

Anthelmintic. Drug for eradicating intestinal worms. Example: thiabendazole (Mintezol)

Anti-infective. Drug that kills microorganisms and sterilizes wounds. Example: hexachlorophene liquid soap

Anti-inflammatory. Drug that reduces inflammation. Example: ibuprofen (Advil)

Antiacne Drug. Drug taken for control of acne vulgaris. Example: isotretinoin (Accutane)

Antiamebic. Drug for eradication or inhibition of amebic parasites. Example: metronidazole (Flagyl)

Antiandrogen. Drug that reduces response to male hormones. Example: cyproterone

Antianginal. Drug that dilates blood vessels; used to treat angina pectoris, pain in chest and left arm. Example: nitroglycerin (Nitrostat Sublingual)

Antiarrhythmic. Drug that depresses the action of the heart to combat irregularities in its rhythm. Examples: procainamide (Pronestyl)

Antiarthritic. Drug for reducing inflammation of joints in arthritic patients. Example: prednisolone (Key-Pred Injection)

Antibacterial. Drug that kills bacteria. Example: bacitracin (AK-Tracin)

ic. Drug used to kill bacteria or otherwise fight or prevent infection. Example: penicillin g athine (Bicillin L-A)

lesterol Drug. Drug that lowers cholesterol levels. Example: colestipol hydrochloride lestid)

agulant. Drug that slows the clotting of blood; for treatment of thrombosis and embolism or storage of collected blood. Examples: heparin (for internal use); anticoagulant citrate trose solution (for collected blood)

nvulsant. Drug given to prevent or arrest seizures. Example: phenytoin (Dilantin)

epressant. Drug that elevates mood. Example: amitriptyline hydrochloride (Elavil)

iabetic. Drug used to treat diabetes. Example: insulin (Humulin L)

iarrheal. Drug used to treat diarrhea. Example: diphenoxylate (Lomotil)

liuretic. Drug that reduces volume of urine produced. Example: desmopressin acetate Stimate Nasal)

dote. Drug given to reverse effects of poisoning. Examples: activated charcoal (general ntidote); dimercaprol (antidote for arsenic and mercury poisoning)

iemetic. Drug given to suppress vomiting. Example: prochlorperazine (Compazine)

iepileptic. Drug that prevents epileptic seizures. Examples: ethosuximide (Zarontin)

tiflatulent. Drug that reduces gastrointestinal gas. Example: simethicone (Maalox Anti-Gas)

tifungal. Drug that eradicates or suppresses fungi. Examples: griseofulvin (systemic); tolnaftate (local)

tiglaucoma Drug. Drug given for treatment of glaucoma. Example: methazolamide (Neptazane)

tihemophilic. Drug given for treatment of hemophilia, to allow blood to clot. Example: antihemophilic factor (Bioclate)

ntiherpes Drug. Drug given to treat genital herpes. Example: acyclovir (Zovirax)

ntihistaminic. Drug for treatment of allergies. Example: chlorpheniramine maleate (Chlor-Trimeton)

Antihypertensive. Drug that lowers blood pressure. Example: guanethidine monosulfate (Ismelin)

Antihypoglycemic. Drug for treating hypoglycemia. Example: glucagon

Antimalarial. Drug for treating malaria. Example: chloroquine phosphate (Aralen Phosphate)

Antimanic. Drug for treating manic psychosis. Example: lithium (Lithane)

Antimigraine Drug. Drug for treating migraine headaches. Example: methylergonovine maleate (Methergine)

Anti-Motion Sickness Drug. Drug for treating motion sickness. Example: dimenhydrinate (Dramamine Oral)

Antinarcotic Drug. Drug that reverses effects of a narcotic. Example: naloxone hydrochloride

Antinauseant. See *Antiemetic.*

Antineoplastic Drug. Drug that attacks and destroys malignant cells. Example: chlorambucil (Leukeran)

Antipruritic. Drug that suppresses itching. Examples: hydrocortisone (Procort), diphenhydramine hydrochloride (Benadryl Oral)

Antipsychotic. Drug that reduces effects of psychotic disorders. Example: haloperidol (Haldol)

Antipyretic. Drug that reduces fever. Example: acetaminophen (Tylenol)

Antispasmodic. Drug that reduces spasms. Example: baclofen (Lioresal)

Antithyroid Drug. Drug that reduces amount of thyroid hormone produced. Example: methimazole (Tapazole)

Antitubercular. Drug that fights tuberculosis. Example: isoniazid (Laniazid)

Antitussive. Drug that suppresses coughing. Example: dextromethorphan (Vicks Formula 44)

Antiviral. Drug that kills or suppresses viruses, or drug that prevents viral infection. Example: amantadine (Symmetrel)

Anxiolytic. Drug that reduces anxiety. Example: diazepam (Valium)

Astringent. Drug that toughens and strengthens tissues. Example: aluminum acetate solution (Boropak)

Barbiturate. A kind of sedative. Example: pentobarbital (Nembutal)

Beta Blockers. Drugs used to relieve angina pectoris, cardiac arrhythmias, postmyocardial hypertension, and migraines. Example: propranolol (Inderal)

Bronchodilator. Drug that expands the bronchial passages, for treating asthma. Example: isoproterenol (Isuprel)

Calcium Channel Blocker. Drug used to block flow of calcium ions in the heart for treatment of angina pectoris, arrhythmia, and hypertension. Example: verapamil (Isoptin)

Cardiotonic. Drug that strengthens heartbeat; for treatment of congestive heart failure. Example: digoxin (Lanoxin)

Cathartic. See *Purgative*.

Chelating Agent. A kind of drug used in treatment of poisoning. Example: edetate calcium disodium (for lead poisoning) (Calcium Disodium Versenate)

Choleretic. Drug that increases secretion of bile by liver. Example: dehydrocholic acid (Cholan-HMB)

Contraceptive. Drug that prevents conception. Example: norethindrone (Micronor)

Corticosteroid. Drug applied topically to relieve itching, vasodilation, and inflammation due to skin disorder. Example: desoximetasone (Topicort)

Diagnostic Drug. Drug given to determine functioning of body or to discover presence of a disease. Example: pentagastrin (Peptavlon)

Digestive. Drug that aids digestion. Example: pancreatin (Creon)

Diuretic. Drug that increases production of urine. Example: furosemide (Lasix)

Emetic. Drug that causes vomiting. Example: ipecac syrup

Estrogen. Hormone affecting female reproductive functions and sexual characteristics. Example: ethinyl estradiol (Estinyl)

Expectorant. Drug that increases secretions of the respiratory tract and lowers their viscosity. Example: potassium iodide (Pima)

Fertility Drug. Drug that promotes ovulation or creation of sperm. Example: clomiphene citrate (Clomid)

Galactokinetic. Drug that begins production of milk after childbirth. Example: oxytocin (Pitocin)

Gonadotropin. A type of fertility drug. Example: luteinizing hormone

Growth Hormone. Hormone that stimulates growth. Example: somatrem (Genotropin Injection)

...tic. Drug that stops bleeding. Examples: oxidized cellulose (local); aminocaproic acid (...mic)

...c. Drug that causes sleep. Example: flurazepam (Dalmane)

...zation. See *Vaccine*.

...le Hydrolytic. Injectable drug that aids in the diffusion of other injected drugs.

...ytic. Drug applied topically to soften and remove superficial skin layer. Example: salicylic (Compound W)

...e. Drug that promotes evacuation from bowel. Example: methylcellulose (Citrucel)

... Drug that constricts the pupils of the eyes. Example: pilocarpine (Adsorbocarpine ...hthalmic)

...e Relaxant. Drug that inhibits muscle contraction. Example: dantrolene (Dantrium)

...iatic. Drug that dilates the pupils of the eyes. Example: phenylephrine hydrochloride (AK-...ilate Ophthalmic Solution)

...otic. Drug, often addictive, used to relieve pain and induce sleep, including opium and its ...erivatives. Example: codeine

...l Decongestant. Drug that constricts vessels in nasal passages. Example: ...phenylpropanolamine and brompheniramine (Dimetapp Elixir)

...ate. A narcotic derived or related to opium. Example: morphine sulfate (Astramorph PF Injection)

...asiticide. Drug that destroys parasites on the skin. See *Scabicide* and *Pediculicide*.

...liculicide. Drug for killing lice. Example: lindane (G-well)

...ychotherapeutic. Drug for treatment of psychological disorder. Example: chlorpromazine hydrochloride (Thorazine)

...diopharmaceutical. Drug containing a radioactive isotope; used for diagnosis or for therapy.

...cabicide. Drug that destroys skin mites and their eggs. Example: lindane (G-well)

...edative. A drug that depresses the central nervous system, causing relaxation. Example: phenobarbital (Luminal)

...ystemic Acidifier. Drug that lowers internal pH (level of acidity or alkalinity), making the blood and tissues more acidic. Example: ammonium chloride

...Tranquilizer. Drug that reduces anxiety or disturbance. Example: trifluoperazine hydrochloride (Stelazine)

Vaccine. Drug that introduces an antigen into the body to stimulate the production of antibodies for protection against a disease-causing microorganism. Example: tetanus immune globulin

Vasoconstrictor. Drug that narrows vessels and increases blood pressure. Example: norepinephrine bitartrate (Levophed Injection)

Vasodilator. Drug that expands vessels and lowers blood pressure. Example: nitroglycerin (Nitroglyn Oral)

Vitamin. Chemical or mineral necessary in small amounts for proper metabolism. Example: vitamin C, present in citric acid

appendix C

COMMONLY PRESCRIBED DRUGS

Brand Name	Manufacturer	Generic Name
Accupril	Parke-Davis	quinapril
Acetaminophen/Codeine	Lemmon	acetaminophen/codeine
Adalat CC	Bayer Pharm	nifedipine
Albuterol Aerosol	Warrick	albuterol
Alprazolam	Purepac	alprazolam
Altace	Hoechst Marion Roussel	ramipril
Ambien	Searle	zolpidem
Amoxicillin	Biocraft	amoxicillin
Amoxil	SmithKline Beecham	amoxicillin
Atenolol	Mylan	atenolol
Ativan	Wyeth-Ayerst	lorazepam
Atrovent	Boehringer-Ingelheim	ipratropium
Augmentin	SmithKline Beecham	amoxicillin/clavulanate
Axid	Lilly	nizatidine
Azmacort	Rhone-Poulenc Rorer	triamcinolone aerosol
Bactroban	SmithKline Beecham	mupirocin
Beconase AQ	Glaxo Wellcome	beclomethasone
Bentyl	Lakeside Pharmaceutical	dicyclomine
Biaxin Susp	Abbott	clarithromycin
BuSpar	Bristol-Myers Squibb	buspirone
Calan SR	Searle	verapamil
Capoten	Bristol-Myers Squibb	captopril
Cardizem CD	Hoechst Marion	diltiazem
Cardura	Pfizer	doxazosin
Carisoprodol	Schein	carisoprodol
Catapres	Boehringer-Ingelheim	clonidine
Ceclor	Lilly	cefaclor
Cefaclor	Zenith	cefaclor
Ceftin	Glaxo Wellcome	cefuroxime
Cefzil	Bristol-Myers Squibb	cefprozil
Cephalexin	Apothecon	cephalexin
Cimetidine	Mylan	cimetidine
Cipro	Bayer Pharm	ciprofloxacin
Claritin	Schering	loratadine
Claritin D	Schering	loratadine/pseudoephedrine
Clonidine	Mylan	clonidine
Coumadin	Du Pont Pharm	warfarin
Cozaar	Merck & Co	losartan
Cyclobenzaprine	Major	cyclobenzaprine
Cycrin	ESI Led Gen	medroxyprogesterone
Darvocet-N 100	Lilly	propoxyphene-N/APAP
Daypro	Searle	oxaprozin
Deltasone	Pharmacia/Upjohn	prednisone
Demulen 1/35	Searle	ethynodiol/Ethinyl Estradiol
Depakote	Abbott	divalproex

c	Organon	desogestrel/Ethinyl Estradiol
ine	Major	diazepam
	CibaGeneva	diclofenac
ɪR	Rugby	dicyclomine
	Pfizer	fluconazole
line Hyclate	Rhone-Poulenc Rorer	diltiazem
	Parke-Davis	phenytoin
	Rachelle	doxycycline
ɪm	Bristol-Myers Squibb	cefadroxil
	SmithKline Beecham	hydrochlorothiazide/triamterene
	Smith-Kline-Beecham	triamterene/HCTZ
)	Wyeth-Ayerst	venlafaxine
ɔcin Stearate	Schering	mometasone
	Abbott	erythromycin
ɇ	Abbott	erythromycin
erm	Ciba	hydrochlorothiazide
	Mead-J Lab	estradiol
ɪil	Ciba/Geneva	estradiol
se	Beecham	phentermine
ɪ	Merck	cycrobenzaprine
nax	Glaxo Wellcome	fluticasone
semide	Ortho Pharm	ofloxacin
fibrozil	Merck & Co	alendronate
ora 1/35	Mylan	furosemide
izide	Warner Chiloott	gemfibrozil
cophage	Rugby	norethindrone/Ethinyl Estradiol
cotrol XL	Mylan	glipizide
buride	Bristol-Myers/Squibb	metformin
nase PresTab	Pfizer	glipizide
aifenesin/PPA	Greenstone	glyburide
ımulin 70/30	Pharmacia/Upjohn	glyburide
ımulin N	Duramed	guaifenesin/Phenylpropanolamine
umulin R	Lilly	human Insulin 70/30
ydrochlorothiazide	Lilly	human Insulin-NPH
ıydrocodone w/APAP	Lilly	human Insulin Regular
ɪytrin	Zenith	hydrochlorothiazide
buprofen	Watson	hydrocodone w/APAP
mdur	Abbott	terazosin
mitrex	Par Pharm	ibuprofen
Insulin Syringe	Schering	isosorbide Mononitrate S.A.
Isoptin	Glaxo Wellcome	sumatriptan
K-Dur-20	Becton	dikinson
Keflex	Knoll	verapamil
Klonopin	Key Pharm	potassium chloride
Klor-Con	Dista	cephalexin
Lanoxin	Roche	clonazepam
Lasix	Upsher-Smith	potassium chloride
Lescol	Glaxo Wellcome	digoxin
	Hoechst-Roussel	furosemide
	Sandoz	fluvastatin

Levoxyl	Daniels	levothyroxine
Lo/Ovral	Wyeth-Ayerst	norgestrel/ethinyl estradiol
Lodine	Wyeth-Ayerst	etodolac
Loestrin-FE 1.5/30	Parke-Davis	norethindrone/ethinyl estradiol
Lopid	Parke-Davis	gemfibrozil
Lopressor	CibaGeneva	metoprolol
Lorabid	Lilly	loracarbef
Lorazepam	Purepac	lorazepam
Lotrisone	Schering	clotrimazole/betamethasone
Macrobid	Procter & Gamble	nitrofurantoin
Medroxyprogesterone	Greenstone	medroxyprogesterone
Methylphenidate	MD Pharm	methylphenidate
Methylprednisolone	Duramed Ph	methylprednisolone
Metoprolol Tartrate	CibaGeneva	metoprolol
Mevacor	Merck	lovastatin
Micronase	Upjohn	glyburide
Monopril	Bristol-Myers Squibb	fosinopril
Motrin	McNeil	ibuprofen
Naproxen	Mylan	naproxen
Naprosyn	Syntex	naproxen
Neomycin/Polymx/HC	Schein	neomycin/Polymx/HC
Nitro-Dur	Key	nitroglycerin
Nitrostat	Parke-Davis	nitroglycerin
Norvasc	Pfizer	amlodipine
One Touch Test-Strip	Lifescan	
Ortho Tri-Cyclen	Ortho Pharm	norgestimate/Ethinyl Estradiol
Ortho-Cept	Ortho Pharm	desogestrel/Ethinyl Estradiol
Ortho-Cyclen	Ortho Pharm	norgestimate/Ethinyl Estradiol
Ortho-Novum 1/35	Ortho Pharm	norethindrone/Ethinyl Estradiol
Ortho-Novum 7/7/7	Ortho Pharm	norethindrone/Ethinyl Estradiol
Oruvail	Wyeth-Ayerst	ketoprofen
Paxil	SmithKline Beecham	paroxetine
Pepcid	Merck	famotidine
Phenergan	Wyeth-Ayerst	promethazine
Phenergan/Codeine	Wyeth-Ayerst	promethazine/codeine
Pondimin	Wyeth Ayerst	fenfluramine
Potassium Chloride	Ethex	potassium Chloride
Pravachol	Bristol-Myers Squibb	pravastatin
Prednisone	Schein	prednisone
Premarin	Wyeth-Ayerst	conjugated estrogens
Prempro	Wyeth-Ayerst	conj estrogens/medroxyprogesterone
Prevacid	Tap Pharm	lansoprazole
Prilosec	Astra/Merck	omeprazole
Principen	Apothecon	ampicillin
Prinivil	Merck & Co	lisinopril
Procardia XL	Pfizer	nifedipine
Propacet 100	Lemmon	propoxyphene N/APAP
Propulsid	Janssen	cisapride
Proventil Aerosol	Schering	albuterol
Prozac	Dista	fluoxetine

Relafen	SmithKline Beecham	nabumetone
Restoril	Sandoz	temazepam
Retin-A	Ortho Derm	tretinoin
Risperdal	Janssen	risperidone
Ritalin	CibaGeneva	methylphenidate
Roxicet	Roxane	oxycodone/APAP
Seldane	Marion Merrell Dow	terfenadine
Seldane-D	Hoechst Marion Roussel	terfenadine/Pseudoephedrine
Septra	Burroughs Wellcome	trimeth/sulfameth
Serevent	Allen & Hanburys	salmeterol
Sumycin	Apothecon	tetracycline
Suprax	Wyeth-Ayerst	cefixime
Synthroid	Knoll	levothyroxine
Tegretol	Basel	carbamazepine
Tenormin	Zeneca Pharm	atenolol
Terazol 7	Ortho Pharm	terconazole
Timoptic	Merck & Co	timolol
Toprol-XL	Astra	metoprolol
Trental	Hoechst Marion Roussel	pentoxifylline
Tri-Levlen	Berlex	l-norgestrel/ethinyl estradiol
Trimeth/Sulfameth	Lemmon	trimeth/sulfameth
Trimox	Apothecon	amoxicillin
Triphasil	Wyeth-Ayerst	l-norgestrel/ethinyl estradiol
Trusopt	Merck & Co	dorzolamide
Ultram	McNeil	tramadol
Valium	Roche	diazepam
Vancenase AQ	Schering	beclomethasone
Vanceril	Key Pharm	beclomethasone
Vasotec	Merck & Co.	enalapril
Veetids	Pothecon	penicillin VK
Ventolin	Glaxo Wellcome	albuterol
Verelan	Lederie Rx	verapamil
Vibramycin	Pfizer	doxycycline
Xanax	Pharmacia/Upjohn	alprazolam
Zantac	Glaxo Wellcome	ranitidine
Zestril	Zeneca Pharm	lisinopril
Ziac	Wyeth-Ayerest	bisoprolol/HCTZ
Zithromax	Pfizer	azithromycin
Zocor	Merck	simvastatin
Zoloft	Pfizer	sertraline
Zovirax	Glaxo Wellcome	acyclovir
Zyrtec	Pfizer	cetirizine

index

Career
    clarifying goals for, 242 (Chart 12.2)
    management of, 241 (Chart 12.1)
    of pharmacy technician, 235
Cathartics, 76
Catheter: of IV administration set, 105, 210
CD-ROMs: references available on, 124
Cell theory, 200
Central processing unit (CPU), 154, 156 (Fig. 8.6)
Certification, 114, 235
    and national certification examination, 236-239
    for pharmacy technicians, 5, 12
    reference works on, 121-122. *See also*
        Recertification
Certification Review for Pharmacy Technicians (Reifman),
    122
Certified Pharmacy Technician (CPhT), 1, 6, 114,
    235, 236, 250
*Charles Press Handbook of Current Medical Abbreviations,
    The,* 53 (Tab. 3.2), 115
Checking prescription, 160-161
Chemicals: disposal of, 222
Chemical sterilization, 202
Chemist, 2
Chemotherapy preparation and dispensing guidelines,
    A-65
Chewable tablets, 81 (Chart 4.2)
Child-resistant containers, 157
    exceptions to requirement for, 26-27 (Tab. 2.2)
Chlorhexidine gluconate, 210
Cholera, 202
Chronic conditions/illnesses, 37, 48, 60
    and long-term care facilities, 10
Cider House Rules, The (Irving), 23
Civil actions: against pharmacists and pharmacy
    technicians, 19, 20
Civil law, 15
Civil penalties, 19
Civil War (American): surgery practices during, 202
Clamps: and IV sets, 209
Class A prescription balance. *See* Class III prescription
    balance
Class III prescription balance, 171, 172 (Fig. 9.1), 184
Cleaning
    after compounding, 183
    of laminar flow hood, 204-205
    and parenteral preparation, 211
Clinical pharmacy, 1
Clinical drug investigations, 198
Clinical era: pharmacist's role in, 2
Clinical functions: of hospital pharmacy, 9
Clinical pharmacists, 10
Clinical pharmacology, 49 (Chart 3.1), 60
Clinical pharmacy, 3, 49 (Chart 3.1), 60, 187
Clinical trials, 24
    and investigational drugs, 163

Coarse powder size, 77
Coated tablets, 80 (Chart 4.2)
"Code of Ethics for Pharmacists of the American
    Pharmaceutical Association," 21-22 (Chart 2.2)
Code of Ethics for Pharmacy Technicians, 112
"Code of Ethics of the American Association of
    Pharmacy Technicians," 22 (Chart 2.3)
*Code of Federal Regulations (CFR), Title 21, Food and
    Drugs,* 15, 20, 120
Collodions, 82 (Chart 4.3), 92
Colloidal dispersion, 84
Comminution, 83 (Chart 4.3), 180
    and blending of drugs, 180
Common law, 15, 16, 32
Common measure, 130-131, 142
    units in, with metric equivalents, 130-131
        (Tab. 7.4)
Communication: by pharmacy technicians, 7 (Chart
    1.1). *See also* Human relations and communications
Community (or retail) pharmacies, 1
    operations, 145-146
    personal service in, 187-190
    pharmacist in, 4
    pharmacy technicians in, 5, 8
Comparative negligence, 18
Compensatory damages, 15, 18
"Competency Statements for Pharmacy Practice," 20
Compliance, 97
    and route of administration, 98 (Chart 5.1), 107
    and sugar-coating, 80 (Chart 4.2)
Compound fractions, 132
Compounding, 1, 4
    date, 183
    equipment for, 172-176
    extemporaneous, 156
    slab, 171, 174, 184
Compound W, 82 (Chart 4.3)
Comprehensive Drug Abuse Prevention and Control
    Act of 1970, 19, 32
    drug schedules under, 25-26 (Tab. 2.1)
Computerized inventory control systems, 164
Computerized patient profile, 150, 152 (Fig. 8.4)
Computer systems, 153-155
    desktop, 156 (Fig. 8.6)
    parts of, 154
    pharmacy, 155
Congenital, 37, 47
Conical graduates, 175, 176 (Fig. 9.7), 184
Conjunctiva: ocular inserts for, 89
Conjunctival, 97
    discs, 249
    route of administration, 101 (Chart 5.2), 107
Consultant Pharmacist, The, 112
Consumer Product Safety Commission, 26
Containers
    child-resistant, 157

Mannitol, 81 (Chart 4.2)

Manual for Hospital Pharmacy Technicians: A Programmed Course in Basic Skills, 121

Manual for Pharmacy Technicians, 121, 236

Manual for the Pharmacy Technician (Keresztes), 121

Manufacturers: regulations on pharmaceuticals returned to, 163

MAR administration times: most frequent, A-94

Master formula sheets, 171, 176, 177 (Fig. 9.8), 183, 184

Materia medica box, 23 (Fig. 2.1)

Mathematics

    decimals, 134-135

    fractions, 132-134

    percentages, 136

    ratios and proportions, 135-136

Means, 136

Measurements and measuring

    balance for, 173

    equipment for, 172-176

    of liquid volumes, 179 (Chart 9.2)

    symbols for, 60

    and syringe dose, 211 (Fig. 11.10)

    and technique for liquid volume, 179

Measurement systems

    conversion of quantities within or between, 137-138 (Chart 7.1)

    on prescription forms, 51

Mechanical sterilization, 202

MedCoach CD-ROM, 117

Medicaid

    and drug use review, 27

    and OBRA-90, 28

Medical Abbreviations: 12,000 Conveniences at the Expense of Communications and Safety (Davis), 115

Medical and pharmaceutical terminology: common Greek and Latin roots, prefixes, and suffixes in, 38-47 (Tab. 3.1)

Medical history: in patient profile, 152 (Chart 8.2)

Medical/pharmaceutical advice, 190

Medical Sciences Bulletin, 122

Medical software developer, 10

Medicated syrups, 84 (Chart 4.3)

Medication cart, 229

Medication delivery: to patients' rooms, 198

Medication fill list, 227

Medication orders, 38, 48, 198, 223-226 (Fig. 11.15), 230

    abbreviations in, 48-58

    forms of, 51

    and unit dose distribution, 223-229

Medication record: computerized, A-92-A-93

Medications: commonly confused names of, 59

Medicine: reference works on, 115

Medicine Shoppe, The, 8

MedWatch News, 122

Meldrum, Helen: *Interpersonal Communication in Pharmaceutical Care*, 122

Meniscus, 172

    and measurement, 180 (Fig. 9.9)

Menu-driven database management systems, 154

Merck Manual of Diagnosis and Therapy, The, 115

Merck Manual of Medical Information, The: Home Edition, 115

Metabolism, 50 (Chart 3.1)

Meter, 128, 142

Metric: apothecary measure converted to, 137 (Chart 7.1)

Metric measurements: on prescriptions, 51

Metric system, 127-130, 128, 142

    measurements of distance, area, and volume using, 128 (Fig. 7.1)

Metric units: common, 129 (Tab. 7.2)

Metric volume, 137 (Chart 7.1)

Metric weights, 173

Michigan Court of Appeals, 59

Michigan Pharmacists Association, 6, 236

Microbial-free product, 211

Microemulsions, 84, 85 (Chart 4.4), 92

Microorganisms, 200

    destroying, 202

    and disease, 201-202

Military services, 10

Milks, 85 (Chart 4.4), 92

Mill, John Stuart: *On Liberty*, 15

Milligrams, 128, 129, 142

    conversion of, 130 (Tab. 7.3)

Milliliters, 128, 129, 142

    conversion of, 130 (Tab. 7.3)

Milliosmoles (mOsm), 98

Millis, John S., 2, 3

Millis Report, 2, 3, 187

Mill's Doctrine, 15

Mineral sources: drugs from, 2

Minibag: label for, 220 (Fig. 11.14)

Minibag administration protocol, 215-217 (Tab. 11.2), A-36

Minicomputers, 154

Misbranded drugs, 24

Mitchell-Hatton, Sarah Lu: *The Davis Book of Medical Abbreviations: A Deciphering Guide*, 53 (Tab. 3.2)

Mitigation, 38, 48, 60

Modem, 154

    billing via, 161

Moderately coarse powder size, 77

Modified block style: in cover letters, 235, 245

Molded tablets, 80 (Chart 4.2)

Monitor: computer, 154, 156 (Fig. 8.6)

"Monitoring Prescriptions for Legitimacy" (Vivian and Brushwood), 121

Robotics, 249, 250
Rod-shaped bacteria, 201
Roller clamp: IV tubing, 209
ROM. *See* Read-only memory
Roman numerals, 128
    on prescriptions, 52
    understanding, 131 (Tab. 7.5)
Roots, 60
    in medical and pharmaceutical terminology, 38-
      44 (Tab. 3.1)
Roster of Faculty and Professional Staff, 111
Routes of drug administration, 98, 107
    and applicable dosage forms, 100-102 (Chart 5.2)
    and characteristics of parenteral preparations, 98,
      103-105
    choosing, 97, 107
    factors influencing choice of, 98-100 (Chart 5.1)
    infusions, 105
    injections, 103-104
    parenteral administration, 97-98
    possible routes of, 97
Routes of exposure: to hazardous substances, 221
Royal Society of London, 200
RPM. *See* Random Path Membrane
Rubber spatulas, 174
Rudeness, 190, 191
Rudman, Jack: *Pharmacy Technician*, 122
℞ area: of community pharmacy, 145
℞ symbol: on prescription, 147 (Chart 8.1)
RxTrek, 122
    Web site for, 242 (Chart 12.2)

Sabin vaccine, 71 (Chart 4.1)
Safe Handling of Cytotoxic and Hazardous Drugs (video), 223
Salary: for certified pharmacy technicians, 236
Salk vaccine, 71 (Chart 4.1)
Satellites, 155
Scabicides, 101 (Chart 5.2)
Schedule I drugs, 25 (Tab. 2.1), 68
Schedule II drugs, 25 (Tab. 2.1)
    dating of, 148
    labels for, 160 (Chart 8.3)
    purchase of, 163
Schedule III drugs, 25 (Tab. 2.1)
    labels for, 160 (Chart 8.3)
    prescription refills for, 149
Schedule IV drugs, 26 (Tab. 2.1)
    labels for, 160 (Chart 8.3)
    prescription refills for, 149
Schedule V drugs, 26 (Tab. 2.1), 68
    labels for, 160 (Chart 8.3)
    refill guidelines for, 149
Scientific era (20th century): pharmacist's role in, 2
Scope of Pharmacy Practice Project, 237 (Tab. 12.2)

Screw clamp: IV tubing, 209
Sebaceous glands, 101 (Chart 5.2)
Sebum, 101 (Chart 5.2)
Semigaseous dosage forms, 73
Semiliquid dosage forms, 73
Semisolid dosage forms, 73
Semisynthetic drugs, 69
Semisynthetic penicillins, 70
Sensitivity requirement (SR), 173
Sexual harassment, 191
Shaft: of syringe needle, 87
Shelving: and inventory management, 163
Shepherd, Robert D.: *Introduction to Computers and Technology*, 153
Short-term care, 8
Sifting, 77
Signa: on prescription label, 148 (Chart 8.1), 149
Signature lines: on prescription, 149
Signatures
    on prescription, 53 (Chart 3.2), 148 (Chart 8.1)
    on prescriptions for Schedule II controlled
      substances, 148
Single-compression tablets (CT), 80 (Chart 4.2), 92
Single Photon Emission Computed Tomography
    (SPECT), 71 (Chart 4.1), 90
Site of action: and route of administration, 99 (Chart
    5.1), 107
Site of administration: and size/shape of suppository,
    78 (Fig. 4.11)
Sites of administration/parts of body:
    prescription/medication order abbreviations for,
      57 (Tab. 3.2)
Skin contact (direct): with hazardous substances, 221
Slide clamp: IV tubing, 209
Smallpox, 202
Smallpox inoculation, 200
Small volume parenterals (SVPs), 212
Smith, C. G.: *The Process of New Drug Discovery and Development*, 118
Smith, Mickey: *Pharmacy Ethics*, 121
Snap-fit design, 74
Soft gelatin shells, 76
Soft-shell capsules, 92
Software programs, 154
Solid dosage forms, 73-81
    capsules, 73-76
    effervescent salts, 76
    implants/pellets, 76
    lozenges/troches/pastilles, 76
    pills, 77
    plasters, 77
    powders and granules, 77
    suppositories, 77-78
    tablets, 78-79
    types of, 92